Lecture Notes in Compute

Edited by G. Goos, J. Hartmanis, ar

Springer
Berlin
Heidelberg
New York
Barcelona
Hong Kong
London
Milan
Paris
Tokyo

Jose Crespo   Victor Maojo
Fernando Martin (Eds.)

Medical
Data Analysis

Second International Symposium, ISMDA 2001
Madrid, Spain, October 8-9, 2001
Proceedings

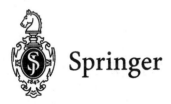 Springer

Series Editors

Gerhard Goos, Karlsruhe University, Germany
Juris Hartmanis, Cornell University, NY, USA
Jan van Leeuwen, Utrecht University, The Netherlands

Volume Editors

Jose Crespo
Victor Maojo
Polytechnical University of Madrid
Artificial Intelligence Laboratory, Medical Informatics Group
28660 - Boadilla del Monte (Madrid), Spain
E-mail: {jcrespo/vmaojo}@fi.upm.es

Fernando Martin
Institute of Health Carlos III, Health Bioinformatics Unit
Ctra. de Majadahonda-Pozuelo Km.2
28220 Majadahonda (Madrid), Spain
E-mail: fmartin@isciii.es

Cataloging-in-Publication Data applied for

Die Deutsche Bibliothek - CIP-Einheitsaufnahme

Medical data analysis : second international symposium ; proceedings /
ISMDA 2001, Madrid, Spain, October 8 - 9, 2001. Jose Crespo ... (ed.). -
Berlin ; Heidelberg ; New York ; Barcelona ; Hong Kong ; London ; Milan ;
Paris ; Tokyo : Springer, 2001
    (Lecture notes in computer science ; Vol. 2199)
    ISBN 3-540-42734-1

CR Subject Classification (1998): I.2, H.3, G.3, I.5.1, I.4, J.3, F.1

ISSN 0302-9743
ISBN 3-540-42734-1 Springer-Verlag Berlin Heidelberg New York

Springer-Verlag Berlin Heidelberg New York
a member of BertelsmannSpringer Science+Business Media GmbH

http://www.springer.de

© Springer-Verlag Berlin Heidelberg 2001
Printed in Germany

Typesetting: Camera-ready by author, data conversion by DA-TeX Gerd Blumenstein
Printed on acid-free paper   SPIN 10840680   06/3142   5 4 3 2 1 0

Preface

The 2nd International Symposium on Medical Data Analysis (ISMDA 2001) was the continuation of the successful ISMDA 2000, a conference held in Frankfurt, Germany, in September 2000. The ISMDA conferences were conceived to integrate interdisciplinary research from scientific fields such as statistics, signal processing, medical informatics, data mining, and biometrics for biomedical data analysis. A number of academic and professional people from those fields, including computer scientists, statisticians, physicians, engineers, and others, realized that new approaches were needed to apply successfully all the traditional techniques, methods, and tools of data analysis to medicine.

ISMDA 2001, as its predecessor, aimed to provide an international forum for sharing and exchanging original research ideas and practical development experiences. This year we broadened the scope of the conference, to included methods for image analysis and bioinformatics. Both are exciting scientific research fields and it was clear to the scientific committee that they had to be included in the areas of interest.

Medicine has been one of the most difficult application areas for computing. The number and importance of the different issues involved suggests why many data analysis researchers find the medical domain such a challenging field. New interactive approaches are needed to solve these problems.

In ISMDA 2001 we tried to enhance this interdisciplinary approach. Scientists from many areas submitted their papers. After a thorough peer-review process, 46 papers were selected for inclusion in the final program. We evaluated the 72 submitted papers according to their scientific originality, clear methodology, relevance, and results. All the papers were reviewed by at least two reviewers from the scientific committee and by additional reviewers. In addition, the volume contains three keynote lectures written by relevant invited speakers in areas of special interest. We did not include posters or "short papers" in the conference program. Thus, it was our aim that all the approved papers selected by the reviewers had a significant scientific content for their inclusion within the symposium proceedings.

We would like to thank all the people, institutions, and sponsors that have contributed to this symposium. Authors, members of the conference committees, additional reviewers, keynote speakers, and organizers collaborated in all aspects of the conference. Finally, we are specially grateful to SEIS, the Spanish Health Informatics Society, and its Executive Board, whose members have enthusiastically supported the conference from the very beginning.

October 2001

Jose Crespo
Victor Maojo
Fernando Martin

Organization

Executive Committee

Chair: Victor Maojo (Polytechnical Univ. of Madrid, Spain)

Scientific Committee Coordinator: Fernando Martin (Institute of Health Carlos III, Spain)

Steering Committee

Rüdiger Brause (J.W. Goethe Univ., Germany)
José María Barreiro (Polytechnical Univ. of Madrid, Spain)
Jose Crespo (Polytechnical Univ. of Madrid, Spain)
Marcial García-Rojo (Hosp. Alarcos, Spain)
Carlos Jimenez (Hospital Gregorio Marañón, Spain)

Scientific Committee

A. Babic (Linköping Univ., Sweden)
A. Colosimo (Univ. of Rom "La Sapienza", Italy)
N. Ezquerra (Georgia Tech, U.S.A.)
A. Giuliani (Nat. Inst. of Health, Italy)
J. Hasenkam (Aarhus Univ., Denmark)
E. Keravnou (Univ. of Cyprus, Cyprus)
P. Larrañaga (Univ. of the Basque Country, Spain)
N. Lavrac (J. Stefan Institute, Slovenia)
R. Lefering (Univ. of Cologne, Germany)
A. Macerata (Institute of Clinical Physiology, Italy)
E. Neugebauer (Univ. of Cologne, Germany)

C. Ohmann (Heinrich-Heine-University of Düsseldorf, Germany)
L. Ohno-Machado (Harvard Univ., U.S.A.)
A. Pazos (Univ. of A Coruña, Spain)
L. Pecen (Academy of Sciences, Czech Republic)
W. Sauerbrei (Univ. of Freiburg, Germany)
B. Sierra (Univ. of the Basque Country, Spain)
B. Silverman (Univ. of Pensylvannia, U.S.A.)
J. Sima (Academy of Sciences, Czech Republic)
H. Sitter (Univ. of Marburg, Germany)
B. Zupan (Univ. of Ljubljana, Slovenia)

Local Committee

Members of the Executive Board of SEIS, the Spanish Society of Health Informatics

Table of Contents

Medical Analysis and Diagnosis by Neural Networks

Rüdiger W. Brause

J.W. Goethe-University, Computer Science Dept.,
Frankfurt a. M., Germany.
Brause@cs.uni-frankfurt.de

Abstract. In its first part, this contribution reviews shortly the application of neural network methods to medical problems and characterizes its advantages and problems in the context of the medical background. Successful application examples show that human diagnostic capabilities are significantly worse than the neural diagnostic systems. Then, paradigm of neural networks is shortly introduced and the main problems of medical data base and the basic approaches for training and testing a network by medical data are described. Additionally, the problem of interfacing the network and its result is given and the neuro-fuzzy approach is presented. Finally, as case study of neural rule based diagnosis septic shock diagnosis is described, on one hand by a growing neural network and on the other hand by a rule based system.

Keywords: Statistical Classification, Adaptive Prediction, Neural Networks, Neurofuzzy Medical Systems

1   Introduction

Almost all the physicians are confronted during their formation by the task of learning to diagnose. Here, they have to solve the problem of deducing certain diseases or formulating a treatment based on more or less specified observations and knowledge. Certainly, there is the standard knowledge of seminars, courses and books, but on one hand medical knowledge outdates quickly and on the other hand this does not replace own experience. For this task, certain basic difficulties have to be taken into account:

- The basis for a valid diagnosis, a sufficient number of experienced cases, is reached only in the middle of a physician's career and is therefore not yet present at the end of the academic formation.
- This is especially true for rare or new diseases where also experienced physicians are in the same situation as newcomers.
- Principally, humans do not resemble statistic computers but pattern recognition systems. Humans can recognize patterns or objects very easily but fail when probabilities have to be assigned to observations.

J. Crespo, V. Maojo, and F. Martin (Eds.): ISMDA 2001, LNCS 2199, pp. 1-13, 2001.

These principal difficulties are not widely known by physicians. Also studies who revealed that about 50% of the diagnoses are wrong do not impede the self-conscience of some physicians. It is not by chance that the disease AIDS which manifests by a myriad of infections and cancer states was not discovered directly by treating physicians but by statistical people observing the improbable density of rare cancer cases at the U.S. west coast.

An important solution for the described problem lies in the systematic application of statistical instruments. The good availability of computers ameliorate the possibilities of statistically inexperienced physicians to apply the benefits of such a kind of diagnosis:

- Also physicians in the learning phase with less experience can obtain a reliable diagnosis using the collected data of experienced colleagues.
- Even in the case of rare diseases, e.g. septic shock, it is possible to get a good diagnosis if they use the experience of world-wide networked colleagues.
- New, unknown diseases can be systematically documented even if this induces complex computations which are not known to the treating physician.
- Also in the treatment of standard diseases a critical statistical discussion for the use of operation methods or medical therapies may introduce doubts in the physicians own, preferred methods as it is propagated by the ideas of evidence based medicine EBM16.

A classical, early study 8 in the year 1971 showed these basic facts in the medical area. At the university clinic of Leeds (UK) 472 patients with acute abdominal pain where examined and diagnosed. With simple, probability-based methods (Bayes classification) the diagnostic decision probabilities were computed based on a data base of 600 patients. Additionally, a second set of probabilities were computed by using a synthetic data base of patients build on the interviews of experts and questionnaire sheets about 'typical' symptoms.

Then, the 472 cases were diagnosed by an expert round of 3 experienced and 3 young physicians. The results of this experiment was as follows:

- Best human diagnosis (most experienced physician): *79.7%*
- Computer with expert data base: *82.2%*
- Computer with 600 patient data: *91.1%*

The conclusion is clear: humans can not ad hoc analyze complex data without errors. Can neural networks help in this situation?

2   The Prognostic Capabilities of Neural Networks

Let us shortly review the prognostic capabilities of adaptive systems like those of neural networks. There is a long list of successful applications of neural networks in medicine, e.g. 13,27. Examples are given below:

Myocardial Infarction [1]

From 356 patients of a heart intensive care unit 120 suffered from acute myocardial infarction. Based on these data, Baxt (1990) trained a network and obtained a sensitivity of 92% and a specificity of 96% for heart attack prediction.

Back Pain [3]

145 responses of a questionnaire represented the input, 4 possible diagnosis results were the output (simple lower back pain SLBP, root pain RP, spinal pain SP, abnormal illness behavior AIB). After training with 50 example cases the following correct percentage for 50 test cases were observed (Table 1):

Table 1   Diagnostic correctness of back pain

Method	SLBP %	RP %	SP %	AIB %	average %
Network	63	90	87	95	83
Neuro-surgeon	96	92	60	80	82
orthoped. surg.	88	88	80	80	84
common phys.	76	92	64	92	81

For this application, the network has (in the average) roughly the same success as the human, experienced experts. Nevertheless, for the non-critical case of simple lower back pain the network was worse than the physicians; for the important case of spinal symptoms where a quick intervention is necessary the network was better than the experts.

- **Survival probability** after severe injury [21]
- For 3 input variables (Revised Trauma Score RTS, Injury Severity Score ISS, age) and 2 output variables (life, death) a network was trained with 4800 examples. Compared to the traditional score method TRISS and a variant ASCOT which separate special risk groups before scoring, resulted in the following diagnostic scores for juvenile patients (Table 2):

Table 2 Diagnostic success for severe injury of juvenile patients

Diagnose	TRISS	ASCOT	NNet
sensitivity %	83,3	80,6	90,3
specificity %	97,2	97,5	97,5

The significant higher sensitivity of the neural network can be deduced to the superiority of the adaptive approach of the neural net compared to the fixed linear weighting of the scores (as e.g. APACHE). A linear weighting corresponds to only one layer of linear neurons (e.g. the *output layer*); the categorical score input corresponds to fixed nonlinear neurons (e.g. the *hidden units*).

Beside the high number of successful medical applications (MedLine [18] listed about 1700 papers for the keywords "artificial neural network" in spring 2001) there are many reviews for the use of artificial neural networks in medicine, see e.g. [9,24,26]. In this contribution, only the basic principles of neural networks will be presented in the next section in order to set the base for applications like the one in section 4.

3   Basic Principles of Neural Networks

Let us start by modelling the artificial neurons. Like in nature neural networks consist of many small units, the formal neurons. They are interconnected and work together. Each neuron has several inputs and one output only. In Fig. 1 a biological neuron and an artificial neuron are shown.

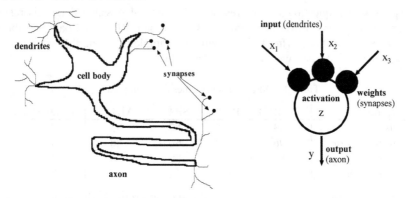

Fig. 1 A biological neuron and an artificial one

Our formal neuron has inputs x_i, each one weighted by a weight factor w_i. We model all of the neural inputs from the same neighbour neuron by just one weighted input. Typically, the activation z is modelled by a weighted sum of the n inputs

$$z = \sum_{i=1}^{n} w_i x_i \qquad (1)$$

The output activity y is a function S of the activation, generally a nonlinear one.

Nonlinear predictions are provided by nonlinear neurons, i.e. neurons with a nonlinear function $S_i(z)$ for the i-th neuron, e.g. a radial basis function (RBF)

$$S_i(z) = e^{-z^2} \text{ with } z^2 = \frac{(c_i - x)^2}{2\sigma_i^2} \qquad (2)$$

This bell-shaped function provides a local sensitivity of each neuron i for an area of width σ_i centred at point c_i.

If we arrange several neurons in parallel and then in different layers, we get a mapping from input to output ("feedforward network"). Given a certain task, what kind of network should we choose? To resolve this question, we should know: what is in general the power of a network? For a two layer network (Fig. 2) containing at least one nonlinear layer we know that we can approximate any function as close as desired. For a more precise notation of this property, see e.g. [15].

For our purpose, we have to decide whether we want to solve a classification or prediction task, based on a number of known cases, or if we want to make a kind of data mining approach, discovering new proportions of the data. In the first case we should take a multi-layer decision network with a learning algorithm based on the classification probability, not on a distance measure like the mean square error of approximation. The classification might be done either by a multi-layer-perceptron MLP or a radial basis function network RBF, see [12]. In either case, the network is trained to do a certain classification job by presenting the patient data and the correct classification to the network. It is the task of the network to predict the class of an unknown patient from the presented data, giving rise to appropriate treatments.

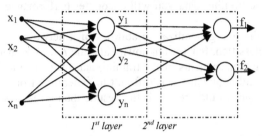

Fig. 2 A two-layer network

Preprocessing the Data

Very important for medical data analysis, especially for retrospective evaluations, is the preprocessing of the data, see [23]. The problems are listed below.

- The **data set** in single studies is often **too small** to produce reliable results.
- Often, medical data material is very **inhomogeneous**, coming from multivariate time series with irregularly measured time stamps.
- **Typing errors** are detected by checking bounds of the variables.
- A lot of variables shows a high number of **missing values** caused by faults or simply by seldom measurements.
- **Feature variables** should be **selected** to avoid the so called "curse of dimensionality"

For our task we heavily rely on the size of the data and their diagnostic quality. If the data contains too much inaccurate or missing entries we have no chance of building up a reliable system even if it is principally possible.

Training and Testing

In general, the networks have to be trained in order to get the parameters set for a proper function. We distinguish between two modes: the *supervised training* where we add to each training sample input (patient data) also the desired network output information (e.g. the correct classification), and the *unsupervised training* which is used to extract statistical information from the samples. The latter is often used for signal preprocessing, e.g. PCA and ICA, see [12].

How do we get the parameters of the chosen network, e.g. σ_i and c_k of eq.(2) ? 1 **Changing the parameters** at fixed network: The parameters are updated such that an objective function $R(w)$ is optimised. 2 **Growing networks** with fixed parameters: Starting with one neuron, for each data sample which causes a high error in the prediction a new neuron is added to the network. All parameters are set such that the error is decreased.

It is well known that the performance of learning systems on the training data often does not reflect the performance on unknown data. This is due to the fact that the system often adapts well on training to the particularities of the training data. Therefore, the training data should be randomly chosen from all available data. It should represent the typical data properties, e.g. the probability distribution. If you have initially a bias in the training data you will encounter performance problems for the test data later.

In order to test the real generalization abilities of a network to unknown data, it must be tested by classified, but yet unknown data, the *test data* that should not contain samples coming from patients of the training data. We have to face the fact that patient data is very individual and it is difficult to generalize from one patient to another. Ignoring this fact would pretend better results than a real system could practically achieve.

Interfacing the Results

One of the most important questions for diagnosis is the design of the user interface. Why?

Neural networks are seldom designed to explain what they have learned. The approach of using the experience of the physician and explaining the diagnosis by proper medical terms is crucial for the question whether a diagnostic system is used or ignored. In general, all diagnostic systems, even the most sophisticated ones, are worthless if they are not used. So, the importance of acquiring the necessary knowledge and presenting the results in a human understandable, easy way can not be overestimated.

Now, with the appearance of fuzzy systems which use vague, human-like categories [20] the situation for knowledge-based diagnosis has changed. Based on the well-known mechanisms of learning in RBF networks, a neuro-fuzzy interface can be used for the input and output of neural systems. The intuitive and instructive interface is useful in medical applications, using the notation and habits of physicians and other medically trained people. In Fig. 3 this concept is visualized.

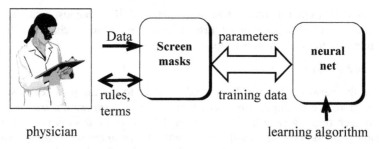

Fig. 3 Interactive transfer of vague knowledge

Here, the user interface must use the typical human properties and formulate the diagnosis by the vague, inexact language of physicians. The following notational habits of physicians for variables and possible outcomes have to be reflected by the user interface:

- Exact notation, e.g. blood sugar = 120 mg/dl.
- Semi-quantitative notation,   e.g. 120 to 130 mg/dl   or ++ , + , 0 , - , -- .
- Qualitative, categorical notation,   e.g. test result = red.

To support these notations, we might use the idea of fuzzy terms, called "vague terms", described by membership functions. As example, in Fig. 4 the assignment of the vague linguistic terms of the medical variable SGOT to the vague variable x (concentration IE/l) is shown. This results in a vague set of membership functions showed in Fig. 4. For each function, the set $\{x \mid \mu(x)=1\}$ is called the *core*, whereas the whole set $\{x \mid \mu(x)>0\}$ is called the *support* of function μ. To each term of a vague set, we have to attach a name or a label.

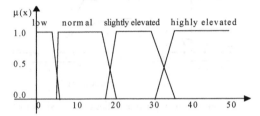

Fig. 4 The vague set of the linguistic variable SGOT

For the sake of an easy, robust interface for network initialization purposes (information stream from left to right in Fig. 3) it is wise not to assume any knowledge about appropriate membership functions by the user which is certainly true for most of the physicians. Instead, let us use the most simple membership function which is in coherence with the medical expert intuition: a simple trapezoidal bell shaped function which is directly assigned to the Radial Basis Function of a RBF neuron.

In conclusion, by using a trapezoidal function as standard membership function we can easily satisfy all the demands of the medical interface. As free parameters the lower and upper core limits [min,max] are chosen as the medical range limits while the ramps are assumed standard. An application of this kind of rule based system is presented in section 4.2.

In [7] a prototype implementation *Analyst1* [16] of such an interface is described.

4   Case Study: Diagnosing Septic Shock Patients

In intensive care units (ICUs) there is one event which only rarely occurs but which indicates a very critical condition of the patient: the septic shock. For patients being in this condition the survival rate dramatically drops down to 40-50% which is not acceptable.

Up to now, there is neither a successful clinical therapy to deal with this problem nor are there reliable early warning criteria to avoid such a situation. The event of sepsis and septic shock is rare and therefore statistically not well represented. Due to this fact, neither physicians can develop well grounded experience in this subject nor a statistical basis for this does exist. Therefore, the diagnosis of septic shock is still made too late, because at present there are no adequate tools to predict the progression of sepsis to septic shock. No diagnosis of septic shock can be made before organ dysfunction is manifest.

By the analysis of septic shock data we want to change this situation.

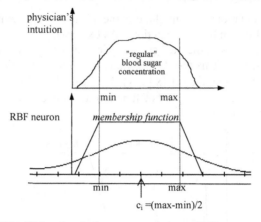

Fig. 5 Mapping the human association to RBF output

The Data

In our case, the epidemiology of 656 intensive care unit patients was elaborated in a study made between November 1995 and December 1997 at the clinic of the J. W. Goethe-University, Frankfurt am Main [28]. The data of this study and another study made in the same clinic between November 1993 and November 1995 is the basis of our work.

We set up a list of 140 variables, including readings (temperature, blood pressure, ...), drugs (dobutrex, dobutamin, ...) and therapy (diabetes, liver cirrhosis, ...). Our data base consists of 874 patients. 70 patients of all had a septic shock. 27 of the septic shock patients and 69 of all the patients deceased.

With only a small amount of data in each study we had to fuse the two studies to one. Additionally, the variables had to be resampled in order to fit into a common time frame. For our data, not the typing errors but the missing values was the main problem.

The data base contains about 140 variables of metric nature, only partially usable. In our case, for analysis the physicians gave us recommendations which variables are the most important ones for a classification, based on their experience. The chosen variable set V is composed of n=16 variables: pO_2 (arterial) [mmHg], pCO_2 (arterial) [mmHg], pH, leukocytes [1000/μl], thromboplastin time (TPZ) [%], thrombocytes [1000/μl], lactate [mg/dl], creatinin [mg/dl], heart frequency [1/min], volume of urine [ml/24h], systolic blood pressure [mmHg], frequency of artificial respiratory [1/min], inspiratorical O_2-concentration [%], medication with antithrombine III AT3 [%], medication with dopamine and dobutrex [μg/(kg·min)].

4.1 Diagnosis by Growing Neural Networks

The neural network chosen for our classification task is a modified version of the supervised growing neural gas (abbr. SGNG, see [10]). Compared to the classical multilayer perceptron trained with backpropagation (see [12]) which has reached a wide public, this network achieved similar results on classification tasks but converges faster, see [14]. The algorithm with our improvements and additional benchmark results are noted in detail in [11]. It is based on the idea of radial basis functions. Its additional advantage is the ability to insert neurons within the learning process to adapt its structure to the data.

In our case we had only 70 patients with the diagnosis "septic shock". Our classification is based on 2068 measurement vectors (16-dimensional samples) from variable set V taken from the 70 septic shock patients. 348 samples were deleted because of too many missing values within the sample. With 75% of the 1720 remaining samples the SGNG was trained and with 25% samples from completely other patients than in the training set it was tested. The variables were normalized (mean 0, standard deviation 1) for analysis.

The network chosen was the one with the lowest error on the smoothed test error function. Three repetitions of the complete learning process with different, randomly selected divisions of the data were made. The results are presented in Table 3.

Table 3 Correct classifications, sensitivity, specificity with standard deviation, minimum and maximum in % from three repetitions

measure	mean value	standard deviation	minimum	maximum
correct classification	67.84	6.96	61.17	75.05
Sensitivity	24.94	4.85	19.38	28.30
Specificity	91.61	2.53	89.74	94.49

To achieve a generally applicable result ten repetitions would be better, but here it is already clear: with the low number of data samples the results can only have prototypical character, even with more cleverly devised benchmark strategies.

On average we have an alarm rate (= 1 − specificity) of 8.39% for survived patients showing also a critical state and a detection of about 1 out of 4 critical illness states. For such a complex problem it is a not too bad, but clearly no excellent result. An explanation for this low number is grounded in the different, individual measurements of each patient.

4.2 Diagnosis by Rule Based Networks

Results of classification procedures could provide a helpful tool for medical diagnosis. Nevertheless, in practice physicians are highly trained and skilled people who do not accept the diagnosis of an unknown machine (black box) in their routine. For real applications, the diagnosis machine should be become transparent, i.e. the diagnosis should explain the reasons for classification. Whereas the explanation component is obvious in classical symbolic expert system tools, neural network tools hardly explain their decisions. This is also true for the SGNG network used in the previous section.

Therefore, as important alternative in this section we consider a classification by learning classification rules which can be inspected by the physician. The details of the network structure and the learning algorithm can be found in [5,19].

The result of the training procedure are rules of the form (belonging to the core or support rectangle)

if variable 1 **in** (−∞, 50) **and**
if variable 2 **in** (20,40) **and**
if variable 3 **in** (−∞,∞)
then *class 1*   (3)

in addition with a classification. Here, variable 3 could be omitted.

Now we present the results of the rule generation process with our previously introduced septic shock data set. The data set is 16-dimensional. A maximum of 6 variables for every sample was allowed to be missing. The missing values were replaced by random data from normal distributions similar to the original distributions of the variables. So it was assured that the algorithm can not learn a biased result due to biased replacements, e.g. class-dependent means. We demand a minimum of 10 out of 17 variables measured for each sample, so there remained 1677 samples out of 2068 for analysis.

The data we used in 5 complete training sessions – each one with a different randomly chosen training data set – was in mean coming from class 1 with a percentage of 72.10% and from class 2 with a percentage of 27.91%. In the mean 4.00 epochs were needed (with standard deviation 1.73, minimum 3 and maximum 7). Test data was taken from 35 randomly chosen patients for every training session, containing no data sample of the 35 patients in the training data set. In Table 4 the classification results are presented.

Table 4 Mean, standard deviation, minimum and maximum of correct classifications and not classifiable data samples of the test data set. In %

	mean	standard deviation	minimum	maximum
correct classifications	68.42	8.79	52.92	74.74
not classified	0.10	0.22	0.00	0.48

Average specificity ("deceased classified / all deceased") was 88 % and average sensitivity ("survived classified / all survived") was 18.15 %. The classification result is not satisfying, although similar to the results in section 4.1 but with the benefit of explaining rules and less training epochs. Deceased patients were not detected very well. Reasons for this can be the very individual behavior of the patients and the data quality (irregularity of measurements, missing values). In this way it seems not possible to classify *all* the patients correctly, but it could be that in some areas of the data space the results are better (*local rules*). In the mean 22.80 rules were generated for the class *survived* and 17.80 rules were generated for class *deceased*.

5   Discussion and Outlook

After a short introduction and review of existing medical applications, the typical problems in analyzing medical data were presented and discussed.

In general, results of a patient classification or prediction task are true only with a certain probability. Therefore, any prognostic system can not predict always the correct future state but may just give early warnings for the treating physician. These warnings should constitute an additional source of information; the backward conclusion that, if there is no warning there is also no problems, is not true and should be avoided.

Two of the most typical and important neural network approaches were presented: the black-box and the neuro-fuzzy rule based system approach. The first approach for medical diagnosis by neural network is the black-box approach: A network is chosen and trained with examples of all classes. After successful training, the system is able to diagnose the unknown cases and to make predictions. The advantage of this approach is the adaptation of all parameters of the system for a (hopefully) best prediction performance.

Another diagnostic approach by neural networks is adaptive rule generation. By this, we can explain the class boundaries in the data and at the same time find out the necessary variables for a rule of the prediction system, see eq.(3). By using a special approach of rectangular basis networks we achieved approximately the same classification results as by the growing neural gas. Additionally, the diagnosis was explained by a set of explicitly stated medical rules.

One of the unresolved questions not only in this contribution is the application of the diagnostic results. Who should apply them when? Although a good test of the network provides the statistical means for the evaluation of the prediction performance, in clinical research this is not sufficient. A widely accepted procedure is a randomized double-blind study. Therefore, in order to make a prediction or classification system acceptable and usable in the medical world, after creating a successful neural network diagnosis system or deducing good rules a new clinical trial has to be conceived and performed with the final network state. Only after such an controlled study the results should be used, eventually taking the classification base and feasibility of such a system into account.

Even when the clinical trial was successful, you will encounter a problem: the problem of ignorance. As long as physicians can come along with their clinical routine in treating patients, they will do it. Nowadays, nearly for each disease there exist an international renowned standard procedure, but most physicians will not use it. Why? First, they have to know it and second, most physicians rely on their own expertise. To overcome this, one have to include diagnostic expertise into the clinical standard software. Here, clinical information systems with the possibility of plug-in software are very rare, but we are on the way. Future administrative necessities for complete input of patient data (e.g. TISS score) will also enhance the possibility for automatic diagnosis by such paradigms as neural networks.

Acknowledgements

The author would like to thank his coworkers of the MEDAN group F. Hamker for the results of section 4.1 and J. Paetz for the work of section 4.2.

References

1. Baxt W. (1990): Use of an artificial neural network for data analysis in clinical decision making: the diagnosis of acute coronary occlusion, Neural Computation; 2: 480-489
2. Bottaci L., Drew P., Hartley J., Hadfield M., Farouk R., Lee P., Macintyre I., Duthie G., Monson J. (1997): *Artificial neural networks applied to outcome prediction for colorectal cancer patients in separate institutions;* Lancet, 350: 469-472
3. Bounds D., Lloyd P. J.(1988): *A multi-layer perceptron network for the diagnosis of low back pain*; Proc. IEEE Int. Conf. on Neural Networks, Vol.II: 481-489
4. Brause R. (1995): *Neuronale Netze*; Teubner Verlag, Stuttgart, 2nd edition
5. Brause R., Hamker F., Paetz J.: *Septic Shock Diagnosis By Neural Networks And Rule Based Systems*; in: L.C. Jain: Computational Intelligence Techniques In Medical Diagnosis And Prognosis, Springer Verlag 2001, *in press*
6. Brause R., Hanisch E. (Eds.) (2000), *Medical Data Analysis ISMDA 2000*. Springer Lecture Notes in Comp.Sc., LNCS 1933, Springer Verlag, Heidelberg
7. Brause R., Friedrich F. (2000): *A Neuro-Fuzzy Approach as Medical Interface*, European Symp. On Neural Networks, ESANN 2000, pp. 201-206, D-Facto, Brussels
8. de Dombal F. T., Leaper D. J., Staniland J. R., McCann A. P., Horrocks J. C. (1972): *Acute Abdominal Pain*, Brit. Med. J. 2: 9-13
9. Forsstrom J. J., Dalton K. J. (1995): Artificial neural networks for decision support in clinical medicine. Ann Med. Oct; 27(5):509-17.
10. Fritzke B. (1995): *A Growing Neural Gas Network Learns Topologies*, Proc. Advances in Neural Information Processing Systems (NIPS 7), in G. Tesauro, D. S. Touretzky, T. K. Leen, MIT Press, Cambridge, MA, 625-632
11. Hamker F., Paetz J., Thöne S., Brause R., Hanisch E. (2000): *Erkennung kritischer Zustände von Patienten mit der Diagnose "Septischer Schock" mit einem RBF-Netz*. Interner Bericht 04/00, Fachbereich Infor*matik*, J. W. Goethe-Universität Frankfurt a. M., http://www.cs.uni-frankfurt.de/fbreports/fbreport04-00.pdf
12. Haykin S. (1999): *Neural Networks, A Comprehensive Foundation*. Prentice Hall, 2nd edition, Upper Saddle River, NJ 07458
13. Heden B., Edenbrandt L., Haisty W. K. jr., Pahlm O. (1994): Artificial neural networks for the electrocardiographic diagnosis of healed myocardial infarction; Am. J. Cardiol. 74(1): 5-8
14. Heinke D., Hamker F. (1998), Comparing Neural Networks, A Benchmark on Growing Neural Gas, Growing Cell Structures, and Fuzzy ARTMAP. *IEEE Transactions on Neural Networks* 9(6), 1279-1291

15. Hornik K., Stinchcombe M., White H. (1990): Universal Approximation of an Unknown Mapping and Its Derivatives Using Multilayer Feedforward Networks; Neural Networks, Vol 3, pp. 551-560
16. http://hiru.mcmaster.ca/
17. http://www.cs.uni-frankfurt.de/~brause/software/Analyst1.exe
18. http://www.ncbi.nlm.nih.gov:80/entrez/query.fcgi?db=PubMed
19. Huber K.-P., Berthold M. R. (1995): *Building Precise Classifiers with Automatic Rule Extraction.* IEEE International Conference on Neural Networks 3, 1263-1268
20. Zadeh L. A., Kacprzyk J. (1992): *Fuzzy logic for the management of uncertainty,* John Wiley & Sons Inc., New York
21. McGonigal M. (1994): *A New Technique for Survival Prediction in Trauma Care Using a Neural Network,* Proc. World Conference on Neural Networks, pp.3495-3498
22. Miller P. L. (1986): Expert Critiquing Systems: *Practice-based Medical Consultation by Computer*; Springer Verlag, New York
23. Paetz J., Hamker F., and Thöne S. (2000): *About the Analysis of Septic Shock Patient Data*, in:6
24. Penny W., Frost D. (1996): *Neural networks in clinical medicine.* Med. Decis. Making. Oct-Dec; 16(4):386-398
25. Sharpe P. K. Solberg H. E. Rootwelt K. Yearworth M. (1993): *Artificial neural networks in diagnosis of thyroid function from in vitro laboratory tests;* Clin. Chem. 39(11 Pt 1): 2248-2253
26. Sharpe P. K., Caleb P. (1994): *Artificial neural networks within medical decision support systems.* Scand J Clin Lab Invest Suppl.;219:3-11.
27. Snow P. B., Smith D. S. (1994): Artificial neural networks in the diagnosis and prognosis of prostate cancer: a pilot study; J. Urology. 152(5 Pt 2): 1923-1926
28. Wade, S., Büssow, M. Hanisch, E. (1998): Epidemiology of Systemic Inflammatory Response Syndrome, Sepsis and Septic Shock in Surgical Intensive Care Patients, Chirurg;69(6):648-655

On Applying Supervised Classification Techniques in Medicine

Basilio Sierra, Iñaki Inza, and Pedro Larrañaga

Dept. of Computer Science and Artificial Intelligence, University of the Basque
Country
P.O. Box 649, E-20080 San Sebastián, Spain
ccpsiarb@si.ehu.es (Basilio Sierra)
http://www.sc.ehu.es/isg

Abstract. This paper presents an overview of the Supervised Classification Techniques that can be applied in medicine. Supervised Classification concerns to the Machine Learning area, and many paradigms have been used in order to develop Decision Support Systems that could help the physician in the diagnosis task. Different families of classifiers can be distinguished based on the model used to do the final classification: Classification Rules, Decision Trees, Instance Based Learning and Bayesian Classifiers are presented in this paper. These techniques have been extended to many research and application fields, and some examples in the medical world are presented for each paradigm.

Keywords: Supervised Classification, Model Search, Machine Learning, Decision Support System, Pattern Recognition.

1 Introduction

Traditionally, medical practice has been guided by empirical observation, in the form of anecdotes, case reports, or well designed clinical trials. With the generalization of the use of computers, health care actions made in the different health services of the world have collected a huge amount of data, having a big number of different databases that contain rich medical information, which would be available to the health care experts if generalization of the knowledge contained could be possible.

In order to develop computer programs that could serve the physicians, a lot of work has been done in hospital and health services; databases containing patients medical histories, information about diseases, pills and medicines, and so one became a normal tool in every medical desk. Traditional manual data analysis has become inadequate, and methods for efficient computer based analysis indispensable. Next step was to develop programs to help in the diagnosis decision. This has be done in the Artificial Intelligence area in the form of Expert Systems, Decision Support Systems, and other kind of computer programs that have in common the capacity of doing an optimal management of the data in order to extract the knowledge contained in the data.

J. Crespo, V. Maojo, and F. Martin (Eds.): ISMDA 2001, LNCS 2199, pp. 14–19, 2001.

Expert Systems (ES) are one of the most developed areas in the field of Artificial Intelligence; ES are computer programs designed to help or replace humans tasks where the human experience and knowledge are scarce and unreliable. Medical domain is characterized by inherent uncertainty, and a great number of paradigms have been developed to deal with patient information.

Some of these paradigms belong to the so called Supervised Classification (CS) area, in which the goal is to decide, based on the information of a given case (the symptoms of a patient, for example) the most likely classification we should consider that it has (the disease (S)he probably has, or the decision about the patient having some determined illness or not). In this paper Supervised Classification is presented, and an overview of the application of the different CS techniques to the medical world is done. See [3] for a good review.

The rest of the paper is organized as follows: Supervised Classification Techniques are introduced in Section 2, while section 3 presents some extensions that can be applied to the basic methods. Section 4 presents some real medical databases that have been used in order to do Supervised Classification. Section 5 presents a brief summary of the work.

2   Supervised Classification Techniques

The main task in Supervised Classification is the application of a learning algorithm (or inducer) to obtain a classifier (or classification model) [4]. The learning algorithm needs a dataset of labelled N examples (or patient information records) $E = \{\mathbf{Patient_1}, ..., \mathbf{Patient_N}\}$, each one characterized by n descriptive features (variables or symptoms) $\mathbf{X} = \{Symptom_1, ..., Symptom_n\}$ and the class label (or disease) $Disease = \{D_1, ..., D_N\}$ to which they belong, where the class label of each instance is part of a discrete set of R values: $D_j \in \{D^1, ..., D^R\}$. The learning algorithm uses the set of labelled examples to induce a classifier which will be used to classify unlabelled examples. An overview of the needed dataset of cases can be seen in Table 1.

Starting from the dataset of labelled examples, the class label *supervises* the induction process of the classifier, which is used in a second step to predict, the most accurately as possible, the class label for further unlabelled examples. Thus, a bet is performed, *classifying* the unlabelled example with the label that the classifier predicts for it.

Table 1. An overview of the needed dataset for supervised classification task

	$Symptom_1$ ... $Symptom_n$		$Disease$
Patient₁	x_1^1	... x_1^n	D_1
Patient₂	x_2^1	... x_2^n	D_2
...	... ...	...	...
Patient_N	x_N^1	... x_N^n	D_N

A structured supervised learning algorithm is able to induce a classifier, which can be seen as a function that maps an unlabelled example to a specific class label. Nowadays, this process can be done automatically by a computer program.

2.1   Decision Trees

A *decision tree* consists of nodes and branches to break a set of samples into a set of covering decision rules. In each node, a single test or decision is made to obtain a partition. The starting node is usually referred to as the root node. In the terminal nodes or leaves a decision is made on the class assignment. In each node, the main task is to select an attribute that makes the best partition between the classes of the samples in the training set.

2.2   Instance-Based Learning

Instance-Based Learning (IBL)[1] has its root in the study of the Nearest Neighbor algorithm in the field of Machine Learning. The simplest form of Nearest Neighbor (NN) or k-Nearest Neighbor (k-NN) algorithms, simply store the training instances and classify a new instance by predicting that it has the same class as its nearest stored instance or the majority class of its k nearest stored instances according to some distance measure. The core of this non-parametric paradigm is the form of the similarity function that computes the distances from the new instance to the training instances, to find the nearest or k-nearest training instances to the new case.

2.3   Rule Induction

One of the most expressive and human readable representations for learned hypothesis is sets of *IF-THEN rules*. In this kind of rules, the *IF* part contains conjunctions and disjunctions of conditions composed by the predictive attributes of the learning task, and the *THEN* part contains the predicted class for the samples that carry out the *IF* part.

2.4   Bayesian Classifiers

Naive Bayes Paradigm The *Machine Learning* community has studied one simple form of Bayes' rule that assumes independence of the observations of feature variables $X_1, X_2, ..., X_n$, which lets us use the equality

$$P(\wedge X_i | Y_j) = \prod_i P(X_i | Y_j)$$

where $P(X_i | Y_j)$ is the probability of an instance of class Y_j having the observed attribute value X_i.

In the core of this paradigm there is an assumption of independence between the occurrence of features values, that in many tasks is not true; but it is empirically demonstrated that this paradigm gives good results in medical tasks.

Bayesian Networks Bayesian Networks (BNs) constitute a probabilistic framework for reasoning under uncertainty. From an informal perspective, BNs are directed acyclic graphs (DAGs), where the nodes are random variables and the arcs specify the independence assumptions that must be held between the random variables.

BNs are based upon the concept of conditional independence among variables. Once the network is constructed it constitutes an efficient device to perform probabilistic inference. This probabilistic reasoning inside the net can be carried out by exact methods, as well as by approximate methods.

2.5 *Neural Networks*

Neural Networks[4] are a statistical analysis tool, that is, they let us build behavior models starting from a collection of examples (defined by a series of numeric or textual "descriptive variables") of this behavior. The neural net, ignorant at the start, will, through a "learning" process, become a model of the dependencies between the descriptive variables and the behavior to be explained.

The model is automatically and straightforwardly built from the data : no skilled (and costly) technician, such as an expert, statistician or "knowledge engineer" is needed.

3   Extending Standard Paradigms

Although presented paradigms can be used separately, experience in the use of them could give us the idea of extending or combining some of them in order to obtain better classification accuracy. Most usual extensions are presented in the following paragraphs.

- *Feature Subset Selection* The main goal is, given a set of candidate features, to select the best subset under some learning algorithm. This dimensionality reduction made by a FSS process can carry out several advantages for a classification system in a specific task [2]:
  - a reduction in the cost of acquisition of the data,
  - improvement of the compressibility of the final classification model,
  - a faster induction of the final classification model,
  - an improvement in classification accuracy.
- *Prototype Selection*
  As it is done with the features, a selection of cases can be done ion order to obtain faster learning and classification[6]. Usually, three main approaches are used to develop Prototype Selection Algorithms:
  1. Filtration of cases.
     This approaches are introduced in the first research works about prototype selection, and use some kind of rule in order to incrementally determine which cases of the training database will be selected as prototypes and which of them discarded as part of the model.

2. Stocastical search.

   Among the stocastical search methods, some of them make use of Genetic Algorithms to select prototypes.

3. Case weighing.

   In these approaches a computation is done to weight the cases based on well classified or on more abstract concepts.

- *Classifier Combination*

   Combining the predictions of a set of component classifiers has shown to yield accuracy higher than the most accurate component on a long variety of supervised classification problems (Sierra et al. [5]).

4   Medical Examples

Supervised Classification Techniques have been applied to many medical domains. The following paragraphs provide a short description of the nature and reality aspects covered by each medical domain. These files can be found in the existing repositories an can be use to do some experimental work and comparisons about the accuracy of different paradigms.

- *Echocardiogram* dataset's task is to predict whether a patient survived for at least one year following a heart attack.
- *Hepatitis* dataset's task is to predict whether a patient will die from hepatitis.
- *Audiology* dataset is obtained from the Baylor College of Medicine. Thanks go to Professor Jergen for providing the data.
- *Heart disease* dataset comes from the Cleveland Clinic Foundation (USA) and was supplied by R. Detrano.
- *Breast cancer* dataset is obtained from the University Medical Centre, Institute of Oncology, Ljubljana, Slovenja. Thanks go to M. Zwitter and M. Soklic for providing the data.
- *Liver (BUPA)* dataset was created at BUPA Medical Research Ltd. As each instance describes a male patient's medical data, the task is to determine whether the patient suffers from liver disorder, that might arise from excessive alcohol consumption.
- *Arrhythmia* dataset was created by H. A. Guvenir, at Bilkent University, Turkey. The aim is to distinguish between the presence and absence of cardiac arrhythmia and to classify it in one of the 15 classes of arrhythmia;
- *Breast cancer (Wisconsin)* dataset concerns medical diagnosis applied to breast cytology. The task is to predict whether a breast tumour is benign or malignant.
- *Diabetes (Pima)* dataset was collected by the USA National Institute of Diabetes and Digestive and Kidney Diseases.
- *Contraceptive* dataset is donated by T.S. Lim and it is a subset of the 1987 National Indonesia Contraceptive Prevalence Survey.
- *Sick-euthyroid* dataset was collected at the Garavan Institute in Sidney, Australia. Its task is to identify a patient as having sick-euthyroid disease or not;

- *Hypothyroid* dataset was collected at the Garavan Institute in Sidney, Australia, and it has the same data format and attributes as *Sick-euthyroid*. Thus, *Hypothyroid* task is to identify a patient as having hypothyroid disease or not;
- *DNA* domain is drawn from the field of molecular biology. Splice junctions are points on a DNA sequence at which 'superfluous' DNA is removed during protein creation.

5   Summary

The aim of this paper is to present a variety of Supervised Classification Techniques while showing the possible use of all of them medical problem solving. All the paradigms have been introduced in a brief manner, and different versions of the presented methods exists, as well as different classification approaches that can be found in the literature.

The main idea the authors would like to transmit is that this kind of algorithms should be used in the medical practice, not as substitute of the physicians, but as a help tool the doctor have in order to help taking the final decision, in the same way that medical people look to medicine databases in order to decide which pills should take the patient.

Acknowledgements

This work was supported by the Gobierno Vasco – Instituto Vasco de Meteorología and the grant UPV 140.226-EB131/99 from University of the Basque Country.

References

1. D. Aha, D. Kibler and M. K. Albert (1991): Instance-Based learning algorithms. *Machine Learning* **6**, 37-66. 16
2. I. Inza, M. Merino, P. Larrañaga, J. Quiroga, B. Sierra and M. Girala (2001): "Feature subset selection by genetic algorithms and estimation of distribution algorithms. A case study in the survival of cirrhotic patients treated with TIPS" *Artificial Intelligence in Medicine* In press. 17
3. N. Lavrač (1999): Machine Learning for Data Mining in Medicine. *Lecture Notes in Artificial Intelligence*, **1620**. 47-62. 15
4. T. Mitchell (1997): *Machine Learning*. McGraw-Hill. 15, 17
5. B. Sierra, N. Serrano, P. Larrañaga, E. J. Plasencia, I. Inza, J. J. Jiménez, J. M. De la Rosa and M. L. Mora (2001): Using Bayesian networks in the construction of a multi-classifier. A case study using Intensive Care Unit patient data. *Artificial Intelligence in Medicine.* **22** 233-248. 18
6. D. B. Skalak (1994): Prototipe and feature selection by Sampling and Random Mutation Hill Climbing Algortithms. *Proceedings of the Eleventh International Conference on Machine Learning*, NJ. Morgan Kaufmann. 293-301. 17

Methods and Criteria for Detecting Significant Regions in Medical Image Analysis

Jose Crespo, Holger Billhardt, Juan Rodríguez-Pedrosa, and José A. Sanandrés

Grupo de Informática Médica, Laboratorio de Inteligencia Artificial, Facultad de
Informática, Universidad Politécnica de Madrid
28660 Boadilla del Monte (Madrid), Spain
jcrespo@fi.upm.es

Abstract. This paper studies the problem of detecting significant regions in medical image analysis. The solution of this non well-defined problem requires in general several criteria to attempt to measure the relevance of an input image features. Criteria properties are important in medical imaging in order to permit their application in a variety of situations. We adopt in this paper the morphological framework, which facilitates the study of the problem and, in addition, provides useful pre-processing and image analysis techniques.

1 Introduction

A central problem in medical image analysis is to detect *significant* regions of an input image [1,2,3]. However, we should note that, in fact, this important problem is not well defined, since the meaning of the term "significant" can greatly depend on the application. Sometimes the primary goal is to locate a pathology within a body organ, whereas in other situations what is important is to abstract to a greater extent the scene and to find the precise boundaries of that organ. Some image analysis techniques use multi-resolution information in order to assess the significance of a feature (attempting to imitate some aspects of the human visual system, which can be considered as a multi-resolution visual system). After significant areas have been detected, an important subsequent objective is often to perform a parition of the input image.

We will address these issues within a specific discipline of image analysis, which is mathematical morphology [4,5,6,7,8]. The strong mathematical foundations of mathematical morphology facilitate the investigation of the properties of operators and the study and comparison of methods and criteria to select significant regions. Nevertheless, most of the ideas covered in this work apply also to other types of image analysis approaches.

The paper is organized as follows. Section 2 treats the image simplification performed by the pre-processing or filtering stage. The segmentation methods that most relate to the significant region detection problem are commented in Section 3. Then, methods and criteria to detect significant regions in medical images are treated in Section 4. Finally, a conclusion section ends the paper, and an appendix provides some basic definitions of mathematical morphology notions.

J. Crespo, V. Maojo, and F. Martin (Eds.): ISMDA 2001, LNCS 2199, pp. 20–27, 2001.

2   Input Image Simplification

The simplification of an input image is an important step, and it can greatly facilitate the significant region extraction task. Medical images present small variations in intensity value and, in general, it is desirable to smooth them away. This stage is often called a pre-processing stage, and the goal is to compute an output image that has *all* significant features of the input image but where un-meaningful and spurious variations have been eliminated.

We normally use at this stage morphological connected filtering [9,10,11], [12,13], which preserves successfully the shapes of the features that have not been smoothed away by the filtering. The idea behind this type of filtering is that if a feature is present in the output image, then its shape should be that of the input image; on the other hand, if a feature is filtered out, then it should not appear at all in the output image. This is achieved because this type of filters impose an inclusion relationship between the piecewise-connected regions of the input image and those of the output regions. This inclusion relationship ensures that the shape of features that are not eliminated is preserved. In particular, we employ compositions of alternating filters by reconstruction. An alternating filter by reconstruction is the sequential composition of a closing $\tilde{\varphi}$ and an opening $\tilde{\gamma}$ by reconstruction: $\tilde{\varphi}\tilde{\gamma}$ or $\tilde{\gamma}\tilde{\varphi}$. When different scales are used, the openings and closings belong to a granulometry $\{\tilde{\gamma}_i\}$ and an anti-granulometry $\{\tilde{\varphi}_i\}$, respectively. For multi-resolution filtering, we use either the so called alternating sequential filters $\tilde{\varphi}_i\tilde{\gamma}_i...\tilde{\varphi}_j\tilde{\gamma}_j...\tilde{\varphi}_1\tilde{\gamma}_1$ (or its dual $\tilde{\gamma}_i\tilde{\varphi}_i...\tilde{\gamma}_j\tilde{\varphi}_j...\tilde{\gamma}_1\tilde{\varphi}_1$) where $i \geq j \geq 1$, or compositions under the the the sup and inf operators of alternating filters by reconstruction, i.e., $\bigwedge_{i=1}^{n} \tilde{\varphi}_i\tilde{\gamma}_i$ and $\bigvee_{i=1}^{n} \tilde{\varphi}_i\tilde{\gamma}_i$. All these filters possess a robustness property against small variations of the input image (such as noise) that is called the *strong* property (a filter ψ is *strong* if and only if $\psi = \psi(I \bigwedge \psi) = \psi(I \bigvee \psi)$).

In Figure 1, a comparison of the effect of three different filters on a medical image is shown. It can be noticed that the morphological connected filter (in particular, an alternating filter by reconstruction $\tilde{\varphi}\tilde{\gamma}$) successfully preserves the shapes of the features of the input image.

3   Partition Methods

Our interest focuses on approaches that can be considered "homogeneity-based", since the first objective is to detect and locate regions whose component pixels share some property. At this step, it is not important to compute the precise shapes of these regions, since their boundaries arise after a pixel assignment method assigns the remaining pixels to one of the selected significant regions. An alternative approach would be the dual one: to detect and to extract first the non-homogeneities of the input image, and then to define significant regions as those sets of connected pixels surrounded by closed contours. However, it is an extremely difficult problem to find the precise location of an input image edges and to ensure that those edges are not broken (i.e., that they form closed contours). These edge-based approaches perform in general worse than

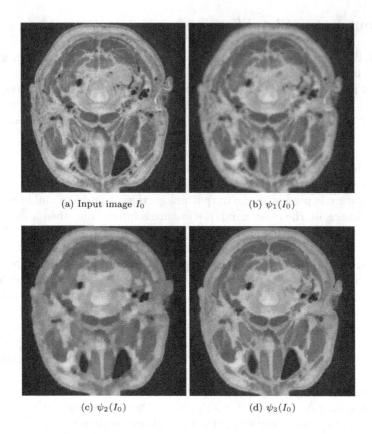

(a) Input image I_0 (b) $\psi_1(I_0)$

(c) $\psi_2(I_0)$ (d) $\psi_3(I_0)$

Fig. 1. Pre-processing stage comparison. ψ_1 is a linear filter, ψ_2 is a morphological non-connected filter, and ψ_3 is a morphological connected filter. In all cases, the size of the window (in (b)) and of the structuring elements (in (c) and (d)) used has been 9×9. (Image size: 600×600.)

homogeneity-based methods, since it is usually the case that is is easier to know where the significant regions are and to find some "safe" region pixels (i.e., pixels that are known to be within homogeneous regions), than to depend on edge information (which is quite sensitive to the presence of noise) to compute the precise boundaries of the image regions at the first stage [14].

In our work we use the significant regions detected as "seeds" of pixel assignment methods that will assign the rest of the pixels to one of the significant regions. In the resulting image, the regions will form a partition (i.e., a set of disjoint connected components that cover the whole image space), and the number of regions will be the same as the number of significant regions. We use mainly morphological segmentation approaches, in particular the watershed approach [15] and a flat zone segmentation method [16]. Nevertheless, the presented ideas apply in general to related techniques such as pixel growing methods. In the morphological framework, the significant regions that constitute the "seeds" of the final regions are denominated *markers*.

4   Significant Regions Detection and Extraction

What constitute a significant feature cannot in general be defined precisely in an objective manner. For example, sometimes size or shape are important whereas in other cases the contrast of a region is the characteristic that determines its significance. And considering contrast, there are several ways to measure it, resulting in similar but different results. A combination of criteria is then normally recommended, since it is not then possible in general to find a single characteristic that successfully locates significant features in a variety of situations. In fact, several multi-criterion approaches can be found in the literature, not only applied for medical imaging [17,16]. Because of the type of filtering used, in this work we consider that features are piecewise-constant regions (or flat zones). This is a restrictive definition but has proven its utility in most applications (besides, it facilitates the study and comparison of different techniques, and piecewise-constant regions relate closely to connected filtering).

Some important criteria to measure the significance of a feature (a piecewise-constant region at the output of connected filtering) are the following:

(a) Whether the feature is a maximum or a minimum
(b) Area (or number of pixels)
(c) Gradient
(d) Gradient-to-area ratio (a combination of (b) and (c))

Features that rank highest in each of the criteria would be selected (a certain number). Some desirable properties of the above mentioned criteria is that they can be defined to be invariant under certain changes of the intensity value. For example, if the dynamic range of an input image were expanded by a factor of 2, the feature ranking for each criterion would not change. This is important especially in medical imaging since dynamic ranges often suffer a great variability. Concerning shape, this characteristic is taken into account in the filtering stage, since morphological filters can be adjusted to remove (or emphasize) certain shapes.

Multi-resolution (or multi-scale) techniques can be an attractive way to compute several sets of features. These approaches provide more information, but correspondences between features obtained at different scales must be established in some way. The pre-processing stage treated in this work facilitate the solution to this problem, since there exist some inclusion relationships between features (piecewise-constant regions) located at different scales. to assess the significance of a feature. A problem that arises using some families of filters is the broken feature problem, displayed in Figure 2. This problem exist when there is not an inclusion relationship between a feature F computed at a certain scale (Fig. 2(b)) and the piecewise-constant regions obtained at a coarser scale

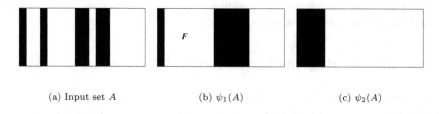

(a) Input set A (b) $\psi_1(A)$ (c) $\psi_2(A)$

Fig. 2. Broken feature problem in multi-scale analysis (binary case)

(Fig. 2(c)). In those cases, further processing of the features at the coarser scale is necessary to avoid this problem.

Nevertheless the utilization of different criteria, in many medical imaging applications used in clinical practice the automatic method to locate significant regions should be supplemented with manual or semiautomatic marker extraction. The reasons are the extreme consequences that can have the failure to locate a significant pathological feature, and that, in general, it cannot be assured that automatic methods will work 100 % of the time. Therefore we have found that in practice most application should offer the possibility to check the markers computed automatically and, if necessary, to add additional markers. Using the segmentation methods commented previously, this is easily performed just by letting physicians to click with the mouse and touch the feature of interest, since it is not necessary to delineate its shape and contours (which, in fact, will be extracted by the segmentation method). The efficiency of the methods involved allows a satisfactory interactivity. Figure 3 displays the extrema piecewise-constant regions (criterion (a)) in white at the output of multi-scale connected filtering (the input image is a part of the image in Fig. 1(a)). This criterion is quite useful in medical image analysis since pathological areas are normaly brighter or darker than their neighboring regions. Multi-scale analysis can be performed considering the extrema region at several scales.

The previous techniques and concepts can be used as well for volumetric 3D images (such as in CT and MRI) The only important modification is the connectivity of the space, which must consider the neighborhood relations between adjacent slices. The extension to 3D image analysis is therefore straightforward. The analysis of multi-modal causes other types of problems. In this case, we have in general one resolution level (although this is not always the case), but there are several bands. In medical imaging this situation arises when, for example, CT and MR slices are available of the same body part. Significant regions must be extracted from the images of each modality and be integrated in a final set of significant regions. The problem is similar to some extent to that of color image analysis, in which the information existent at each band can be quite different.

5   Conclusion

This paper has studied the problem of the detection of significant regions in medical image. Although most ideas apply to other type of processing, we have focused in mathematical morphology approaches because they possess a solid mathematical foundation which facilitates the study of the properties of operators and techniques. A single criteria is not in general sufficient to detect significant regions in a variety of medical imaging situations. Therefore, the usage of several criteria should be normally the case in automatic and semi-automatic medical image applications. Multi-resolution approaches facilitate the assessment of the the significance of features. Once significant regions have been located at several scales, there is the problem of establishing the correspondence between same features at different scales. Connected morphological filtering facilitates this problem because the are some inclusion properties that are satisfied in some situations. However, if that is not the case, further processing of the extracted significant regions is necessary to avoid missing some of them in the final segmentation.

Concerning our medical image analysis and visualization software, we use a mixture of languages. The Python language interpreter is utilized for high-level modules, whereas computational intensive image operations are implemented in C/C++. In addition, we use mainly Java to build GUI for applications that provide both image analysis and 3D visualization capabilities.

Acknowledgements

This work has been supported in part by "Fondo de Investigación Sanitaria" of the Spanish Ministry of Health.

A   Appendix: Basic Concepts in Mathematical Morphology

A basic set of notions on mathematical morphology can be the following.

- Mathematical morphology deals with *increasing* mappings defined on a complete *lattice*. In a complete lattice there exists an ordering relation, and two basic operations called *infimum* and *supremum* (denoted by $\wedge$ and $\vee$, respectively).
- A transformation ψ is *increasing* if and only if it preserves ordering.
- A transformation ψ is *idempotent* if and only if $\psi\psi = \psi$.
- A transformation ψ is a *morphological filter* if and only if it is increasing and idempotent.
- An *opening* γ (or respectively a *closing* φ) is an anti-extensive (respectively extensive) morphological filter.
- An ordered set of openings $\{\tilde{\gamma}_i\}$ (or respectively closings $\{\tilde{\varphi}_i\}$) is called a *granulometry* (respectively *anti-granulometry*).

– An *opening by reconstruction* $\tilde{\gamma}$ can be defined as $\bigvee_{x \in E} \gamma_o \gamma_x$, where γ_x is the operation that extracts the connected component to which x belongs, and where γ_o is a *trivial opening* that leaves unchanged an input set that satisfies an increasing criterion. The dual operator would be a *closing by reconstruction* $\tilde{\varphi}$. These filters are normally computed iterating *geodesic* operators until idempotency.

References

1. Coster, M., Chermant, J.: Précis d'Analyse d'Images. Presses du CNRS (1989) 20
2. Haralick, R., Shapiro, L.: Computer and Robot Vision. Vol. I. Reading, Massachusetts: Adison-Wesley Publishing Company (1992) 20
3. Haralick, R., Shapiro, L.: Computer and Robot Vision. Vol. II. Reading, Massachusetts: Adison-Wesley Publishing Company (1992) 20
4. Serra, J.: Mathematical Morphology. Volume I. London: Academic Press (1982) 20
5. Serra, J., ed.: Mathematical Morphology. Volume II: theoretical advances. London: Academic Press (1988) 20
6. Giardina, C., Dougherty, E.: Morphological Methods in Image and Signal Processing. Englewood Clliffs: Prentice-Hall (1988) 20
7. Beucher, S., Meyer, F.: The morphological approach to segmentation: the watershed transformation. In Dougherty, E., ed.: Mathematical morphology in image processing. New York: Marcel Dekker (1993) 433–481 20
8. Soille, P.: Morphological Image Analysis: Principles And Applications. Springer-Verlag Berlin, Heidelberg, New York (1999) 20
9. Salembier, P., Serra, J.: Flat zones filtering, connected operators, and filters by reconstruction. IEEE Transactions on Image Processing 4 (1995) 1153–1160 21
10. Crespo, J., Serra, J., Schafer, R.: Theoretical aspects of morphological filters by reconstruction. Signal Processing 47 (1995) 201–225 21
11. Crespo, J., Schafer, R.: Locality and adjacency stability constraints for morphological connected operators. Journal of Mathematical Imaging and Vision 7 (1997) 85–102 21
12. Crespo, J., Maojo, V.: New results on the theory of morphological filters by reconstruction. Pattern Recognition 31 (1998) 419–429 21
13. Crespo, J., Maojo, V.: Shape preservation in morphological filtering and segmentation. In: XII Brazilian Symposium on Computer Graphics and Image Processing, IEEE Computer Society Press. (1999) 247–256 21
14. Crespo, J., Schafer, R., Maojo, V.: Image segmentation using intra-region averaging techniques. Optical Engineering 37 (1998) 2926–2936 22
15. Vincent, L., Soille, P.: Watersheds in digital spaces: An efficient algorithm based on immersion simulations. IEEE Trans. Pattern Anal. Machine Intell. 13 (1991) 583–598 22
16. Crespo, J., Schafer, R., Serra, J., Gratin, C., Meyer, F.: The flat zone approach: A general low-level region merging segmentation method. Signal Processing 62 (1997) 37–60 22, 23
17. Salembier, P.: Morphological multiscale segmentation for image coding. Signal Processing 38 (1994) 359–386 23

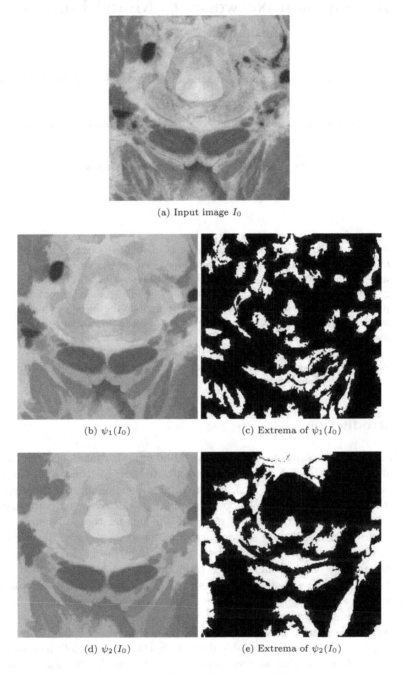

(a) Input image I_0

(b) $\psi_1(I_0)$

(c) Extrema of $\psi_1(I_0)$

(d) $\psi_2(I_0)$

(e) Extrema of $\psi_2(I_0)$

Fig. 3. Extrema regions. The outputs of multi-scale connected filtering at two scales are shown in (b) and (d); their extrema are displayed, respectively, in (c) and (e). (Image size: 256 × 256.)

Using Bayesian Networks to Model Emergency Medical Services

Silvia Acid[1], Luis M. de Campos[1], Susana Rodríguez[2], José María Rodríguez[2], and José Luis Salcedo[2]

[1] Dpto de Ciencias de la Computación e I.A., Universidad de Granada
18071 - Granada, Spain
`acid@decsai.ugr.es,lci@decsai.ugr.es`
[2] Hospital Universitario Virgen de las Nieves
18014 - Granada, Spain
{`susana,joser`}`@hvn.sas.cica.es`

Abstract. Due to the uncertain nature of many of the factors that influence on the performance of an emergency medical service, we propose using Bayesian networks to model this kind of systems. We use an algorithm for learning Bayesian networks to build the model, from the point of view of a hospital manager, and apply it to the specific case of a spanish hospital. We also report the results of some preliminary experimentation with the model.

Keywords: Bayesian networks, Learning algorithms, Emergency medical services, Management problems.

1 Introduction

Health-care systems are complex and depend on organizational, economical and structural factors. The availability of appropriate tools for their representation would allow to study and understand the interactions among the different elements that determine their behaviour, as well as to analyze some alternatives to improve their performance. As many of the factors that influence on the performance of a health-care system are of a uncertain nature, Bayesian networks [Pea88] could play an important role in their study. In this paper we introduce a representation model, based on Bayesian networks, applied to the specific case of an emergency medical service. This model has been obtained, from real data recorded at the hospital "Virgen de las Nieves", using an algorithm for learning Bayesian networks.

The paper is structured as follows: In Section 2 we describe the problem we are going to study and the available data. In Section 3 we briefly comment on the learning algorithm that we have used to build the model. Section 4 describes the network obtained and the results of several experiments, which try to assess the quality of the model from a classification-oriented perspective. In Section 6 we offer some conclusions and proposals for future work.

J. Crespo, V. Maojo, and F. Martin (Eds.): ISMDA 2001, LNCS 2199, pp. 28–34, 2001.

Table 1. Variables

Variable	n. of values	Variable	n. of values
Financing	11	Identification	6
Day	7	Duration of the Stay	3
Shift	3	Cause of Discharge	11
Cause of Admission	8	Medical Service	36
Pathology	7	Centre	3
P10	2		

2   The Problem and the Data Set

As we have already commented, we want to model some aspects of the health-care system for patients that arrive to the emergency department of a hospital. Our first objective is to better understand the interactions between some of the factors that shape this system, and obtain a model that describes reasonably these interactions. Afterwards, the model could be used to estimate the different probability distributions of some variables of interest in different contexts, or even to make predictions about these variables given some partial evidence. Our point of view is not clinical but management oriented, i.e., we try to assist to the hospital manager in organizational and economical questions (e.g., possible redistribution or reinforcement of personnel and infrastructure).

From the set of variables which are collected when a patient enters in the emergency department, the eleven variables displayed in Table 1 were selected. The number of possible values for each variable is also shown in the table. We used a database containing 31937 records, corresponding to all the arrivals to the emergency departments of the hospital "Virgen de las Nieves" at Granada, from 01/01/2001 to 20/02/2001.

Financing represents the type of entity that supports the expenses (Social Security, Insurance companies, International agreements, ...). *Day* is the day of the week in which the patient arrives to the emergency department. *Shift* corresponds to the arrival time of the patient, discretized into 3 values, representing the three different horary periods of the day: morning (8:01-15:00), evening (15:01-22:00) and night (22:01-8:00). *Cause of Admission* codifies 8 different values[1]. *Pathology* includes Common Disease, Common Accident, Industrial Accident, Traffic Accident, Aggression, Self-inflicted Lesion and Other. *P10* represents whether the patient was sent to the emergency medical service by a family doctor. *Identification* codifies the type of identification document of the patient (Identity Card, Social Security Card, Passport, Oral Identification, Other and Unidentified). *Duration of the Stay* is the lenght of time (in hours) that the patient stayed in the emergency department, discretized into 3 values, considered meaningful by the physicians (from 0 to 8 hours, from 8 to 72 hours, and more than 72 hours, which correspond to normal, complicated and anomalous

---

[1] Considered as confidential by the hospital staff.

cases, respectively). *Cause of Discharge* represents several reasons (Return to duty, Death, Hospitalization, Transfer to another hospital, ...). *Medical Service* includes all the different emergency units at the hospital. Finally, *Centre* represents the three different emergency departments corresponding to the three centres that compose the hospital (Maternity hospital, Orthopedic Surgery and General hospital).

3   The Algorithm for Learning Bayesian Networks

There are many algorithms for learning the structure of a Bayesian network from a database, although they may be categorized in only two methods, those based on *independence criteria* [SGS93] or on *scoring metrics* [CH92,HGC95].

The learning algorithm that we have applied to our problem is a version of the BENEDICT (BE) algorithm[2] [AC]. This algorithm, which searches in the space of equivalence classes of directed acyclic graphs (dags)[3], is based on a hybrid methodology that shares with the methods based on scoring metrics the use of heuristic search methods to build a model and then evaluate it using a scoring metric. At the same time, the method has some similarities with those based on independence tests: it explicitly uses the conditional independencies embodied in the topology of the network to elaborate the scoring metric, and carries out conditional independence tests to limit the search effort.

The basic idea of this algorithm is to measure the discrepancies between the conditional independences represented in any given candidate network G (d-separation statements) and those displayed by the database (probabilistic conditional independences). The lesser these discrepancies are, the better the network fits the data. The aggregation of all these local discrepancies results in a measure of global discrepancy between the network and the database. The local discrepancies are measured using the Kullback-Leibler cross entropy, $Dep(x, y|Z)$, which measures the degree of dependence between two variables x and y, given that we know the values of the subset of variables Z. To evaluate a network G, only the values $Dep(x, y|Z)$ for pairs of non-adjacent variables in G, given a d-separating set for x and y of minimum size, Z [AC96], are calculated. The main search process is greedy and only addition of arcs is permitted, although a final refining process (reinsertion of discarded arcs and pruning of inserted arcs) mitigates the irrevocable character of the whole search method.

To compute the conditional (or marginal) probability distributions stored at each node in the network, thus obtaining a complete Bayesian network, we used a maximum likelihood estimator (frequency counts).

---

[2] Acronym of BElief NEtwork DIscovery using Cut-set Techniques.

[3] Other versions of BENEDICT, that search in the space of dags with a given ordering of the variables, and use a slighty different metric, can be found in [AC01].

4 Results

After running the learning algorithm we obtained the network displayed in Figure 1. We want to remark that we do not assume a causal interpretation of the arcs in the network (although in some cases this could be reasonable). Instead, we interpret the arcs as direct dependence relationships between the linked variables, and the absence of arcs means the existence of (conditional) independence relationships.

Due to space limitations, we will not comment on all the 16 arcs included in the network, but only about some of them. The dependence between *Pathology* and *Financing* is explained because the expenses are charged to different entities depending on the type of pathology (traffic accident, industrial accident,...). *Financing* also depends on *Identification* (obviously the expenses will be charged to some entity or company only if the patient can be identified as a member of this entity). The dependence between *Pathology* and *Cause of Admission* is quite evident. The relation between *Cause of Admission* and *Shift* may be due to the fact that the reason to go to the emergency department is not homogeneous across the different hours (Shifts). The arc going from *Medical Service* to *Centre* is justified because Centre is a variable functionally dependent on Medical Service (each Centre has its own emergency medical units). The *Duration* of the stay at the emergency department essentially depends only on the medical unit that tended the patient and the *Cause of Discharge* (the seriousness of the diseases, which is strongly related with the duration of the stay, probably varies from one unit to another). In turn, these two variables are also correlated: For example, a decease as being the cause of discharge is much more unlikely for some medical units than for others.

The learned network can be used with predictive purposes, by using the inference methods (propagation of evidence) available for Bayesian networks. More precisely, from the perspective of a classification problem, we want to use the network to predict the values of some variable of interest given some evidence,

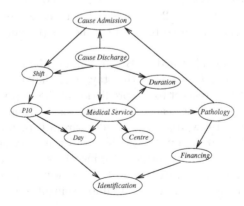

Fig. 1. Structure obtained by the BENEDICT algorithm

Table 2. Success percentages of classification

	Training Set				Test Set			
	BE	$\emptyset_{em}$	NB	C4.5	BE	$\emptyset_{em}$	NB	C4.5
D %	89.9	86.1	86.5	90.1	91.6	96.1	86.3	92.0
MS %	75.9	30.4	76.0	75.9	75.0	31.9	76.0	76.1
P %	85.5	79.6	85.5	85.5	85.6	80.7	85.6	85.6

and compare the predictions obtained with the true values of this variable, thus obtaining the corresponding percentages of success. We have considered three different situations:

- Predicting the values of *Duration* (D %), given evidence about the values of all the other variables, except *Cause of Discharge*. In this way, we try to determine the most probable duration of the stay at the emergency department before the patient is effectively discharged. This information could be useful to redistribute some resources.
- Predicting the values of *Medical Service* (MS %), given evidence relative to all the remaining variables, except *Pathology*, *Cause of Discharge* and *Duration*, which would be unknown at the arrival time of the patient. If accurate, this prediction could serve to direct the arriving patient to the appropriate emergency unit.
- Predicting the values of *Pathology* (P %) given *Medical Service* and *Cause of Admission*.

These experiments may also give us an idea of the robustness of the Bayesian network as a general classifier, as opposed to have to manage a different model for each different problem. We have computed the success percentages obtained for the network learned by BENEDICT and the empty network ($\emptyset_{em}$), which is obviously a poor model (no interaction among the variables), as well as those obtained by the Naive Bayes (NB) classifier [DH73] and C4.5 [Qui93] (a classifier based on decision trees). Table 2 displays the percentages of success obtained for classifying the same data used to build the models (training set) and also for a separate test set[4].

In general, the results obtained by BE, NB and C4.5 are quite similar. With respect to predicting the *Duration* of the stay, note that the percentage of improvement obtained with respect to the prediction of the empty network is rather small for the training set. The reason is that the distribution of the duration of the stay is quite biased towards its first value (from 0 to 8 hours) and therefore the default rule that assigns to all the cases the 'a priori' most probable class gets a high percentage of correct classifications (in fact, in the test set, the proportion of cases with a duration of the stay from 0 to 8 hours is even greater). Similarly, we also get a moderate improvement in the prediction of the

---

[4] containing 12292 arrivals of patients, from 21/02/01 to 10/03/01.

Table 3. Posterior distribution of Shift given P10 and Day

Configuration	Morning	Evening	Night
P10=no, ∀ Day	0.34	0.47	0.18
P10=yes, Day=Weekday	0.47	0.36	0.17
P10=yes, Day=Weekend	0.44	0.37	0.18

Pathology, when using any of the models instead of the 'a priori' distribution. In this case the distribution of pathology is also quite biased towards its first value (common disease). The problem of predicting the *Medical Service* involved is more difficult, and in this case BE, NB and C4.5 considerably outperform the prediction of the empty network.

The network model can also be used to compute the posterior probability of any variable in different contexts. For example, we have calculated the posterior probability distribution of *Shift* given *P10* and *Day* for all the possibles values of these two variables. Table 3 summarizes the results.

It is interesting to note how the arrival pattern to the emergency medical services is quite homogeneous across the different days (including weekend), but this pattern is different depending on patients having a P10 document or not. As expected, patients having a P10 document arrive more frequently in the morning.

5   Concluding Remarks

The complexity of the health-care systems requires appropriate tools for their representation, study and optimization. Bayesian networks constitute a very attractive formalism for representing uncertain knowledge that has been successfully applied in different fields. However, Bayesian networks have been used in medicine essentially to assist in the diagnosis of disorders and to predict the natural course of disease after treatment (prognosis). A novelty of this work is the application of Bayesian networks to other, more management oriented, medical problems. The preliminary results obtained are encouraging, because the learned network is able to manage in a robust way, using a single model, a variety of different prediction problems.

For future works, we plan to extend and refine our model, including more variables, validate it taking into account expert knowledge and use it as a tool to assist to the hospital manager. We also plan to apply Bayesian networks to other management medical problems.

References

AC96.   S. Acid, L. M. de Campos. An algorithm for finding minimum d-separating sets in belief networks. in: E. Horvitz, F. Jensen (Eds.), *Proceedings of the Twelfth Conference on Uncertainty in Artificial Intelligence*, Morgan Kaufmann, San Mateo, 3–10, 1996. 30

AC01.   S. Acid and L. M. de Campos. A hybrid methodology for learning belief networks: BENEDICT. *Int. J. Approx. Reason.*, 27(3):235–262, 2001. 30

AC.   S. Acid and L. M. de Campos. An algorithm for learning probabilistic belief networks using minimum d-separating sets. Submitted to *J. Artif. Intell. Res.* 30

CH92.   G. F. Cooper and E. Herskovits. A Bayesian method for the induction of probabilistic networks from data. *Mach. Learn.*, 9(4):309–348, 1992. 30

DH73.   R. Duda, P. Hart. *Pattern Classification and Scene Analysis.* John Wiley and Sons, New York, 1973. 32

HGC95.   D. Heckerman, D. Geiger, D. M. Chickering. Learning Bayesian networks: The combination of knowledge and statistical data. *Mach. Learn.*, 20:197–243, 1995. 30

Pea88.   J. Pearl. *Probabilistic Reasoning in Intelligent Systems: Networks of Plausible Inference.* Morgan Kaufmann, San Mateo, 1988. 28

Qui93.   J. R. Quinlan. *C4.5 Programs for Machine Learning.* Morgan Kaufmann, 1993. 32

SGS93.   P. Spirtes, C. Glymour, R. Scheines. *Causation, Prediction and Search.* Lecture Notes in Statistics 81. Springer Verlag, New York, 1993. 30

Analysis of Strength Data Based on Expert Knowledge

Fernando Alonso[1], África López-Illescas[2], Loïc Martínez[1],
Cesar Montes[3], and Juan P. Valente[1]

[1] Dept. Languages & Systems, Univ. Politécnica de Madrid
Campus de Montegancedo s/n, Boadilla, Madrid
{falonso,loic,jpvalente}@fi.upm.es
[2] High Performance Centre, Madrid, Spanish Council for Sports
africa.lopez@csd.mec.es
[3] Dept. Artificial Intelligence, Univ. Politécnica de Madrid
Campus de Montegancedo s/n, Boadilla, Madrid
cmontes@fi.upm.es

Abstract. Isokinetics systems are now a leading technology for assessing muscle strength and diagnosing muscle injuries. Although expensive, these systems are equipped with computer interfaces that provide only a simple graphical display of the strength data and do not interpret the data. This paper presents the I4 System (Interface for Intelligent Interpretation of Isokinetic Data), developed as a knowledge-based system, which provides an expert knowledge-based analysis of the isokinetic curves. The system was later extended with a KDD architecture for characterising injuries and creating reference models.

1 Introduction

The assessment of muscle function has been a primary goal of medical and sports scientists for decades. The main objectives are to evaluate the effects of training and the effectiveness of rehabilitation programs [1, 2]. An isokinetics machine is used for the purpose of evaluating and diagnosing a possible injury. This machine consists of a physical support on which patients perform exercises using any of their joints (knee, elbow, ankle, etc.) within different ranges of movement and at constant velocity. The machine records the strength applied throughout the exercise. The data measured by the isokinetic dynamometer are presented to the examiner by means of a computer interface. This interface sets out given parameters, which are used to describe the muscle function tested (e.g., maximum strength peak, total effort, etc.).

The mechanical component of the isokinetics systems now on the market generally meets the demands of muscle strength assessment. However, the performance of the software built into these systems (e.g., LIDO) still does not make the grade as far as isokinetic test interpretation is concerned. This means that the massive data flow supplied by these systems cannot be fully exploited.

J. Crespo, V. Maojo, and F. Martin (Eds.): ISMDA 2001, LNCS 2199, pp. 35–41, 2001.
© Springer-Verlag Berlin Heidelberg 2001

The I4 project, developed in conjunction with the High Performance Centre at the Spanish Council for Sports and the Spanish National Organisation for the Blind's School of Physiotherapy, aimed at providing a more comprehensive analysis of the data output by the isokinetics machine. This project is sponsored by the CICYT, through contract number TIC98-0248-C02-01

2   Overview of the System

The isokinetics machine includes the LIDO^{TM} Multi-Joint II system, which supplies the data from the isokinetic tests run on patients. Seated patients extend and flex their knees, moving their right or left leg within a 0 to 90°C flexion/extension arc. The system records the angle, as well as the strength exerted by the patient (Fig. 1a).

As shown in Fig. 1b, after the isokinetic tests have been run by the LIDO system, I4 first decodes, transforms and formats the LIDO output into a standard format and corrects any inaccurate or incomplete data. This is the only I4 module that depends on the LIDO isokinetics system.

These transformed data are stored in a separate database for later processing. The Visualisation Module can display stored exercises either individually or jointly as graphs. So, this module can be used to analyse an individual exercise, to compare any pair of exercises or even to compare an exercise with a pattern or model that is representative of a particular population group.

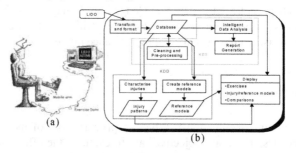

Fig. 1. I4 system and I4 architecture

The Data Cleaning and Pre-processing Module automatically processes the data stored in the database in order to correct and remove any inconsistencies between the isokinetic tests. These data are processed on the basis of the expert knowledge stored in the knowledge-based system (KBS). The data are then ready for analysis by the KBS and by the KDD (knowledge discovery in databases) architecture.

The Intelligent Analysis Module is the core of the KBS. Its job is to interpret the isokinetic data stored in the database using the system expert knowledge. It aims to provide an assessment of the numerical parameters and morphology of the isokinetic curves. The Report Generator Module is responsible for editing and printing the reports that describe the KBS inference process on the processed exercises.

The above three modules -Data Cleaning and Pre-processing, Intelligent Data Analysis and Report Generation- are what make up the system's KBS architecture.

Finally, the Create Reference Models Module processes all the exercises of a given patient population and gets a reference curve for the group. To do this, it has to assure that the curves of the patient population are similar and discard any atypical curves.

3   Intelligent Test Interpretation

The KBS provides an expert knowledge-based analysis of the isokinetic curves related to both their numerical parameters and their morphology. It lightens the workload of experienced physicians in isokinetics and provides support for non-specialists. This knowledge is vital for data cleaning and pre-processing in the KDD process.

Expert knowledge is formalised in the system using three different structures: *functions*, *rules* and *isokinetic models*. Each of these structures, and therefore the knowledge they contain, plays a different, though complementary, role in expert analysis.

3.1   Functions

The objective of this representation structure is to assess the morphology of each isokinetic curve and to eliminate any irregularities in the curves for which the patient is not responsible. The functions evaluate the curve characteristics and implicitly contain the expert knowledge required for this task.

Firstly, the strength curves are pre-processed in order to eliminate flexion peaks, that is, maximum peaks produced by machine inertia rather than by the actual strength of the patient. I4 also detects exercise extensions and flexions that are invalid because the patient exerted much less strength than in others and movements that can be considered atypical as their morphology is unlike the others.

The analysis of the strength curves also involves the assessment of different characteristics of the extension/flexion curve morphology, which are themselves of interest to the specialist, such as uniformity, regularity, maximum peak, troughs, etc.

The analysis of these morphological aspects of the curves may seem straightforward for an experienced physician. However, their automated assessment is important for inexperienced physicians and crucial for visually impaired physicians.

The development of these functions can be described as interactive human induction. Given a number of curves, the expert evaluated each one and assessed its characteristics. Tentative functions were then implemented. These functions were applied to a new set of tests, and the results were shown to the expert for evaluation. This led to changes in function implementation, and so on. This process ended when the methods provided the correct value in a high percentage of the cases (over 98%). It took 3 to 5 iterations, to evaluate each characteristic.

3.2   Rules

It was obvious from the very start of the design that functions alone were insufficient. They represent procedural knowledge very well, especially if it involves calculations, but they are not suited for representing fine grain knowledge, like heuristic assertions such as "If there are many invalid exercises, repeat the test". Fine grain knowledge for test validation and analysis is therefore represented in I4 by production rules.

There are over 480 rules in the system. They output conclusions on three concerns in isokinetics analysis: *protocol validation* (to determine whether the protocol has been applied correctly), *numerical analysis of data* (every numerical feature of the curve is expertly analysed and conclusions are presented to the user), *morphological analysis of data* (the rule-based subsystem analyses the morphology of the strength curve of each leg and their comparison and tries to identify dysfunctions).

3.3   Isokinetic Models

One of the processes most commonly performed to evaluate patient strength is to compare the test results against a standard. This third structure, called *isokinetic model*, aims to reflect the normal isokinetic values for a given population group. It is composed of an average isokinetic curve and a set of attributes (common irregularities, mean value, etc.). These attributes were added to return the information needed to compare a new patient against a model. Some of the attributes are calculated automatically from the set of tests performed on the population group (i.e. standard deviation), whereas others, like how close a curve should be to the model for it to be considered as normal, are defined by the expert.

The curve is automatically calculated from a set of tests. The user selects a group of tests, usually belonging to patients of similar ages, the same sex, similar sport if any and/or same injury, and the system calculates the reference curve for the group in question. This requires some sort of pre-processing (to discard poor exercises, standardise the curve, etc.), for which purpose functions are used. However, there may be some heterogeneity even among patients of the same group. Some patients will have a series of particularities that make them significantly different from the others. Take a sport like American football, for instance, where players have very different physical characteristics. Here, it would make no sense to create just one model, and separate models would have to be built for each subgroup of players having similar characteristics. Therefore, exercises have to be sifted, and the reference model has to be built using exercises among which there is some uniformity.

The discrete Fourier transform, whose use for comparing time series is widely documented [3,4], is used to perform this process efficiently. This technique sharply reduces the number of comparisons to be made, which is very important in this case, since there are a lot of exercises in the database and comparison efficiency is vital.

The process for creating a new reference model from a set of exercises is as follows.

- Calculate the discrete Fourier transform of all the exercises.
- Class these exercises, using some sort of indexing to rapidly discard all the exercises that deviate from the norm. The system creates a variation on the R* search tree [5]. The exercises are classed, and groups of similar exercises are clearly identified. Users generally intend to build a reference model for a particular group. In this case, there is a clear majority group of similar exercises, which represents the standard profile that the user is looking for, and a disperse set of groups of one or two exercises. The former is used to create a reference model.

Comparison with models

For comparison, the isokinetic model curve and the patient curve are translated to the frequency domain by the Fourier transform [4]. The automatic comparison algorithm visually displays similar parts for the user and presents a global measure of similarity. Similarities between curves or parts of curves is calculated by means of the Euclidean distance between the respective Fourier transforms.

Isokinetic models play an important role in the isokinetic assessment of patients, as they allow physicians to compare each new patient with standard groups. For example, it is possible to compare a long jump athlete with a group of elite long jumpers, compare a promising athlete with a set of models to determine which is the best suited discipline, assess strength dysfunctions in apparently normal patients, etc.

The interface (Fig. 2) that represents model/exercise comparison provides the following comparison options:

- *Normal:* outputs a full comparison of each curve.
- *Extensions:* compares the extension regions of the curves for the knee joint. A similar option is available for flexions.
- *Windows:* compares the windows into which the user has divided the curves. This would output all similar windows. Fig. 2 shows an example: four windows were selected by the user, and the algorithm calculates that window 2 of the model is similar to window 2 of the exercise.
- *Selection:* searches regions of a curve similar to the region marked by the user.

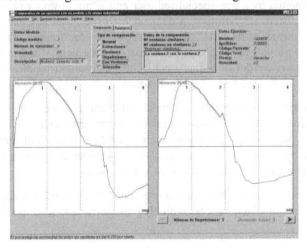

Fig. 2 Model/exercise comparison interface

The system provides the possibility of modifying advanced options for exercise/exercise and model/exercise comparison: 1) Comparison accuracy can be: "Very Accurate", "Fairly Accurate", "Accurate", "Normal" and "Not Very Accurate"; 2) Sample size chosen for comparison: number of data for time series; 3) Number and size of the windows for comparison; 4) Window grid selection.

3.4   Co-operation between the Three Formalisms

One of the reasons for implementing the system with three different structures is that each comprises the different types of knowledge provided by the expert more intuitively. The individual tasks needed to perform a full analysis of the patient required different knowledge representation structures. The knowledge of which each structure is composed can be used separately to provide conclusions on particular questions and can also be employed together to provide more general conclusions.

As mentioned above, these three types of knowledge are related and are complementary to each other. The rule-based subsystem needs the results supplied by running the expert functions on the curves. The output of these functions is an important input for the rule preconditions. Functions also play a major role in the creation of isokinetic models, as they provide the values of some model attributes. The conclusions supplied by the rule-based subsystem are also important for this task.

However, the relations between these structures for representing expertise are not one way. The models also input facts into the rule-based subsystem for assessing comparisons between a patient and a model.

4   Conclusions and Future Work

Most technological systems nowadays output a huge collection of information that cannot be interpreted by a non-specialised user and is not always easy to understand for a specialist. There is, therefore, a demand for expert systems that interpret this information by means of an intelligent analysis of the data output. The goal of the I4 project was to provide one such system, focused on the field of isokinetics.

For this purpose, we developed an intelligent system, built by means of an incremental KBS, which has the following peculiarities:

* A modular system architecture: a) data cleaning and pre-processing; b) intelligent data analysis; c) data and results display and report generation.
* An expert system for the intelligent analysis of data, which structures procedural knowledge by means of functions, declarative knowledge by means of rules and structural knowledge by means of an isokinetic model.

The system was built into two applications, one for the blind and another for elite athletes, the results of which have been highly praised by isokinetic specialists [6].

References

1. Gleeson, N. P. and Mercer, T. H.: The utility of isokinetic dynamometry in the assessment of human muscle function. Sports Medicine, Vol. 21 (1), (1996)
2. López-Illescas A.: Estudio del balance muscular con técnicas isocinéticas. In: Proceedings of the I Curso de Avances en Rehabilitación, Seville, (1993)
3. Berndt, D. and Clifford, J.: Finding patterns in Time Series in Advances in Knowledge Discovery and Data Mining, U. Fayyad et al. (Eds.), MIT Press (1996).

4. Agrawal, R. and Strikant, R.: Mining sequential patterns In: Proc. 1994 Int. Conf. Very Large Data Bases, Santiago, Chile, (1994) 487-499
5. Alonso, F., Lopez-Chavarrías, I., Valente, J. P. and Montes, C.: Knowledge Discovery in Time Series Using Expert Knowledge in Medical Data Mining and Knowledge Discovery, K. J. Cios (Ed.) Physica-Verlag Heidelberg New York, (2001)
6. Valente, J. P, López-Chavarrías, I., and Montes, C., "Functions, rules and models: three complementary techniques for analyzing strength data," *Proc. of the simposium of the ACM for Applied Computing,* (2000).

A Computational Environment
for Medical Diagnosis Support Systems

Victor Alves [1], José Neves [1], Moreira Maia [2], and Luís Nelas [2]

[1] Universidade do Minho
{jneves,valves}@di.uminho.pt
[2] Centro de Tomografia de Braga
Braga, Portugal
{lnelas,mmaia}ctb@ctbraga.pt

Abstract. As more health-care providers invest on computerised medical records, more clinical data is made accessible, and more of clinical insights will become reliable. As data collection technologies advance, a plethora of data is available in almost all domains of one's lives, being of particular interest to this work that of *Medicine*. Indeed, *Intelligent Diagnosis Systems* (IDS) with built-in functions for knowledge discovery or data mining, concerning with extracting and abstracting useful rules from such huge repositories of data, are becoming increasingly important for purposes such as of offering better service or care, or obtaining a competitive advantage over different problem's solving strategies or methodologies [1]. In particular, embedding *Machine Learning* technology into IDS' systems seems to be well suited for medical diagnostics in specialized medical domains, namely due to the fact that automatically generated diagnosis rules slightly outperform the diagnostic accuracy of specialists when physicians have available the same information as the machine.

1 Introduction

The time has come for the global medical practice constituency to deliberate the case for international standards in medical practice, and reach consensus about better healthcare of populations through medical programmes suited to societal needs. This goal conforms a problem that may be approached in terms of learning agent's shells and methodologies for building knowledge bases and agents and their innovative application to the development, among others, of *Intelligent Medical Diagnosis Support Systems*. Building upon this perspective to problem solving, a Computational Environment that supports Medical Diagnosis based Systems (MEDsys) was developed, making the amalgam of knowledge discovery and data mining techniques via an hybrid theorem prover that combines the potential of an extension to the language of Logic Programming, with the functionalities of a connectionist approach to problem solving using Artificial Neural Networks. The majority of *Computer*

J. Crespo, V. Maojo, and F. Martin (Eds.): ISMDA 2001, LNCS 2199, pp. 42–47, 2001.

Vision applications used in diagnosis processes in *Medical Imaging* involve real time analysis and description of object behaviour from image sequences. *Computer Vision* is also one of the main subfields of *Artificial Intelligence (AI)*, dealing with problems related to recognition, evaluation and manipulation of conceptual descriptions of the world. Indeed these Extended Logic Programming *(ELP)* programs define the extension of an input-output mapping relation, that make the building blocks of the so-called *Artificial Neural Networks (ANNs)*; i.e., proving *ELP* goals one may define *ANNs* topologies. *ANNs* that present properties such as non-linearity learning, input-output mapping, adaptability and noise tolerance, being therefore perceived as natural candidates as diagnosis tools. The recognition of more abstracts conceptual descriptions involves the recognition of events in terms of *ELP* programs, which are considered as primitives and that can be accepted directly by the lower layers of an image evaluation system, in terms of *ANNs*.

2   A Computational Environment that Supports Medical Diagnosis Based Systems

An architecture that is envisaged to support the computational environments for the *MEDsys* is a model of an intelligent information processing system, in terms of its major subsystems, their functional roles, and the flow of information and control among them. Indeed, many complex systems are made up of specialised subsystems that interact in circumscribed ways. The benefits of this architecture also applies to the design of intelligent agents, entities that interact with their environments in flexible, goal-directed manners, and are understood as logical theories or logical programs in their own right. The intelligence of the system as a whole arises from the interactions among all the system's agents. The system's interfaces are based on Web-related front-ends using *HTML* pages, that can be accessed using a standard Web browser. The system structure or architecture is depicted in Figure 1, in terms of the entities:

The Server Agents, which were mainly developed using the *C (GTK)* language for the *LINUX* operating system, being responsible for acquiring Information from the *DICOM* devices *(DICOM server)* and from the Hospital Information system;

The Knowledge agents, which present themselves as *LINUX* supported applications, were developed using the *C (GTK)* language and implement the system's *ANN's*;

The Monitor agent, that was mainly developed with *CGI* and *PERL*. This module provides a front-end to the administrator and is used for system configuration;

The Physician Diagnostic Support Agents, which were mainly developed with *CGI* and *PERL*. This module provides the physician front-end to the system, either for image consultation, or in terms of diagnosis; and

The Resource agent, that was mainly developed using the *C (GTK)* language for the *LINUX* operating system, and is responsible to maintain the server's resources at appropriate levels.

Such an approach can provide decision support, with the radiologist conducting a form of dialogue with the technicians to query the knowledge base and test hypothesis. The strategy is to compare a modality independent model with the image via an intermediate symbolic feature space. The system is characterised by the use of explicit anatomical models and for the visualisation of the anatomical structures identified in the image segmentation.

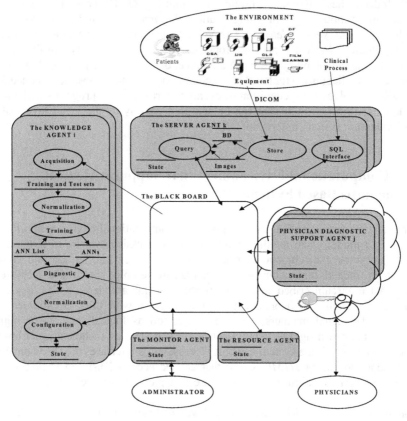

Figure 1 – The System's Architecture

The anatomical model make a major component of the system, and is organised in terms of a semantic network. The inference engine handles the decision making proceedings during the process of segmenting major anatomical landmarks. The primary goal of the work reported in this paper is to emulate the radiologist's expertise in the identification of malfunction regions (e.g., in *Computer Tomography (CT)* through the use of a combination of pure symbolic systems and the use of computational pattern recognition techniques provided by the *ANNs* paradigm). One also aims to minimise the number of unnecessary medical interventions which might otherwise be necessary to make an accurate diagnosis. *CT* has some advantage over other imaging modalities, once it can provide images of tissue with a variety of contrast levels based on a simple adjustment of the window width and level of the image's raw data; i.e., it provides information that is not seen on film [2],[3]. In order to implement this system, distributed by nature, internet technology was used on the side of the end user (i.e., the radiologist), and *LINUX* supported applications on the other side (i.e., the processing one). The intranet was implemented using a *PC* with *LINUX* as operating system, and an *Apache WEB server*. Outside connections were achieved via a *ISDN* router with *RAS* (*Remote Access Service*). The image server uses a *PC* with *LINUX* as operating system, and a *ODBC SQL*-compliant *RDBMS* for database support. Browsing is done with *Netscape's* browser with a *DICOM* viewer plug-in running on a *PC* with *Windows* as the operating system. The *DICOM* image server supports the m*edical interface* – this window sets the via for the visualisation and exploration of original *DICOM 3.0* data from *CT, MRI,* etc. It provides the user with interactive image visualisation functions (e.g., graylevel windowing).

3   A Computer Tomography Diagnostic System – A Case Study

The process of development, analysis and use of one's *Computational Environment* that supports *Medical Diagnosis based Systems* for *Computer Tomography* is now depicted below, and some results are presented. One modality was used, the *Axial Computed Tomography* one, under a *GE prospeed* equipment. The images were in *RAW* data (*DICOM*) format, and 188 images were selected. The selected images refer to the section of the head that passes through the apex of the squamous part

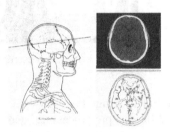

Figure 2 – The selected body's section under study

of the occipital bone and the frontal sinus (Figure 2). The knowledge agent was configured as a multilayered feedforward ANN with one hidden layer, bias connections, the logistic activation function and RPROP training. 25% of the selected images were used as test cases. The input layer of the ANN is made of the normalized values for each image, plus the patients sex and age. The output layer is made of its diagnostic. The images, the patients sex and age were presented to two physicians that pronounced their own judgment according to what is depicted in Table 1 (notice that some of the images point to more than one pathology). It is interesting to note that under the same circumstances and based on the same information, judgments of the two physicians only match on 78% of the cases (Table 2), which points to the necessity of further judgements or opinions, something that can be at the doorstep by using intelligent medical systems of type *MEDsys*.

	Physician A		Physician B	
Normal	125	125	111	111
Atrophy	48		62	
Isquemic Lesions	12		24	
Hemorragy	6	73	7	101
Malign Tumour	3		3	
Normal Variants	4		5	

Table 1 - The physician's judgments.

	Cases	
Agree	147	78%
Partially agree	15	8%
Disagree	26	14%

Table 2 - The physician's match or agreement.

The images of Figure 3 were pre-processed and normalized. In Figure 4 this information is given in a graphical mode. Notice the difference between images that revealed no pathologies and images that revealed atrophy.

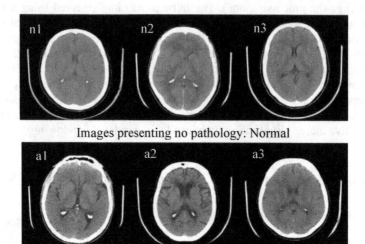

Images presenting no pathology: Normal

Images presenting a pathology: Atrophy

Figure 3 – Sample images

The results from the *ANN* for three different pre-processing and normalization techniques, leading to three different *ANN's* topologies and given as output one or more out of five possible pathologies as diagnosis, were quite good (e.g., when using the first technique, in 47 test cases the system presents 31 correct results with a standard deviation (*std*) of 2,46). Changing the configuration of the *ANN* so that the output is binary, an indication of the existence or not of a pathology, then the results get much better. In

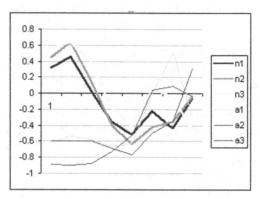

Figure 4 – The graphical representation.

47 test cases the system gave 39 correct results with a *std* of 1,5. The golden standard the ANNs are trained upon and based on scientific methods which aims to derive mathematical models that may be useful to understand and exploit phenomena, whether they be natural or human made. Learning with ANNs can be viewed as just such a phenomenon. On the other hand a fuller theoretical analysis and understanding of their machine's performance has been a major research objective for the last decade. Indeed, the results presented in this work follow such a pattern, coming from a computational learning system based on Mathematical Logic, with fewer assumption than the physicians use to do, and make the way to stronger statements than, for example, the frequently used Bayesian analysis. Since the results are presented in terms of a percentage, the system not only gives a diagnostic but also indicates a measure of its accuracy or correctness.

4   Conclusions

The ultimate goal of this work is to increase the awareness and acceptance of *Intelligent Data Analysis* (*IDA*) within the medical community through the development, adaptation or reuse of knowledge based systems to cope with specific medical problems. It is also believed that to increase the chances of utilising these tools within clinical practice, the *IDA's* process gains from interaction with the physicians in all its phases, beginning with the procedures of data gathering and cleansing, to evaluation and exploitation of results. Indeed, one of the interesting aspects of the present work is in the involvement of the physicians in the preparation of data for *IDA's* processes (e.g., data representation, modelling, cleaning, selection, and transformation). All that was stated above is only the beginning of a long story for *IDA's* systems in the portuguese health-care institutions. As a part of the project, pilot projects are being launched involving portuguese counties in the north of Portugal, and suppliers for the health care sector.

Acknowledgements

The work of José Neves was partially supported by a grant from *Centro de Investigação Algoritmi*, the University of Minho, Braga, Portugal. We are also indebted to the CTB (*Centro de Tomografia de Braga, Lda*), in Braga, to SMIC (*Serviços Médicos de Imagem Computorizada, SA*), in Oporto, *Radiconsult, Lda*, in Braga, and *Jogima, Lda*, in Oporto for their help in terms of experts, technicians and machine time.

References

1. Agrawal, R., Mannila, H., Srikant, R., Toivonem, H., and Verkamo, A.I. "Fast Discovery of Association Rules", in U.M.Fayad, G. Piatetsky – Shapiro, P.Smith, and R. Uthurusamy, editors – Advances in Knowledge Discovery and Data Mining, pages 307-328, The AAAI/MIT Press, 1995.
2. Neves, J., Alves V., Nelas L., Maia M., and Cruz R. "A Multi-Feature Image Classification System that Reduces the Cost-of-Quality Expenditure", in Proceedings of the Second ICSC Symposium on Engineering of Intelligent Systems, Paisley, Scotland, UK, 2000.
3. Alves, J. Neves, M. Maia, L. Nelas. "Computer Tomography based Diagnosis using Extended logic programming and Artificial Neural Networks". Proceedings of the NAISO Congress on Information Science Innovations ISI2001, Dubai, U.A.E., March 17-21, 2001.

Automatic Detection of Regions of Interest in Digitized Mammograms for Computer-Aided Diagnosis

José M. Barreiro[1], Alberto Carrascal[1], Daniel Manrique[1], Juan Ríos[1], Amparo Vilarrasa[2]

[1]Artificial Intelligence Dept.
Facultad de Informática. Universidad Politécnica de Madrid, Spain.
[2] Radio-Diagnostic Dept.
Hospital Universitario 12 de Octubre
Madrid, Spain.
{jmbarreiro, dmanrique, jrios}@fi.upm.es

Abstract. This work presents a new system for real time breast abnormalities detection that could be related to a carcinoma, taking as input a digitized mammography, in order to assist radiologists in their mammography interpretation task. The system built has been designed to the parallel detection of microcalcifications and breast masses. Algorithms based on mathematical morphology combined with dynamic statistical methods are employed in microcalcifications detection. Histogram analysis of the digitized mammogram and a modified version of the watershed algorithm have also been used for breast masses localization. The output given by the system consists on a set of suspicious regions of being a carcinoma located in the original digitized image. A clinical database has been built for testing purposes comprising 690 mammographic studies for which surgical verification is available, 392 of them obtained in 1997, and the rest in 1998.

1 Introduction

Broad implementation of screening recommendations to enable the early diagnosis of breast cancer [1] will generate a large volume of mammograms that must be interpreted by radiologists. However, if a computerized detection system could assist radiologists by indicating locations of suspicious abnormalities in mammograms, the effectiveness and efficiency of the screening procedure might be improved. It is also very important, apart from breast masses detection, to be able to detect microcalcifications as soon as they appear since between 30% and 50% of breast carcinomas demonstrate microcalcifications on mammograms [2].

Several investigators have attempted to analyse breast abnormalities with computerized schemes. Threshold segmentation algorithms have been applied with other techniques based on left and right breast comparison [3]. The major problem in many of the algorithms developed is the great amount of parameters needed to be adjusted, so researches for the automatic tuning of these parameters have been carried out [4].

J. Crespo, V. Maojo, and F. Martin (Eds.): ISMDA 2001, LNCS 2199, pp. 48-53, 2001.

Other researches have focused on studying different techniques for automatic local-ization of microcalcifications as a presenting sign in most of breast cancers. Mathe-matical morphology has been widely employed with this aim in both, computerized detection [5] and feature analysis of microcalcifications[6]. Asynchronous dynamics for the iterative computation of morphological image filters has also been applied to improve the convergence efficiency of such operators [7].

A system for automatic real time detection of microcalcifications and breast suspi-cious masses of carcinoma is presented. This system takes a digitized mammogram as its input, and gives as its output the same image where white squares are placed in those suspicious areas of having a carcinoma. The procedure has been developed employing mathematical morphology techniques [8] combined with dynamic thresh-olding algorithms, signal analysis of the image histogram and the watershed algorithm, based on a modified version of the multiscalar gradient algorithm [9].

The structure of the system is modular and it is divided into two subsystems that work in a parallel way: the Microcalcifications Detection Subsystem (MDS) and the Nodule Detection Subsystem (NDS). The outputs given by these two subsystems will feed both microcalcification and nodule classifiers, now in progress stage, in order to give a final diagnosis of the detected abnormalities in the mammography.

A clinical database has been built for test purposes comprising 690 mammographic studies, 392 of them obtained in 1997, and the the rest in 1998 from the Department of Radiology of the University Hospital "12 de Octubre" in Madrid, Spain. 154 mammo-graphic studies have been randomly chosen from the database having microcalcifica-tions in 104 of them to test the MDS. Other 90 clinical studies, having any kind of breast mass in 60 of them, were chosen to test the NDS.

2 Microcalcifications Detection Subsystem

Starting from a whole digitized mammography, microcalcifications detection sub-system employs in first place an initial filtering stage where the top-hat algorithm is used with a squared structuring element of 21x21 pixels. Figure 1 shows a detailed section of a mammography where microcalcifications can be seen inside a nodule an in one of its spiculas, while figure 2 shows the image obtained from this step where small areas appear to be highlighted over the rest of the pixels.

The second step consists on a novel dynamic statistical method is applied to obtain the threshold value h in order to decide which of the pixels of the image obtained in the previous step are really microcalcifications, and which are not. To do this, atypical grey-level values of figure 2 are calculated using the following formulas:

$$U_l = q_3+1.5 \ (q_3-q_1) \qquad\qquad L_l=q_1-1.5(q_3-q_1)$$

Where q_1 is the first quartile of the sample, and q_3 is the third one. Once these val-ues have been obtained, it is considered that a point is atypical if it is greater than the upper limit U_l or lower than the minimum limit L_l. So $h = U_l$. All pixels with a grey-level value greater that h are considered that belong to a microcalcification.

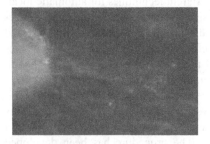

Fig. 1. A detailed section of interest where it can be better seen microcalcifications inside of a nodule on the left and inside of a spicula on the right.

Fig. 2. The results obtained after the morphological top-hat operation has been applied.

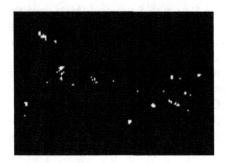

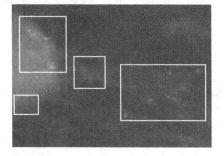

Fig. 3. Points obtained as micro-calcifications after threshold segmentation.

Fig. 4. The results obtained after the morphological top-hat operation has been applied.

Figure 3 shows the same section studied after this thresholding step has been applied. All pixels belonging to microcalcifications appear in white colour (gray-level value of 255) and all of the rest of the points in black colour (value 0).

Finally, those regions where a cluster of microcalcifications (small regions of breast tissue having more than 5 microcalcifications) has been detected, is highlighted by a white square as a breast abnormality that could be a carcinoma. This result is shown in figure 4.

3   Nodule Detection Subsystem

It has been seen that the histograms of all digitized images have a similar shape, as the one showed in the figure 5. Firstly it has a great quantity of pixels close to the value 0, that corresponds to the mammography background (the height of the histogram has been cut in the value 31000 with the purpose of being able to observe the details better). Afterwards, a sudden fall has occurred and the number of white pixels decreases (point 1), until a minimum is reached (point 2), that is a value near the separation between the background of the mammography and the breast tissue. From the

From the point 2, the histogram is increasing again (point 3) until it reaches a maximum (point 4), (it is possible to find one or two maximums depending on the mammography) and it decreases again. All the area corresponding to the points 3,4 and 5 are pixels belonging to breast tissue. If there exists a big quantity of sudden sharp peaks in region 5, due to the existence of atypical white pixels, then it is a histogram concerned with solid tissue breasts. A nodule could be hidden in one of the peaks.

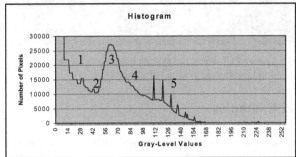
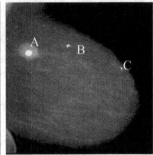

Fig. 5. Points obtained as micro-calcifications after threshold segmentation.

Fig. 6. The input image where the markers have been placed inside the suspicious regions.

As a consequence of what is previously exposed, NDS places *markers* (small white areas) inside those suspicious regions of being a carcinoma due to the presence of an abnormal mass detected by the presence of an unusual peak in region 5.

Due to the sharp irregularities existing in the breast tissue, there ere many more minima in the mammograms than regions of interest. If watershed algorithm is directly applied on image of figure 6 then, the *over-segmentation* effect is produced. In order to avoid this problem, a new previous processing of the image to be segmented has been designed to be used before employing watershed algorithm. This procedure is based on the utilization of the morphological gradient operation, and is called *eroded multiscalar morphological gradient algorithm* (EMMGA).

EMMGA consists on the successively application of the morphological erosion of the gradient operation using a larger structuring element each time until a given size is reached (29x29 pixels for practical considerations). Finally a new image is obtained as the average of all the images obtained in each application of the eroded gradient operation with a different structuring element. Figure 7 shows the output given by the watershed algorithm after EMMGA operation has been applied for each of the three suspicious regions where the system has placed a marker. It can be seen how the masses are perfectly segmented.

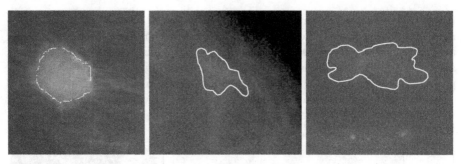

Fig. 7. The three regions of interest (A, B and C) where the system has placed the markers have been now segmented using watersheds and multiscale gradient algorithm.

4 Results and Additional Examples

To test the MDS, 154 clinic cases were studied (taken from the 690 available in the data base), being normal breasts 50 of them and showing microcalcifications in 104. Another set of 90 cases has been taken to test the NDS showing a nodule with or without microcalcifications in 60 of them, and being the remaining 30, normal breasts.

The receiver operating characteristic (ROC) curve is constructed to test the accuracy of the MDS in detecting microcalcifications. The area A_z under the ROC curve measures the expected probability of the correct classification. A value of A_z near to 1 indicates that the algorithm can correctly detect microcalcifications with a small error. The area under the ROC curve obtained by the MDS was calculated by numerical integration giving a result of $A_z=0.83$ which is quite good level.

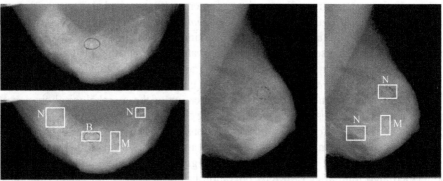

Fig. 9. Two difficult cases are presented, showing one of the views in each case. In both, the original image is presented with a black circle indicating the presence of a nodule, then the final output of the system is also showed. The black circle has not influence in the results.

To test NDS, each of the 90 clinic cases of study were individually presented. The system gave a 16% of false negatives, which is unacceptable. However, radiologists use both mediolateral and craneocaudal mammographic views in order to make a study. The developed system works in the same line: NDS analyses both mammographic views for each breast to obtain all suspicious regions due to abnormal masses in the breast tissue. This way all the false negatives obtained in one of the views were detected as positive in the other one, getting a final 0% of false negatives.

Two additional example cases are shown in figure 9. These cases have been chosen because of their nodule and microcalcification detection complexity as these abnormalities are inside dense regions of the breast and they are harder to see. For each case, the original mammogram used as the input to system and the final output are shown, indicating if there is an abnormal mass (N), a clustered microcalcification (M) or both (B), for each one of the zones defined as suspicious by the system.

5   Conclusions

A new system able to detect cancer suspect areas has been presented, taking as input a digitized mammogram. These suspicious areas can be determined by the system because of the presence of clustered or isolated microcalcifications, or abnormal masses in the breast. So the system bears in mind the two most important factors in early breast cancer detection. The proposed system employs both mediolateral and craneocaudal mammographic views. This feature allows the system to reduce the number of errors in nodule and microcalcification detection.

This system could be actually used to assist the radiologist indicating all these suspicious areas to be studied, reducing the total diagnostic time. Our research is now focused on developing the classification module for microcalcifications and nodules from which a final diagnosis will be obtained.

References

1. Hoffert SP.: New Technology Weighs in on Mammography Debate. The Scientist Vol. 11, No. 23 (1997) 11-14.
2. Goerge SK, Evans J, Cohen GPB.: Characteristics of Breast Carcinomas Missed by Screening Radiologists. Radiology Vol. 204 (1997) 131-135.
3. Pikaz A, Averbuch A.: Digital Image Thresholding, Based on Topological Stable-State. Pattern Recog. Vol 29 No. 5 (1996) 829-843.
4. Murino V, Foresti GL, Regazzoni CS.: A Belief-Based Approach for Adaptive Image Processing. Int. J. of Pattern Recog. and Art. Int. Vol. 11 No 3 (1997) 359-392.
5. Vilarrasa A, Gimenez V, Manrique D, Rios J.: A New Algorithm for Computerized Detection of Microcalcifications in Digital Mammograms. Proc. of the 12th Int. Symp. on Computer Assisted Radiology and Surgery (1998) 224-229.
6. Giménez V, Manrique D, Ríos J, Vilarrasa A.: Automatic Detection of Microcalcificactions Using Mathematical Morphology. 6th Eu. C. in Int. Tech. and Soft. Comp. (1998) 1407-1411.
7. Robin F, Privat G, Renaudin M.: Asynchronous Relaxation of Morphological Operators. Int. J. of Pattern Recog. and Art. Int. Vol. 11 No 7 (1997) 1085-1094.
8. D'Alotto L.A., Giardina CR.: A Unified Signal Algebra Approach to Two-Dimensional Parallel Digital Signal Processing. Marcel Dekker, New York, (1998).
9. Wang D. A.: Multiscale Gradient Algorithm for Image Segmentation Using Watersheds. Pattern Recog. Vol. 30 No 2 (1997) 2043-2052.

A New Method for Unifying Heterogeneous Databases*

Holger Billhardt[1], Jose Crespo[1], Victor Maojo[1],
Fernando Martin[2], and José Luis Maté[1]

[1] Fac. de Informática, Univ. Politécnica de Madrid, Spain
{holger,vmaojo,jcrespo}@infomed.dia.fi.upm.es
jlmate@fi.upm.es
[2] Instituto de Salud Carlos III, Madrid, Spain
fmartin@isciii.es

Abstract. In this article we present a new method for unifying heterogeneous databases. We propose the unification at the level of *conceptual schemas* in a two-step process. First, the internal database schemas
are mapped to conceptual schemas in a user interactive process. These
schemas are then automatically integrated, creating a *virtual repository*.
Virtual repositories give users the feeling of working with single, local
databases and can be used for epidemiological research (e.g. data analysis) or clinical practice. We implemented the proposed method in a
tool for accessing medical information from remote databases located at
different machines with different technological platforms in the Internet.

1 Introduction

The development of Internet has increased dramatically the exchange of information during the last decades. In medicine, the large number of databases (e.g.,
medical records, health services, trials) and the deployment of the Web make
necessary new models to search, and access information from remote sources.

Some models have been proposed to use Internet as the information infrastructure to exchange information among multiple remote sources. In one of these
proposals, national databases could be accessed and fed from multiple remote
sites [5]. Thus, these databases could store national information about topics
such as outcomes research, clinical trials, and so on. The information needed
to maintain and increment this database would come from health sites such as
hospitals, research laboratories, pharmaceutical companies and so on.

The development of the World Wide Web has modified the technical features
that this model should present. Thus, the concept of virtual databases appears.
A virtual database is a database, which is not physically available, but acts like
a real database and can integrate data from different sources.

---

* Financial support for this research was provided in part by an FPI grant from the
Madrid regional government and by "Fondo de Investigación Sanitaria" (Spanish
Ministry of Health).

J. Crespo, V. Maojo, and F. Martin (Eds.): ISMDA 2001, LNCS 2199, pp. 54–61, 2001.

Examples of virtual databases can be found in research projects carried out at different sites. In [6], a consortium of Boston research groups has proposed a virtual medical record. This medical record is the result of an aggregation from previously existing medical records at various Boston hospitals. A physician can retrieve a specific patient record and visualize the record's content using a WWW browser. Patient data have been unified from records located at the different databases and integrated to create a single view. HL7 was used to facilitate exchange of information among different information systems.

Another project at the National Cancer Institute [4] aims to integrate different centres participating in research projects (e.g., clinical trials). This integration is carried out over the Web merging the contents of databases and linking various information systems. Virtual databases are again necessary to facilitate access and use of remote information for research and analysis purposes.

In this report, we present a tool for creating *virtual repositories* (VR) from sets of remote databases. The work is based on the idea that a set of databases builds an information space, which can be described by a single schema and used in tasks like information search, data mining, and data analysis.

When unifying heterogeneous databases, two levels of heterogeneity have to be considered: i) different technological platforms (machines, operating systems, and DBMS), and ii) different database schemas or underlying conceptual data models. While the first two aspects require rather technical solutions the latter is of a more conceptual or theoretical kind. Even though different databases may contain information from the same area or context, they will usually have different internal schemas. Thus, in order to integrate existing databases it is necessary to map their local schemas to a common global schema. Such a global schema constitutes the core of the proposed system.

In Sect. 2 we present our database integration approach. Sect. 3 describes the general architecture of the system. Sect. 4 gives some conclusions and directions for further research.

2   Unifying Heterogeneous Databases

Integrating heterogeneous databases is usually a tedious task that requires a deep analysis of the internal schemas of the databases in order to identify the correspondences of data structures. There, the following aspects have to be taken into account: i) different naming conventions, ii) structuring of the same information in different ways, iii) hierarchical relationships between entities (e.g. tables), iv) different units for values, and v) duplicated and/or inconsistent data. A normal approach is to define a common schema and to map each database's internal schema to this schema ([2], [6]). This approach, however, is very inflexible and new databases can only be integrated if they can be mapped to the common schema. Thus, the systems support only data of a specific domain. We propose a domain independent approach, which is based on the idea that in many occasions a "perfect" integration is not necessary. We do not address the aspects related with the data itself and approach unification at the abstract level of conceptual data models. With this assumption, database integration can be semi-automated. First, we represent each database in form of a *conceptual schema* (*mapping* process) and, then, we unify these schemas obtaining a conceptual schema that reflects the structure of the information space composed by the set of databases (*unification* process).

Conceptual schemas consist of classes, attributes and relationships. Their aim is to reflect the conceptual structure of real world entities rather than the internal structure of data in databases. We say that structured data forms an information space whose structure can be represented by a conceptual schema. We call this information space virtual repository. To describe conceptual schemas formally, we introduce the notion of a domain D. A domain represents the possible descriptors of the structural elements of an information space. A domain D contains a set of class descriptors CN_D, a set of relationship descriptors RN_D, a set of attribute descriptors AN_D, and a relation $CH_D \subset CN_D \times CN_D$. An element (cn_i, cn_j) of CH_D described the fact that the class described by cn_i includes all instances of the class described by cn_j. Thus, CH_D defines a set of hierarchical trees on class descriptors where a class descriptor at a higher node is a generalization of the class descriptors at lower nodes. We assume that CN_D, RN_D, and AN_D are repetition free set, and that they are *synonym-free*, that is, there is only one descriptor for each conceptual entity. We define a conceptual schema for an information space of a given domain D by $CS_D = (C, R)$. C is a set of classes $\{c_1, \ldots, c_n\}$, where each class c_i is a tuple (cn_i, AN_i), with $cn_i \in CN_D$ is the class descriptor and $AN_i \subseteq AN_D$ is the set of attributes of class c_i. $R = \{r_1, \ldots, r_k\}$ is the set of relationships defined on the classes, where $r_i = (rn1_i, rn2_i, c1_i, c2_i)$. $c1_i, c2_i \in C$ are the related classes, $rn1_i \in RN_D$ is the name of the relationship leading from class $c1_i$ to class $c2_i$ and $rn2_i \in RN_D$ is the name of the relationship leading from class $c2_i$ to class $c1_i$.

If two conceptual schemas $CS_D^1 = (C^1, R^1)$ and $CS_D^2 = (C^2, R^2)$ are defined on the same domain they can be unified to a schema $CS_D^u = (C^u, R^u)$ using the following algorithm:

```
Unify(CS_D^1, CS_D^2)
    1. C^u = ∅,  R^u = ∅
    2. Order the classes of C^1 ∪ C^2 into families CF_i, such that:
       ∀c_k, c_j ∈ C^1 ∪ C^2 : c_k and c_j belong to the same family iff.
       their descriptors belong to the same tree in CH_D.
    3. For each family CF_i = {(cn_1, AN_1), ..., (cn_m, AN_m)}:
       create a new class (cn_i, AN_i) in C^u, where:
       i) cn_i is the most general descriptor of {cn_1, ..., cn_m} and
       ii) AN_i = AN_1 ∪ ... ∪ AN_m
    4. Create the set of relationships R^u:
       4.1. R^u = R^1 ∪ R^2
       4.2. For all relationships (rn1, rn2, c1, c2) ∈ R^u:
            substitute c1 and c2 by the classes representing
            c1 and c2 in C^u as specified in step 3.
       4.3. Eliminate duplicate elements from R^u
```

   5. Return $CS_D^u = (C^u, R^u)$
End Unify.

The returned schema CS_D^u represents the structure of the information space composed by the schemas CS_D^1 and CS_D^2. If these schemas correspond to two databases DB^1 and DB^2, then CS_D^u is a VR for the union of DB^1 and DB^2.

It should be noted that database entities might be represented by more general entities in a unification schema and relationships may be 'passed' from specific classes to more general classes. Also, instances of a class in the VR do not necessarily contain values for all attributes. These facts can be seen as limitations of the approach, since they may cause a loss of specificity.

The aim of the mapping process consists of finding the conceptual schema of a particular database and a given domain D. This is done in four steps:

1. Select the tables and fields that provide useful information,
2. Select descriptors for these elements from the sets CN_D and AN_D,
3. Identify the conceptual relationships between the mapped tables and the fields that represent these relationships in the database,
4. Select appropriate descriptors for the relationships from the set RN_D.

While the unification process is fully automated, mapping requires user interaction. In a certain sense, mapping reverses the process of database modelling. A conceptual schema is obtained from an internal database schema. The user should only select those structural elements of a database that provide real world information and that he wants to offer to the system. In the third step, the fields that join tables in the database to reflect relationships have to be identified. (If a conceptual relationship corresponds to a chain of relationships in the database, the chain of field correspondences has to be specified.) All mapping information is stored and can be used later to translate queries the VR receives.

The mapping process requires the existence of the sets of descriptors CN_D, AN_D, and RN_D, and the unification process requires the hierarchical relation on the class descriptors CH_D. This meta information may be fixed before mapping and unification takes place. This, however, requires that all possible entities, attributes and relationships that may exist in the databases are known. We propose another approach, where the domain increases with the incorporation of new databases. Initially the domain is empty. When the first database is mapped the user chooses appropriate descriptors at his one discretion. These descriptors are added to the domain. In each successive mapping the previously chosen descriptors are presented and a user should preferably use them. Only if none of the descriptors represent the concept of an element well enough the user may choose a new descriptor. This is added to the domain. In this way no previous knowledge of the whole information space is necessary and it is assured that the conceptual schemas for all mapped databases are defined on the same domain. Thus, unification can be automated.

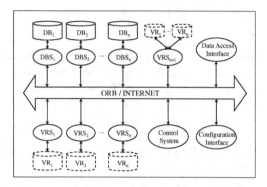

Fig. 1. System architecture based on CORBA

3   System Architecture

The system's architecture is based on CORBA, the *Common Object Request Broker Architecture* [3]. It allows the creation of individual components that each accomplishes a particular task and which are connected over some network. Using CORBA has three basic advantages over traditional client-server architectures: i) separation of the communication part from the components, ii) solving the communication between objects written in different programming languages and located on different technological platforms, and iii) new components can be easily plugged into the system.

Fig. 1 shows the components of the system. For each connected database (DB_i) there exists a *Database Server*, DBS_i, which acts as a bridge to the database for other objects. VRs, obtained through mapping or unification, are controlled by *Virtual Repository Servers*, VRS. VRSs have two basic tasks: i) offering their schemas for unification, and ii) solving queries. The *Control System* provides the mapping and unification facilities and the domain information, and maintains a register of connected objects. Each object inscribes itself in this register when it starts and eliminates its entry when it finishes.

The system offers two basic interfaces: i) configuration, and ii) information access. The configuration interface facilitates the creation of new DBSs, the creation of VRSs via the mapping process, and the creation of VRS's through unification. To create new DBSs a user simply has to select the location of the database and the access mode (currently database access is only possible for ODBC databases). In the mapping process all currently registered DBS are presented and the user is asked to select the database he wants to map. Then, all data elements (tables, fields, and relationships) of the selected database are presented and the user can 'pass' elements to the new conceptual schema. This is done with a graphical interface. For the task of descriptor selection the set of currently available descriptors is presented. If a user chooses a new descriptor it is added to this set. In unification, a list of all registered VRs is presented and the user simply has to select those that he wants to unify. The system creates automatically the server object for the new virtual repository.

All DBSs and VRSs can be stored as persistent objects and launched whenever it is desired. Each VRS stores internally its conceptual schema, a reference to its children (underlying repositories or databases), and the information on the correspondences of its schema to the children's schemas. That is, VRSs created with mapping store the mappings of the conceptual schema to the corresponding internal database schema, and VRSs created with unification store the mappings of their schema to the schema of each child.

The information access interface provides methods for retrieving data from any of the connected VRs. It also provides functions to obtain the list of all currently connected repositories, their descriptions, and their schemas. We defined a query language similar to SQL for querying VRs. When a query is launched for a particular repository it is passed to the corresponding VRS. Each VRS that receives a query translates it to a valid query for each of its children and passes the query to the corresponding child servers. There, each VRS uses its schema mapping information to translate the query. At the lowest level in the hierarchy (VRSs obtained by mapping) the queries are translated to SQL and passed to the corresponding DBS. Results are returned the same way back, and each VRS merges the results received from all of its children. Finally, the data access interface passes the results to the calling application.

The use of the system may be various (e.g. information search tool, data analysis, clinical trials). At the current state we have created an information search and navigation interface, which is accessible from the Web. The user connects to the system and selects an available repository. After selecting a repository its set of classes is shown. The user is asked to select a class and to specify the attributes and/or related classes he is interested in. Filters may be specified for the attributes. Then, a search is started and the results are presented in form of tables. Each column corresponds either to a selected attribute or to a selected relationship. Relationships are presented as links to the related records. In this way the information space can be explored by navigating along the links.

4   Conclusions

Virtual repositories are strategic tools for modern biomedical research. The rapid development of the WWW has facilitated the exchange of information among researchers at different sites. This new environment has been one of the main causes of the success of the human genome project. An enormous amount of genomic information is now available to genetic researchers. Bioinformatics has become an emerging discipline attracting resources and professionals to facilitate the integration and manipulation of genomic information. Thus, new tools are needed to access, integrate, and use genomic information for research purposes.

In this paper, we described a new model for creating virtual repositories that integrate data from heterogeneous remote sources. Our research was motivated by the need of linking data from heterogeneous sources, including genomic and clinical information. This idea has been reported elsewhere [1].

The architecture of the proposed system is very flexible and allows each of the components to be located on a different machine connected over Internet. The integration of new databases into the system is simple and can be done without any changes to the system. The architecture also permits the creation of several virtual repositories where each is composed of a different set of databases. Thus, different views of the accessible information space can be provided. This may be used to specify security levels, or, it may be used to group similar information together in specific repositories, but maintaining at the same time a general view of the whole information space.

Compared to other database integration methods our approach does not require a previous definition of a common schema. By splitting database integration into a unification and a mapping process, manual intervention is only required in the latter. And there, the person that is doing the mapping does not need to know the structure of all connected databases; he just has to know his particular database. A common schema is obtained in the fully automated unification process.

In some scenarios a very specific common schema is required or the schema is known beforehand (e.g. clinical trials). In such cases, the databases can be mapped directly to the defined common schema in the mapping process. Then, unification is straightforward and the previously defined common schema will reflect the structure of the obtained virtual repository.

There are some limitations that we plan to solve in the future. At the current state our tool does not consider hierarchical relations for attributes. Also, attributes and classes are considered as separate entities. In some occasions, however, an attribute-class unification mechanism may be necessary. Finally we plan to apply the tool in a real world case to integrate various databases with genomic information in the Institute of Health Carlos III in Madrid.

References

1. Maojo, V., Martin, F., Ibarrola, N., Lopez-Campos, G., Crespo, J., Caja, D., Barreiro, J. M., Billhardt, H.: Functional definition of the INFOGENMED WORKSTATION: a virtual laboratory for genetic information management in clinical environments. In: Proceedings AMIA'99 Annual Symposium, Washington USA (1999) 1112 60
2. Ohno-Machado, L., Boxwala, A. A., Ehresman, J., Smith, D. N., Greenes, R. A.: A Virtual Repository Approach to Clinical and Utilization Studies: Application in Mammography as Alternative to a National Database. In: Proceedings of the 1997 AMIA Annual Fall Symposium, Nashville USA (1997) 369–373 55
3. Siegel, J.: CORBA Fundamentals and Programming. Wiley & Sons, Inc., New York (1996) 58
4. Silva, J., Wittes, R.: Role of Clinical Trials Informatics in the NCI's Cancer Informatics Infrastructure. In: Proceedings AMIA'99 Annual Symposium, Washington USA (1999) 950–954 55

5. Shortliffe, E. H., Perreault, L. E.: Medical Informatics: Computer Applications in Health Care and Biomedicine. 2nd edn. Springer-Verlag New York (2001) 54
6. Wang, K., van Wingerde, F. J., Bradshaw, K., Szolovits, P., Kohane, I.: A Java-based Multi-Institutional Medical Information Retrieval System. In: Proceedings of the 1997 AMIA Annual Fall Symposium, Nashville USA (1997) 538–542 55

Fatigue Indicators of Drowsy Drivers Based on Analysis of Physiological Signals

Bittner Roman [1,2], Smrčka Pavel [2], Pavelka Miroslav [2],
Vysoký Petr [3], and Poušek Lubomír [2]

[1] Czech Technical University in Prague, Faculty of Electrical Engineering,
Dept. of Cybernetics, Technická 2, 166 27 Prague 6, Czech Republic
Bittner@cbmi.cvut.cz
[2] Czech Technical University in Prague, Centre for BioMedical Engineering,
Bílá 91, 166 35 Prague 6, Czech Republic
{Smrcka,Pousek}@cbmi.cvut.cz
[3] Czech Technical University in Prague, Faculty of Transportation Sciences,
Dept. of Automation in Transportation, Konviktská 20, 110 00 Prague 1,
Czech Republic
Vysoky@fd.cvut.cz

Abstract. The analysis of physiological signals (EEG, ECG EOG) of
drowsy and alert drivers described here is aimed at determining the fatigue level of the driver while driving. We tested possible fatigue indicators: 1. extracted from EEG spectrum; 2. based on blinking frequency,
interval histogram and speed of blinks; 3. fractal properties of RR interval-series. The first group of indicators is assumed to provide information about immediate fatigue level, whereas groups 2 and 3 are more
suitable for determining the driver's global state (alert/drowsy).

1 Introduction

In this paper, we continue on our research on detecting fatigue states of a car driver
[1]. Various technical signals provided by the car (longitudinal and lateral acceleration, steering wheel angle), physiological and behavioural signals of the driver (EEG,
ECG, EOG, video-recording of the driver's face) are recorded during the experiments.
All the experiments are performed in a real on-the-road environment.

The relationship between physiological signals and fatigue while driving have been
studied previously [2], [3], [6]. However, only basic information about the driver's
state was usually known: his/her fatigue level during all the drive (persisting 20 minutes or more). In our research, we focused on the immediate fatigue level measured in
1-minute long intervals.

Currently, the fatigue level of the driver is being determined by a group of 10
evaluators on the basis of 1-minute long segments of video-recordings of the driver's
face. This process is the most time-consuming part of the project, so other ways are

J. Crespo, V. Maojo, and F. Martin (Eds.): ISMDA 2001, LNCS 2199, pp. 62-68, 2001.
© Springer-Verlag Berlin Heidelberg 2001

being sought. We are trying to develop an automatic fatigue level estimator based on analysis of physiological signals. The research is supported by MSM210000012 grant.

2   Spectral Indices of EEG

An EEG signal most probably contains sufficient information for a quality estimate of the driver's fatigue state. The perceptive, cognitive and control processes active during driving visualise themselves through the electrical activity of the brain. However, the complexity of the EEG signal makes this task less than easy. Various authors have proved that it is possible to distinguish between a drowsy driver and an alert driver by analysing large EEG segments (half an hour or more), but we aim to monitor fast fatigue changes (in the scale of minutes).

2.1   Methods

EEG is often analysed for the dominant rhythm and presence of alpha, beta, theta etc. waves. De Waard et al. [2] suggested a relative energy parameter [(alpha + theta) / beta] as an indicator of the activation level of the driver. Kecklund and Akerstedt [3] showed earlier that the energy in the alpha and theta bands decreases rapidly during prolonged drives. The changes in theta to beta ratio for patients with chronic fatigue syndrome was examined in [10].

Here, we investigate the behaviour of 6 spectral indices: *alpha, beta, theta, ind1, ind2* and *ind3*. Parameters *alpha, beta* and *theta* are calculated as the integral of the energy of the corresponding frequency band, *ind1* is defined as [*alpha+theta*]/*beta*, *ind2* is equal to the ratio *alpha*/*beta* and *ind3* is *theta*/*beta*. The window width for the Fourier transform varies in the range from 1 second to 1 minute: the upper limit is equal to the sampling frequency of fatigue, while the lower limit is below the desired minimal resolution. Input EEG contained 19 standard channels sampled at 250 Hz. To reduce noise from eye blinks, additional differential leads were used, which gave 51 leads in all (19 unipolar leads and 32 neighbouring differential leads). Finally, the strength of the relationship between a certain index and fatigue level was examined by the linear correlation coefficient.

2.2   Results

We did not find a significant difference among the 6 tested indices; in some EEG records *ind1* is the best indicator of fatigue, in other cases *ind2*. The highest correlation of all reached value 0.77 (record s14), but the average value of correlations was 0.21, which is a very poor result. As supposed, differential leads gave better results than unipolar leads. It can be concluded that, unfortunately, the information about fatigue is spread over a wide range of frequencies. The region in the neighbourhood of the P3 electrode provided a significantly higher correlation to fatigue than other regions. On the other hand, the region in the frontal cortex is related to fatigue only very weakly. The highest average correlations were reached using bipolar leads a) C3-T3 in combination with index *ind1*; b) C3-P3 and *ind1*; c) P3-O1 and *ind2*.

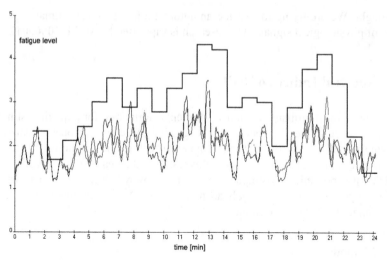

Fig. 1. Indices *alpha* and *ind2*, record s08, drowsy driver

3   Eye Blinking Analysis

Eye movements and blinking are assumed to be a significant indicator of driver fatigue. Blinking is required for lubricating and cleaning the corneal surface, but many blinks are controlled by the central nervous system rather than by environmental processes [7]. Blink amplitude, blink rate, and average closure duration are commonly used indices of fatigue [8].

3.1   Methods

The oculograms of alert and sleep-deprived drivers (after 24-48h sleep deprivation) were compared. The eye blinks were recognised as sharp peaks in the filtered signal. The following properties of eye blinks were measured: frequency of eye blinks, duration between consecutive eye blinks, speed of eye closing and opening. The following properties of eye blinks were measured: a) frequency of eye blinks; b) time interval between consecutive eye blinks; c) speed of eye closing and opening.

3.2   Results

Frequency of eyeblinks. The mean number of eye blinks varied in a broad band between 10-20 eye blinks within a 30s interval. No significant differences were found between alert and drowsy drivers (sleep deprived drivers usually blink more often than alert drivers, but this is not a rule).

Time intervals between consecutive eye blinks. The time intervals between consecutive eye blinks were rounded to the nearest 0.2s, and their frequency polygons were compared. We found that the frequency polygons do not differ in some drivers whether they are drowsy or not. However, other drivers produce a <u>bimodal curve</u> with a small maximum at 0.5s intervals between two consecutive blinks (the mean interval is about 1.6 s) in an alert state, and a unimodal curve when they are sleep deprived. Some of the eye blinks occur in the form of bursts as a symptom of fatigue.

The 'speed' of blinking. A comparison was made of the slope of the rising and sinking edge of the peak representing eye blinks, and differences were found between alert and drowsy drivers. The rising part of the blink peak (= closing of the eyes) is more appropriate for comparison. A drowsy driver blinks "more slowly" than an alert driver. The slopes of the peaks of blinks in the oculograms are sharper in all alert drivers than in drowsy drivers.

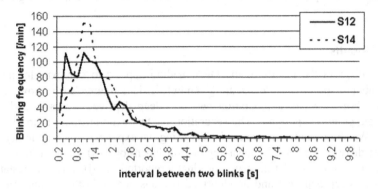

Fig. 2. Frequency polygon of time intervals of consecutive eye blinks in an alert (s12) and a drowsy (s14) driver

4   Distinguishing between Sleep Deprived and Non-deprived Persons from RR Interval-Series Analysis

Motivation. Especially in the last 10 years, statistical and spectral properties of inter-beat interval sequences (measured as the distance between two successive R-waves on an ECG record, RR) have attracted the attention of researchers, and it has been shown heart rate fluctuations carry much more information about neuro-autonomic control than had previously been supposed.

4.1   Methods

In practice, the method of such analysis must be resistant to non-stationarities arising trivially from the environmental conditions and changes in these conditions. On the contrary, it must capture most of the fluctuations in heterogeneous HRV structure which arise from the intrinsic dynamics of the human system itself. One methodology that fulfils our requirements is estimation of selected fractal properties of HRV and observing some scaling differences between sleep deprived and nondeprived groups. There are many ways of doing this. One promising method, which was used in this

work, is so-called Detrended Fluctuation Analysis (DFA). The DFA scaling exponent
d was proved to change with ageing (Iyengar et al., 1996) and to be one of the best
predictors of mortality in a patient after acute myocardial infarction (Makikallio et al,
1999). Using this descriptor, we can measure long-range correlations in highly non-
stationary time-series. It works with „accumulated" time series – accumulation is
a step that can be interpreted as a mapping of the original (bounded) time series to an
integrated signal with a fractal behaviour. Then *d* is a self-similarity measure of this
fractal. If d=0.5 –> RR is uncorrelated (like white noise), if d=1.0 -> RR behaves as
„1/f" noise, if d=1.5-> RR behaves like Brownian noise (random walk). These values
arise from the fact that we are analysing accumulated series – this increases the usual
Brownian noise exponent 0.5 by 1 to 1.5. A detailed method description is given, e.g.,
in [9].

4.2   Results

Figure 3 displays the results of the DFA method applied to our experimental data
(details about experimental design are given in [6]). This figure clearly shows a region
of scales 2<n<3, where a separation between sleep deprived (crosses) and nondeprived (big points) is possible. The separation for this experimental group of persons
is 98 %. We should note that we are in fact using the exponent *d* as a scale-dependent
measure; there are at least 2 linear regions on log n-log y(n) graphs (the crossover
region is at scales around 1.2, as was originally reported in [9]). The manifestation of
changes in sleep-deprived and nondeprived persons occurs in the second region on
higher scales (n>2, 100 and more heartbeats).

We found differences in the scaling properties of accumulated heart interbeat interval time series, from which we are able to classify persons into two groups: sleep
deprived and nondeprived.

We are now carrying out more experiments in order to verify this methodology and,
especially, its accuracy. For our first experimental groups the results are quite promising.

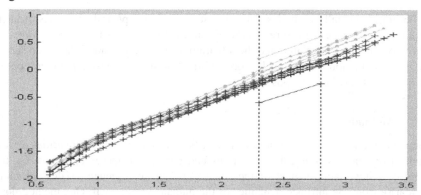

Fig. 3 Log n – log y(n) (sleep deprived – crosses, nondeprived - big points. The exponent *d* is
obtained as the local slope of each curve)

5   Conclusion

The main purpose of our work is to find a sufficient and robust estimator of fatigue level based on physiological and technical signals. In this paper, we present our first experience with EEG, EOG and RR-series analysis based on simple mathematical methods. Most of these "methods" were designed ad-hoc in order to satisfy our technical needs.

Spectral indices of EEG. The results indicate that the linear correlation between spectral indices and fatigue course is weak. Therefore, a neural network for fatigue estimation was designed, and it is at present being tested. We have confirmed the well known fact that an EEG signal is very complex and no simple conclusions can be drawn on the basis of our analysis – however we were able to spot the location of leads with the best results, and found that differential leads give better results than unipolar leads.

Eye blinking analysis. Frequency of blinking itself is not an appropriate indicator of fatigue. We have a hypothesis that the blinking pattern of old drivers is similar to that of young drowsy drivers (but there is not enough data yet to support or deny this statement statistically). A correlation exists between the number of blinks and the mean slope of the rising edge of the peaks in the same time interval.

RR interval-series analysis. It is necessary to investigate the physiological origins of the results based on fractal HRV-analysis. In this field, much more work needs to be done in the future. We speculate that a „simple" general reason (not only in our case of „sleep-deprived" data) lies in the ability of the organism to respond to environmental needs making effective use of its own metabolic resources, and that some „shadows" of underlying complex processes are accessible for example through the fractal scaling properties of biological time series (and we can explain this in terms of persistence, long-term correlation or anticorrelation). However, this methodology is very primitive. We plan to try using multifractal formalism in an attempt to specify the local behaviour of biological time series.

References

1. Bittner, R., Smrčka, P., Vysoký, P., Hána, K., Schreib, P., Poušek, L.: Detecting of Fatigue States of a Car Driver. In: Brause, R.W., Hanisch, E. (eds.): Medical Data Analysis. Lecture Notes in Computer Science. Springer-Verlag, Berlin Heidelberg New York (2000)
2. De Waard, D.: The Measurement of Drivers' Mental Workload. PhD thesis. University of Groningen, Traffic Research Centre (1996), ISBN 90-6807-308-7
3. Kecklund, G., Åkerstedt, T.: Sleepiness in Long Distance Truck Driving: An Ambulatory EEG Study of Night Driving. Ergonomics 36 (1993) 1007-1017
4. Makeig, S., Jung, T. P.: Changes in Alertness are a Principal Component of Variance in the EEG Spectrum, Neuro Report 7 (1995) 213-216
5. Juang, T. P., Makeig, S., Stensmo, M., Sejnowski, T. J.: Estimating Alertness from the EEG Power Spectrum. IEEE Trans. BME, Vol. 44 (1997) No. 1, 60-69

6. Wierwille, W. W., Ellsworth, L. A., Wreggit, S. S., Fairbanks, R. J., Kirn, C. L.: Research on Vehicle-Based Driver Status/Performance Monitoring; Development, Validation, and Refinement of Algorithms For Detection of Driver Drowsiness. U.S. Department of Transp., National Highway Traffic Safety Administration. DOT HS 808 247, Final Report (1994)
7. Ponder, E., Kennedy W. P.: On the act of blinking. Quarterly Journal of Experimental Physiology. 18 (1927) 89-110
8. Stern, A. J., Boyer, D.: Blink Rate: A Possible Measure of Fatigue. Human factors. 36 (1994) No. 2, 285-297
9. Peng, C. K., Havlin, S., et al.: Quantification of scaling exponents and crossover phenomena in nonstationary heartbeat time series. Chaos Vol 5, No 1 (1995), 82-87
10. Billiot K. M., Budzynski T. H., Andrasik F.: EEG Patterns and Chronic Fatigue Syndrome. Journal of Neurotheraphy. No 1 (1997).

Secure and Interoperable Document Management over the Internet – The Generic HARP Cross-Security Platform for Clinical Studies

Bernd Blobel [1], George Stassinopoulos [2], and Petra Hoepner [3]

[1]Otto-von-Guericke University of Magdeburg, Medical Faculty,
Institute of Biometry and Medical Informatics,
Leipziger Str. 44, D-39120 Magdeburg, Germany
`bernd.blobel@mrz.uni-magdeburg.de`
[2]NTUA,
Heroon Polytechniou 9, Zographou, EL-157 73 Athens, Greece
`stassin@cs.ntua.gr`
[3]GMD FOKUS,
Kaiserin-Augusta-Allee 31, 10589 Berlin, Germany
`hoepner@fokus.gmd.de`

Abstract. Due to its legal, ethical, social, and psychological implications, the personal information dealt with in health-related documentation and information systems is highly sensitive and must be recorded, processed, stored and communicated in a trustworthy way. Such documentation and information systems might establish comprehensive Electronic Health Care Record (EHCR) systems or partial aggregation of such data as done, e.g., in the context of clinical studies. Increasingly, such systems are based on the Internet technology. They have to meet approved and emerging protocols and standards of the domain. Within the European HARP project, the HARP Cross-Security Platform has been specified and implemented as an open transparent middleware for providing enhanced services for communication security but especially for application security such as policy enforcement and authorisation of applications. The generic solution has been demonstrated for a multi-centric quality assurance study in paediatric endocrinology.

1 Introduction

Documentation and information systems for health have to respond to the requirements of the domain. Such requirements are the support of shared care as the answer to the challenge for efficient and high quality health care systems on the one hand and the meeting of domain-specific policies on the other hand. Regarding shared care information systems, communication and co-operation must be implemented across organisational, regional and even national borders. Due to its legal, ethical, social, and

J. Crespo, V. Maojo, and F. Martin (Eds.): ISMDA 2001, LNCS 2199, pp. 69–74, 2001.
© Springer-Verlag Berlin Heidelberg 2001

psychological implications, the personal information dealt with in health-related documentation and information systems is highly sensitive and must be recorded, stored, processed, and communicated in a trustworthy manner. The policy agreed on defines the legal, ethical, social, organisational, functional and technical framework to be established for communication and co-operation. An environment meeting the same policy forms a policy domain. Depending on the granularity of system specifications, the domain can be refined into subdomains or aggregated to superdomains. Forming a new domain requires the negotiation of a common policy, also called policy-bridging. Examples for domains are single application components, workplaces, departments, hospitals, regional or even pan-European networks [1].

1.1   Security Models

Regarding security in general, we have to look for the concepts of security, safety and quality. Considering security issues, the concepts of communication security can be distinguished from application security. Quality and safety are related to the latter one. Within one concept, different levels of granularity and abstraction can be defined defining a layered model of services, mechanisms, algorithms, and data [1, 2].

1.2   Security Services

At service level, communication security requires strong mutual authentication, related control access to the other principal's site, and accountability of communicating principals, integrity, availability, and confidentiality of information communicated as well as some notary's functions.

Concerning application security services, authorisation, access control and accountability of the authorised principal for objects as well as integrity, availability, and confidentiality of objects, i.e., data and functions recorded, stored, processed, and communicated have to be guaranteed. Furthermore, proper audit and some notary's functions must be provided.

1.3   The ONCONET Security Infrastructure

The trustworthy environment needed for healthcare communication and co-operation is based on specification and implementation of security services mentioned. Most of these services deploy cryptographic algorithms. For applying asymmetric algorithms such as RSA or elliptic curves, e.g., to provide services for both communication security and application security, such as authentication, accountability, integrity and confidentiality, a security infrastructure has to be established. In Europe, this Public Key Infrastructure (PKI) is based on token for storing the private keys and for processing (signing and verifying) the digital signature mechanism and encoding/decoding as well as on appropriate Trusted Third Party (TTP) services.

At both the European level and the German national level, smart cards for health professionals have been standardised as proper token [3, 4]. These Health Professional Card (HPC) standards specify three key pairs for authentication, digital signature and encoding/ decoding information or symmetric session key as well as corresponding key-related certificates, but also attribute certificates certifying the card holder's role-defining attributes. Also the legal, organisational and functional infrastructure framework has been specified by the European Electronic Signature Directive as well as by the European Electronic Signature Standards Initiative [5].

Supported by several European project's results, the first German demonstrator of an Internet-based secure health network following these standards has been implemented by the Magdeburg Medical Informatics Department. This open network aims to facilitate shared care of cancer patients in the region, therefore called ONCONET Magdeburg / Saxony-Anhalt. More details about ONCONET can be found in [6].

For enhancing the clinical registry's functionality, specification and implementation of clinical studies and measures for quality assurance such as quality assurance studies are currently under development. Like ONCONET, also these applications have to be trustworthy, interoperable and shall run at the open Internet. They have to use the security infrastructure of HPC and TTP services avoiding any proprietary architecture.

Regarding the Internet, interoperability leads to a closer connection of both communication and application security services. The HARP project funded by the European Commission within the Information Society Technologies (IST) Programme deals with enhanced security solutions and TTP services for Internet-based communication and applications [7]. The solutions concern secure authentication as well as authorisation of principals even not registered before deploying proper Enhanced TTP (ETTP) services [8]. Especially, it helps to endorse policies by mapping them on processing components.

2   Methods

Openness, scalability, flexibility, and interoperability of information systems can be provided using a middleware between specific application components and the hardware including communication infrastructure. An example for an open and generic middleware approach is OMG's CORBA specification with health-specific services as CORBA Vertical Facilities specified by the CORBAmed Task Force. One essential service for secure interoperability is the Resource Access Decision (RAD) service specified at the first author's responsibility. The establishment of the security environment needed requires further services, basic protocols and ORB functionalities specified in a comprehensive and therefore expensive way.

The HARP project's objective is building up entirely secure applications in client-server environments over the Web.

To provide platform independence of solutions in HARP, the design pattern approach of developing a middleware-like common cross platform called HARP Cross-Security Platform (HCSP) has been used. In HCSP, platform-specific security features have been isolated. Using an abstraction layer, communication in different environment is enabled. According to the component paradigm, an interface definition of a component providing a platform-specific service specifies how a client accesses a service without regard of how that service is implemented. So, the HCSP design isolates and encapsulates the implementation of platform-specific services behind a platform-neutral interface as well as reduces the visible complexity. Only a small portion has to be rewritten for each platform.

3   Application Environment for Clinical Studies

For sharing clinical study information at each of the co-operating sites, the appropriate application environment needed for recording, presenting and using this information has to be established.

Generic solutions for embedding security into any application to be instantiated over the Web-based environment have to meet the component paradigm [2]. The granularity of components defines their reusability. "Atomic" components enable the open design of any thinkable application scenario. However, the business logic for rational interactions between the components must be managed by a supervisor. This business logic might be established in more complex components, however providing a more specific solution. In the concrete clinical study scenario described above, the extension of a component has been fixed in relation to logic segments of the documents (basic forms) used in conventional paper-based studies.

For enabling communication and especially interoperability based on components in a secure way, the network-centric, the server-centric and the client-centric approach might be distinguished. The network-centric approach transparently provides only communication security services to security unaware business logic such as legacy applications or group communication services, e.g. by Virtual Private Networks (VPN). Due to the need for application security service, it must be combined with both the server-centric and the client-centric approach. Characteristics and usability of the latter approaches in the clinical study context will be discussed in the following sections.

3.1   Server-Centric Approach

In server-centric scenarios, the required business logic is mainly provided in the health telematics provider's domain – in the study context by the centre – deploying, e.g., the Java servlet technology and emerging portal solutions. Therefore, the needed trustworthy functionality is running on authorised users' request at the server site. The server-centric approach establishes the basis for client-server interactions and therefore for the client-centric approach. It is used for provision of applets and ETTP services. Additionally, the server-centric approach is deployed for exploring centralised databases containing, e.g., clinical studies' results held at the study centre.

3.2   Client-Centric Approach

In the user-centric approach which requires that business logic is mainly provided in the user domain (for example by Java applet technology), operational and security services are realised by downloadable components. Integrity and trustworthiness of the components transferred and locally implemented must be assured. This is provided by signing and certifying the components. Structure and behaviour of these components as well as their functionality have to be controlled depending on the user and its roles expressed in attribute certificates, by the way enforcing the policy agreed on.

Such components sharable to authorised parties are, e.g., forms, viewers or more complex applications used for realising clinical studies. Furthermore, these components have to perform comprehensive services for quality assurance (QA) of remote data entry, e.g., plausibility checks and more. The components' functionality must be different according to the different user's roles. Considering clinical studies or quality assurance studies, study partners collecting information, documentation personnel recording data, QA team members checking the information, and the study co-ordinator managing the roles, rules, procedures, etc. fixed in the policy must be served establishing different rights (create, read, write, update, delete) on the one hand and granting rights on the other hand. The policy including the studies objective has to be defined and controlled by the study council.

Applet security from the execution point of view is provided through the secure downloading of policy files, which determine all access rights in the client terminal. This has to be seen on top of the very desirable feature that the local, powerful, and versatile code is strictly transient and subject to predefined and securely controlled download procedures. All rights corresponding to predefined roles are subject to personal card identification with remote mapping of identity to roles and thereby to corresponding security policies with specific access rights. These services are provided by policy repository, policy solver and authorisation manager.

4   The Clinical Study Demonstrator

The first demonstrator for specifying and implementing the HARP ETTP services was an approach for quality assurance in paediatric endocrinology performed at the German national level. After mutual three way authentication between user and server of the study centre based on HPC or HPC-plug-in at the server site respectively, the user's role is checked and interpreted according to the policy established. Then, the authorised user is enabled to download the certified study component needed currently providing the policy-conform functionality.

On the server side, HARP applies servlet technology for modularity and flexible access to legacy components, mainly existing databases. Attribute certificates and a corresponding Authorisation Manager are extensively used in order to map functions to roles and to implement the security policy. HARP views these features as externally provided enhanced Trusted Third Party (TTP) services and provides the necessary interfaces to these.

At the client site, HARP provides an open solution strictly using Internet technology such as browsers and Java applets enabling the actual functionality the user has been authorised for. After establishing the applet, it sets up a secure communication channel for exchanging information requested from the centre or recorded locally.

The exchange of recorded or requested information is performed by XML messaging managed by the XML parser and XML generator subcomponents. Using the revolutionary idea of specifying applications via XML, an easy to use application generator has been developed.

5   Conclusions

The HARP project's objective is building up open and entirely secure applications in client server environments over the Web. The HARP solutions concern secure authentication as well as authorisation of principals even not registered before deploying proper Enhanced TTP (ETTP) services. By associating role profiles and security attributes to standard Web-based interactions, HARP provides an initial degree of 'automation' in building secure medical Internet-based applications. Moreover, it clearly separates and demarcates security and policy related issues according to the component paradigm. This enables administrative bodies acting as 'policy councils' to define off-line and according to the standing legislation all procedural regulations without entering into implementation details.

In the near future, the HARP approach will be improved by adopting other open specifications such as specific CORBA services, by facilitating the specification and implementation of applets and servlets using an XML-specified component generator as well as finally by tools for a model driven "CORBA Lite" application development.

Acknowledgement

The authors are in debt to the European Commission for funding as well as to the HARP project partners for kind co-operation.

References

1.   Blobel B., Roger-France F.: A Systematic Approach for Secure Health Information Systems. Int. J. Med. Inf. 63 (2000) (in print).
2.   Blobel B.: Application of the Component Paradigm for Analysis and Design of Advanced Health System Architectures. Int. J. Med. Inf. 60 (3) (2000) pp. 281-301.
3.   CEN TC 251 prENV 13729: Health Informatics - Secure User Identification – Strong Authentication using Microprocessor Cards (SEC-ID/CARDS). Brussels, 1999.
4.   The German HPC Specification for an electronic doctor's license. Version 1.0, July 1999. http://www.hcp-protocol.de
5.   Council of Europe: 99/93/EC: Directive on Electronic Signatures. Strasbourg, 1999.
6.   Blobel B.: Onconet: A Secure Infrastructure to Improve Cancer Patients' Care. Eur. J. Med. Res. 2000: 5: 360-368.
7.   The HARP Consortium: http://www.ist-harp.org
8.   Blobel, B., Pharow, P., Engel, K.: Enhanced Security Services for Enabling Pan-European Healthcare Networks. In: Bryden, J.S., Roberts, J. (eds.): MEDINFO 2001. Towards Global Health: The Informatics Route to Knowledge. (2001) (in print)

A Generalized Uncertainty Function and Fuzzy Modeling

Arkady Bolotin

Epidemiology and Health Services Evaluation Department
Ben-Gurion University of the Negev, Beersheba, P.O.B. 653, Israel
arkadyv@bgumail.bgu.ac.il

Abstract. In this paper, a new hypothesis concerning the relationship between fuzzy truth values and probabilities is put forward. According to the hypothesis, the possibility distribution function and probability density function are not independent mathematical entities, but only different forms of a generalized uncertainty function.

Keywords: Fuzzy sets, Probability, Possibility theory, Possibility distribution function, Probability density function, Generalized information theory of uncertainty, Fuzzy modeling in medicine and biology.

1 Introduction

A fuzzy set (or, in other words, membership function) is a natural tool for modeling and dealing with uncertainty involved in medical and biological knowledge expressed in natural language.

Attractive as fuzzy modeling may seem at first sight, however, it is open to one serious objection. This objection is that one cannot measure the membership grade directly, and therefore the choice of the curve, describing a link between values of variable (measured physically) and a linguistic term, presents a quite arbitrary ("artificial") move. Furthermore, it should be stressed that the problem of determination of the fuzzy set has nothing to do with technical troubles, which could be surmounted at least theoretically. The fact is any direct measurement of membership values is impossible on principle. Let us show that.

2 Collapse of the Possibility Function

Take, for example, a player playing a chess game. Assume we have a possibility distribution function μ, which allows us to determine all possible moves the player could make[1]. Before the player makes a move, his brain continues to generate possibilities in accordance with objects of the game. All these possibilities exist simultaneously and interfere with each other. As soon as the player makes a move, however, the possibilities change.

---

[1] In the article, we use the fuzzy-set interpretation of possibility theory. According to this interpretation, a possibility distribution r is a fuzzy set μ (see Ref. [3, 8]).

J. Crespo, V. Maojo, and F. Martin (Eds.): ISMDA 2001, LNCS 2199, pp. 75–80, 2001.

Suppose in some episode of the game the player has two pieces to move: a Bishop and Knight. So, in this particular moment the function μ contains two possibilities (which exist all together). The first possibility is that the player will move the Bishop (possibility Pos_B). The second possibility is that the player will move the Knight (possibility Pos_K).

Now suppose that when we examine the game we find that the player has moved the Knight. As soon as we know this, we also know that the player did not move the Bishop (because in accordance with chess rules a player can only make one move at a time). Possibility Pos_B no longer exists.

The graphic representation of the function μ before the player made the move had two humps in it. One of the humps (B) represented Pos_B, and other hump (K) represented Pos_K. When the player moved the Knight, Pos_B ceased to exist. When that happened, hump B changed to a straight line representing 0, and hump K turned to the vertical straight line intercept representing 1. Hence, the whole function μ has changed. We can call this phenomenon "the collapse of the possibility function μ".

The collapse of the possibility function μ makes any effort to measure a possibility distribution an impossible one. At the instant when the player makes a move (i.e. when we make a measurement of the membership function μ) one of the possibilities actualizes (i.e. turns to 1), and all the others vanish (i.e. turn to zero). Consequently, what we measure is not what it was an instant before the measurement. In other words, trying to measure membership values, we completely change them.

3   Possibility vs. Probability

The possibility function μ is that mathematical entity which allows us to determine the possible results of an interaction between an observed system and a measuring device. (In the chess player example, the observed system is the player's way of thinking, and the measuring devise is the board with the chessmen.)

A second mathematical entity necessary to describe uncertainties is a probability density function p. This function gives us the probabilities at a given time(s) of each of the possibilities represented by the possibility distribution function μ. (Let us back to the chess player thinking over his next move. The probability function p can tell us how many players in the episode of the game we are observing make a move with the Bishop, and how many players make a move with the Knight.)

The possibility function μ gives a possibility degree of every event could happen to the observed system. The probability function p determines probabilities of those events actually happen to the system. The possibility function μ cannot be measured. The probability function p is measurable by definition.

It is quite logical to assume that the function μ and function p are connected somehow. Indeed, we can say that events with high degree of possibility occur more often (than events with low degree of possibility). Besides, events, which are impossible, do not occur at all. This means, that high values of the possibility function μ should correspond to high values of the probability function p, and when the function μ is equals to zero the function p must turn to zero too.

If these two functions correlate with each other, one can try to determine membership values μ by using frequency histograms or other probability curves.

As a matter of fact, there is a variety of methods of membership determination through probabilities [4-7]. Each of these methods has its own mathematical and methodological strengths and weaknesses. However, all of them have one thing in common: they treat the function μ and function p as two independent mathematical entities.

4   Generalized Uncertainty Function

The main idea of this paper is that the possibility distribution function μ and probability density function p exist only as different forms of a generalized uncertainty function Ψ:

$$\mu(x) = \frac{|\Psi(x)|}{\sup_{x \in X} |\Psi(x)|} \quad , \tag{1}$$

$$p(x) = |\Psi(x)|^2 \quad , \tag{2}$$

where x denotes all the variables of an observed system, which take values on the universal set X; $\mu(x)$ is the degree of possibility that $x = x'$; $p(x)dx$ is the probability to find x in the interval $x' - dx < x < x' + dx$.

As one can see, the basic requirement of fuzzy sets

$$0 \le \mu(x) \le 1 \tag{3}$$

is trivially satisfied by Eq.(1):

$$0 \le |\Psi(x)| \le \sup_{x \in X} |\Psi(x)| \quad . \tag{4}$$

But the key equality of probability

$$\int_X p(x)dx = 1 \tag{5}$$

presents an additional condition to put on the function $\Psi(x)$.

Let us take, for example, the extreme case when the generalized uncertainty function $\Psi(x)$ is a delta-function:

$$\Psi(x) = \delta(x - x') \quad . \tag{6}$$

Then we get

$$\mu(x) = \frac{\delta(x - x')}{\sup_{-\infty \le x \le +\infty} [\delta(x - x')]} = \begin{cases} 1, & x = x' \\ 0, & x \ne x' \end{cases} \tag{7}$$

and

$$\begin{cases} M = \int\limits_{-\infty}^{+\infty} x[\delta(x-x')]^2 dx = \int\limits_{-\infty}^{+\infty} x'\,\delta(x-x')dx = x' \\[2mm] S^2 = \int\limits_{-\infty}^{+\infty} (x-M)^2[\delta(x-x')]^2 dx = \int\limits_{-\infty}^{+\infty} (M-M)^2\,\delta(x-x')dx = 0 \end{cases} \tag{8}$$

where M and S are the mean and standard deviation. Equalities (7-8) mean that we have the case where any uncertainty is absent: the function $\mu(x)$ describes a classical set [0, 1] (corresponding to classical "either-or" logic), and the function $p(x)$ describes a distribution without statistical "noise".

Now we take another extreme case when the function $\Psi(x)$ is a simple harmonic function:

$$\Psi(x) = A \cdot \exp(-i\omega x) \quad , \tag{9}$$

where A and ω are some real constants. We obtain

$$\mu(x) = \frac{|A \cdot \exp(-i\omega x)|}{\sup_{-\infty \le x \le +\infty} |A \cdot \exp(-i\omega x)|} = 1 \tag{10}$$

and

$$\begin{cases} M = A^2 \int\limits_{-\infty}^{+\infty} x\left|\exp(-i\omega x)\right|^2 dx = 0 \\[2mm] S^2 = A^2 \int\limits_{-\infty}^{+\infty} (x-M)^2\left|\exp(-i\omega x)\right|^2 dx = \infty \end{cases} \tag{11}$$

This means, that now we have the extreme case of total uncertainty: all values of x are possible, and one can find $x = x'$ everywhere on the axis X.

In contrast, let us take the "normal" case of $\Psi(x)$:

$$\Psi(x) = \frac{1}{\sqrt{S \cdot \sqrt{2\pi}}} \cdot \exp\left[-\frac{(x-x')^2}{4S^2}\right] \quad . \tag{12}$$

Then we get

$$\mu(x) = \exp\left[-\frac{(x-x')^2}{4S^2}\right] \quad , \tag{13}$$

$$p(x) = \frac{1}{S \cdot \sqrt{2\pi}} \cdot \exp\left[-\frac{(x-x')^2}{2S^2}\right] \quad . \tag{14}$$

If the random variable z

$$z = \frac{x-x'}{S} \tag{15}$$

submits to function (12), we can describe the distribution of z with the following characteristics:

Table 1. Distribution characteristics in the case of the normal generalized uncertainty function

Y	$P\{|z| \le Y\}$	$\mu(Y)$
0.67	≈0.50	≈0.9
1.96	≈0.95	≈0.4
2.58	≈0.99	≈0.2

where $P\{|z| \le Y\}$ is the probability to find x in the interval $x' - YS \le x \le x' + YS$, $\mu(Y)$ is the degree of possibility that $x = x'$ if x is equal to $x' \pm YS$.

Suppose, for example, that x is the wavelength of the light reflected from an object, and x' is the wavelength of "ideal" red color. Assume that the ability of normal human eye to recognize red color can be represented by random variable (15). Then the figures shown in Table 1 can be interpreted in the following way. When $|z| \le 0.67$, up to 50% of people will say *"the object is definitely red"* $(0.9 \le \mu \le 1)$. When $0.67 < |z| \le 1.96$, some 45% of people will say *"the object is rather red than not"* $(0.4 \le \mu < 0.9)$. And when $|z| > 2.58$, practically all people will answer that *the object is not red at all* $(\mu < 0.2)$.

5   Conclusion

Any direct measurement of membership values is impossible because of the collapse of the possibility function $\mu(x)$ (i.e. an abrupt, discontinuous change of possibility grades caused by the process of measurement). This point was always missing in many works on fuzzy modeling.

Therefore, the only way to determine membership values "physically" is to use frequency histograms or other probability curves (assuming that the possibility function $\mu(x)$ correlates with the probability function $p(x)$).

So far as mathematically fuzzy sets and probability are different parts of a greater generalized information theory of uncertainty[2], the possibility function $\mu(x)$ and probability function $p(x)$ are different forms of the generalized uncertainty function $\Psi(x)$. It is the major assumption of the paper.

According to this assumption, the amplitude of the generalized uncertainty function $\Psi(x)$ gives a possibility degree of every event that could happen to an observed system. Meanwhile, square amplitude of the function $\Psi(x)$ gives probabilities of those events actually happen to the system. In view of that, restoring the generalized uncer-

---

[2] This theory includes many formalisms for representing uncertainty (including random sets, Demster-Shafer evidence theory, probability intervals, possibility theory, general fuzzy measures, interval analysis, etc. (see Ref.[1-2]).

tainty function $\Psi(x)$ by measuring probabilities we can determine the system membership values.

References

1. M. Grabisch, H. Nguyen, E. Walker, Fundamentals of Uncertainty Calculi with Application to Fuzzy Inference, Kluwer, Boston, 1995.
2. D. Harmanec, G. Klir, Measuring total uncertainty in Dempster-Shafer theory: A novel approach, J. General Systems, 22(4) (1994) 405-419.
3. G. Klir, On fuzzy-set interpretation of possibility theory, FSS, 108 (1999) 263-273.
4. G. Klir, Z. Wang, D. Harmanec, Constructing fuzzy measures in expert systems, Fuzzy Set and Systems, 92 (1997) 251-264.
5. G. Klir, Z. Wang, W. Wang, Constructing fuzzy measures by transformations, J. Fuzzy Math., 4(1) (1996) 207-215.
6. Turken, Measurement of Fuzziness: Interpretation of the Axioms of Measure. In: Proc. Conf. on Fuzzy Information and Knowledge Representation for Decision Analysis, Oxford, IFAC (1984) 97-102.
7. J. Wang, Determing fuzzy measures by using statistics and neural networks. In: Proc. 6th IFSA Congress, Sao Paolo, Brazil (1995) 519-521.
8. L. Zadeh, Fuzzy Sets as the basis for a Theory of Possibility, Fuzzy Set and Systems, 1 (1978) 3-28.

Special Time Series Models for Analysis
of Mortality Data

Maria Fazekas

Debrecen University, Department of Agroinformatics and Applied Mathematics
H-4032 Debrecen, Boszormenyi ut 138, Hungary
fazekasm@date.hu

Abstract. The mortality data may be analysed by time series methods such as autoregressive integrated moving average (ARIMA) modelling. This method is demonstrated by two examples: analysis of the mortality data of diseases of digestive system and analysis of the mortality data of bronchitis, emphysema and asthma. Mathematical expressions are given for the results of analysis. The relationships between time series of mortality rates were studied with ARIMA models. Calculations of confidence intervals for autoregressive parameters by three methods: standard normal distribution as estimation, the estimation of the White's theory and the continuous time estimation. Analysing the confidence intervals of the first order autoregressive parameters we may conclude that the confidence intervals were much smaller than other estimations by applying the continuous time estimation model.

1   Introduction

Time series analysis has been a well-known method for many years [1]. In the 1970's Box and Jenkins provided a method for constructing time series models in practice [2,3]. Their method has been well-known for many years and is often referred to as the Box-Jenkins approach and the autoregressive integrated moving average models (ARIMA). These are called Box-Jenkins models. This method was applied earlier in fields such as industry and economics, however later it appeared in medical research as well [4,5,6,7,8,9,10,11,12].

2   Special Time Series

Mortality data often change according to 'time series'. The frequency data of the mortality rates are usually collected at fixed intervals for several age groups and sexes of the population. Let the value of the mortality rates be z_t, z_{t-1}, z_{t-2}, ... in the years t, t-1, t-2, ... For the sake of simplicity let is assume that the mean value of z_t is zero, otherwise the z_t may be considered as deviations from their mean. Denote a_t, a_{t-1}, a_{t-2}, ... as a sequence of identically distributed uncorrelated random variables with mean 0 and variance σ_a^2. The a_t is called a white noise.

J. Crespo, V. Maojo, and F. Martin (Eds.): ISMDA 2001, LNCS 2199, pp. 81-87, 2001.
© Springer-Verlag Berlin Heidelberg 2001

The autoregressive integrated moving average of order p,d,q can be represented by the following expression [2], [13]:

$$z_t = \phi_1 z_{t-1} + \ldots + \phi_p z_{t-p} + a_t + \theta_1 a_{t-1} + \ldots + \theta_q a_{t-q} \tag{1}$$

Where ϕ_1, ϕ_2, ... , ϕ_p and θ_1, θ_2, ... , θ_q are parameters, p means the p order of autoregressive process, q denotes the q order of moving average process and d is the differencing operator. Usually d=0, 1, 2; ∇ is the symbol of the differencing operator. The meaning of the operator is $\nabla z_t = z_t - z_{t-1}$. There are special cases of the ARIMA models: the autoregressive model of order p and the moving average model of order q [2,13]. The special case of autoregressive model of order p, when p=1. This is called first order autoregressive model. The special case of moving average model of order q, when q=1. This is called first order moving average model.

The time series that has a constant mean, variance, and covariance structure, which depends only on the difference between two time points, is called stationary series. Many time series are not stationary series. It has been found that the series of the first differences is often stationary. Let w_t be the series of first differences and if z_t the original time series then $w_t = z_t - z_{t-1} = \nabla z_t$. The Box-Jenkins modelling may be used for stationary time series [2, 13].

The dependence structure of a stationary time series z_t is described by the autocorrelation function. The empirical autocorrelation function is a main tool for the identification of the model [2,13].

The autocorrelation function of the first order autoregressive process changes as if it were an exponential curve and the autocorrelation function of the second order autoregressive process decays exponentially and sinusoid. The autocorrelation function of MA(1) process has a single peak at time lag k=1 [2,13].

To identify an ARIMA model Box and Jenkins have suggested an iterative procedure [2]:

1. a provisional model may be chosen by looking at the autocorrelation function
2. the parameters of the model are estimated
3. the fitted model is checked
4. if the model does not fit the data adequately one goes back to the start and chooses an improved model.

Among different models, which represent the data equally well, one chooses the simplest one, the model with the fewest parameters [2,13].

The relation between two time series z_t and y_t can be given by the crosscorrelation function. This function determines the correlation between the time series as a function of the time lag k [2]. The crosscorrelation function estimated by empirical crosscorrelation function.

3   Estimations for Confidence Intervals

Two methods are well-known for the estimation of the parameter of first order autoregressive model. Apply the standard normal distribution as estimation and the White method. The appropriate estimations we can find in the [14] reference.

These methods above cannot be applied in non-stationary case. The continuous time processes are applied for the estimation of the first order autoregressive parameter as well. This methods are not well know [14,15]. However, this method can be applied in each case properly.

4   Results

A WHO database contains the analysed mortality data. The SPSS program-package was used for the analysis. ARIMA models were identified for some diagnoses of causes of death. The results are demonstrated in two cases from Hungarian mortality rates. Fig. 1. illustrates the mortality rates of digestive system.

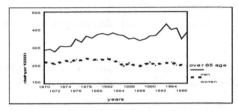

Fig. 1. Mortality rates of digestive system over age 65 for men and women

The autocorrelation functions decay for both data series.

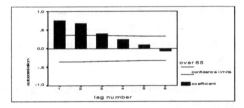

Fig. 2. The autocorrelation function for mortality data of digestive system over age 65 for men

The partial autocorrelation functions have a significance value at k=1 lag. For other lags the values of functions were in the confidence intervals.

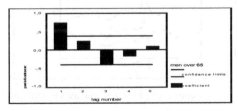

Fig. 3. The partial autocorrelation function for mortality data of digestive system over age 65 for men

The first order autoregressive model can be acceptable on the basis of autocorrelation and partial autocorrelation functions. The estimated parameter of the model gives the empirical autocorrelation coefficient. So the stochastic equation for men: $z_t=0,742z_{t-1}+\varepsilon_t; \sigma_a^2=526,18$. The model for women is the following

$$z_t=0,756z_{t-1}+\varepsilon_t; \sigma_a^2=66,92.$$

When the fitted model is adequate, then the autocorrelation of residuals have χ^2 distribution with (K-p-q) degree of freedom [2,13,16,17]. On the basis of the test the selected models were adequate; as $\chi^2_{over\ 65,men}=8,475$; $\chi^2_{over\ 65,women}=5,794$; $\chi^2_{0,05;5}=11,07$. Fig. 4. demonstrates the crosscorrelation function before fitting the model.

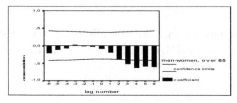

Fig. 4. The crosscorrelation function for mortality data of digestive system over age 65 between men and women

The crosscorrelation function for the residuals can be seen in Fig. 5. after fitting the model. This function has not a significance value on 95% significance level.

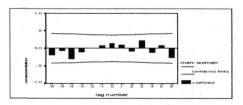

Fig. 5. The crosscorrelation function of residuals for mortality data of digestive system over age 65 between men and women

From the behaviour of residuals we may be conclude that between the examined time series is no "synchronisation".

The change in the mortality data of bronchitis, emphysema and asthma for all age groups between men and women are well illustrated in Fig. 6.

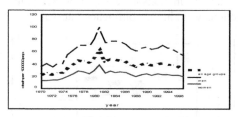

Fig. 6. Mortality rates of bronchitis, emphysema and asthma for all age groups, men and women

The analysis carried out similarly as previously and the autocorrelation and partial autocorrelation functions have a similar shape. So a first order autoregressive model can be acceptable. The stochastic equation for the death rates of women

$z_t=0,702z_{t-1}+\varepsilon_t; \sigma_a^2=14,17$; for the data of men: $z_t=0,78z_{t-1}+\varepsilon_t\ \sigma_a^2=62,95$.

We examined the residuals with the help of a χ^2 test. On the basis of the test the selected models were adequate; because χ^2_{women}=1,3399; χ^2_{men}=0,9983; $\chi^2_{0,05}$=11,07 [2, 13,16,17].

The crosscorrelation function carried out before fitting the model was similar to Fig. 4. The crosscorrelation function for residuals is demonstrated in Fig. 7. It has a significance value at k=0 lag on 95% significance level. It may be concluded that there is "synchronisation" between time series. In years when the death rates for men increased the death rates for women increased as well. It is also true for the decrease.

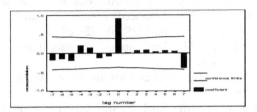

Fig. 7. The crosscorrelation function of residuals for mortality rates of bronchitis, emphysema and asthma between examined groups

The confidence intervals were carried out by the three above-mentioned methods. Applying normal distribution as estimation and the estimation of White's we get larger than one for the upper estimation of confidence bounds. It is not acceptable in a stationary case. Applying the continuous time estimation in each case we get a value for the upper limit that is smaller than one.

For the calculations of the confidence limits we used the table of the known exact distribution of the maximum-likelihood estimator of the damping parameter of an autoregressive process [14,15].

5   Discussion

The Box-Jenkins models may be useful for analysing epidemiological time series. The method described the relationship between the time series of mortality rates. It reveals a strong synchronised behaviour of the bronchitis, emphysema and asthma, between the sexes. This behaviour is not detectable at the plot of the original series. The crosscorrelation function shows a positive peak at time lag k=0 but not at other lags after fitting the model. For time series of mortality data for diseases of digestive system for men and women no such synchronisation is found between subgroups.

The synchronised behaviour of the bronchitis, emphysema and asthma is probably due to exogenous time varying factors. These factors simultaneously influence bronchitis, emphysema and asthma in both sexes but do not have any influence on the mortality rates caused by the diseases of digestive systems.

From the analysis of the first order autoregressive parameters it may be seen that by applying the normal distribution as estimation and the White method the confidence intervals are near equal. These methods cannot be applied when the time series are not stationary [14,15]. For the upper estimations of confidence limits we can get larger than one applying normal distribution and estimation of White's or we can get smaller than zero as well. These are not acceptable in a stationary case [14,15]. Applying the continuous time process for the estimation of the confidence intervals they are much smaller and it can be used in each case.

References

1. Kendall, M.G., Stuart, A.: Design and Analysis and Time Series. In: Kendall, M.G., Stuart, A. (eds): The Advanced Theory of Statistics. Vol. 3. Clarles Griffin&Company Limited, London (1966) 342-504
2. Box, G.E.R., Jenkins, G.M.: Time Series Analysis, Forecasting and Control. Holden-Day, San Francisco (1976)
3. Jenkins, D.M., Watts, D.G.: Spectral Analysis and its Applications. Holden-Day, San Francisco (1968)
4. Allard, R.: Use of Time Series Analysis in Infectious Disease Surveillance. Bull. World Health Organ. **76** (1998) 327-333
5. Box, G.E.P., Tiao, G.C.: Intervention Analysis with Applications to Economic and Environmental Problems. Journal of the American Statistical Association. **70** (1975) 70-79
6. Dimitrov, B.D., Shangova-Grigoiadi, S., Grigoriades, E.D.: Cyclicity in Variations of Incidence Rates for Breast Cancer in Different Countries. Folia Med. **40** (1998) 66-71
7. Helfenstein, U.: Detecting Hidden Relationships between Time Series of Mortality Rates. Methods Inf. Med. **29** (1990) 57-60
8. Helfenstein, U., Ackermann-Liebrich, U., Braun-Fahrlander, C., Uhrs Wanner, H.: The Environmental Accident at 'Schweizerhalle' and Respiratory Diseases in Children: A Time Series Analysis. Statistics in Medicine. **10** (1991) 1481-1492
9. Madrigal, L.: Lack of Birth Seasonally in a Ninetieth-Century Agricultural Population: Escazu, Costa Rica. Hum. Biol. **2** (1993) 235-271
10. Nelson, C.R., Plosser, C.I.: Trends and Random Walks in Macroeconomic Time Series: Some Evidence and Implications. Journal of Monetary Economics. (1982) 139-162
11. Nelson, B.K.: Statistical Methology: V. Time Series Analysis Using Autoregressive Integrated Moving Average (ARIMA) Models. Acad. Emerg. Med. **7** (1998) 739-744
12. Rios, M., Garcia, J.M., Cubedo, M., Perez, D.: Time Series in the Epidemiology of Typhoid Fever in Spain. Med. Clin. **106(18)** (1996) 686-689
13. Csaki, P.: ARMA Processes. In: Tusnady, G., Ziermann, M. (eds): Time Series Analysis. Technical Publishing House, Budapest (1986) 49-84
14. Arato, M., Benczur, A.: Exact Distribution of the Maximum Likelihood Estimation for Gaussian-Markovian Processes. In: Tusnady, G., Ziermann, M. (eds): Time Series Analysis. Technical Publishing House, Budapest (1986) 85-117
15. Arato, M.: Linear Stochastic Systems with Constant Coefficients: A Statistical Approach. Springer, Berlin (1982)

16. Haugh, L.D.: Checking the Independence of Two Covariance Stationary Time Series: a Univariate Residual Crosscorrelation Approach. J. Am. Stat. Assoc. **71** (1976) 378-385
17. Haugh, L.D., Box, G.E.P.: Identification of Dynamic Regression (Distributed Lag) Models Connecting Two Time Series. J. Am. Stat. Assoc. **72** (1977) 121-130

Knowledge Organisation in a Neonatal Jaundice Decision Support System

J. A. Fernández del Pozo[1], C. Bielza[1], and M. Gómez[2]

[1] Technical University of Madrid, Decision Analysis Group, Spain
{jafernandez, mcbielza}@fi.upm.es
[2] University of Jaén, Computer Science Department, Spain
mgomez@ujaen.es

Abstract. The tables containing the optimal decisions obtained when solving real decision-making problems under uncertainty are often extremely large. Tables can be considered as multidimensional matrices (MMs) and computers manage them as lists, where each position is a function of the order chosen (or base) for the matrix dimensions. In this paper, we propose turning the decision tables into minimum storage lists. Evolutionary computation is required to minimise the number of list entries (items). The optimal list includes the same knowledge as the original list, but it is compacted, which is very valuable for explaining expert reasoning. We illustrate the ideas using our decision support system *IctNeo* (Bielza *et al.*, 2000) for neonatal management, outputting excellent results. The methodology is so general that it also applies to any table considered as a knowledge base (KB).

Keywords: Decision Analysis, Neonatal Jaundice, Medical Decision Support Systems, Decision Table, Multidimensional Matrix, Combinatorial Optimisation, Explanation, Dependency Analysis

1 Introduction

Decision Support Systems (DSSs) demanded nowadays are very complex knowledge-based systems since they involve processes of evaluation, analysis, validation, operation and maintenance. DSSs are considered the human user oriented knowledge-based systems par excellence.

IctNeo is a complex DSS for neonatal jaundice management, a very common medical problem in which bilirubin accumulates when it is not excreted by the liver at a normal rate. It represents and solves the problem by means of an influence diagram, a tool which is becoming more and more popular in Decision Analysis. Its first version is already implemented at the Neonatology Service Department of the Gregorio Marañón Hospital in Madrid. The model includes the process of admission, treatment and discharge of a patient.

The main objectives are to include a lot of uncertain factors and decisions, define when it is best to order and/or change the treatment, decrease the costs of diagnostic and therapeutic phases, decrease risks due to, e.g., a blood exchange,

J. Crespo, V. Maojo, and F. Martin (Eds.): ISMDA 2001, LNCS 2199, pp. 88–94, 2001.
© Springer-Verlag Berlin Heidelberg 2001

which is sometimes needed, and take into account the preferences of parents and doctors, see [1].

The development of the diagram was very complex and time consuming, although the inputs were decomposed into small parts: variables, decision stages, joint probabilities factorised in conditional probabilities and additive or multiplicative utility functions. The evaluation of the diagram to obtain the optimal policy was even harder. The conventional evaluation [5] provides, at each decision node, a table with the optimal alternative for *each possible combination* of outcomes of the value node predecessors at that moment. Therefore, the results rely on a combinatorial knowledge representation space because the sizes of these tables are exponential in terms of number of attributes (those predecessors). Once the DSS has generated all these tables, it only needs to look for the combination that matches the patient under consideration.

In our case, our large influence diagram entails computational intractability, mainly because the need for storage space (in those tables) grows enormously during the problem-solving process due to node inheritances at chance node removal and arc reversal operations (requirements of approximately 10^{16} memory positions). For illustration purposes, we will use the first version of IctNeo, with only two decision nodes rather than five. It covers the first 48 hours of a baby's life, which are the most critical ones. The diagram has 41 nodes, 71 arcs, 1451 probability entries, where the biggest table has 225 entries, and an initial table for the value node of size 5400. The diagram evaluation gives rise to an optimal strategy indicating what to do when making both decisions for each combination of the variables in the tables. The first decision depends on nine variables, whereas the second stage, depends on these nine, on the first decision and on another three variables. Taking into account the cardinal of each attribute domain, the number of combinations is $59,719,680$. The table for the non-reduced diagram of five stages is even worse. It considers up to 10^{10} different combinations!

Obviously, it is a tough job to summarise the optimal policy content because of the size of the tables. However, it is very important indeed for doctors. Doctors want DSSs to have an interface and communication close to their domain. They can accept/reject a DSS proposal but it will be better if they receive a good, reasoned, consistent and structured explanation. The explanation should give a description of why the proposed decision is optimal and new insights into the problem solution. Thus, doctors are actively involved not only during the system construction and use but also during its validation.

This is the topic of the paper: how to manage the tables and extract the information that is compact enough to easily provide explanations. A table can be considered as a MM that stores or represents knowledge and therefore it can be managed as a list. We will define one of such lists of a KB MM, and we will call it $KBM2L$, read as $K.B.M.M.to.L$. Once this list is optimised, it will show the implicit rules of the protocol modelled and evaluated by the DSS. It can be used to implement an explanation procedure and it will add important details of validation, affinity and relevance of the attributes of the original table.

2   From Decision Tables to Optimised $KBM2L$ Lists

In general, a decision table can be considered as a set of attributes –relevant variables– that determine an action. Defining an order in the set of attributes (base) and in each discrete domain allows us to consider the decision tables as MMs. The content of the table stored in the cell with coordinates $\vec{c} = (c_0, c_1, ..., c_{n-1})$ will be assigned to the same position in the MM. Then, the values of the MM will be stored successively in a computer as a list. They will be arranged in main memory by means of the typical application $f : N^n \rightarrow N$,

$$f(c_0, c_1, ..., c_{n-1}) = c_0 * \prod_{i=1}^{n-1} D_i + c_1 * \prod_{i=2}^{n-1} D_i + ... + c_{n-2} * D_{n-1} + c_{n-1} = q,$$

where q provides the memory offset of the index $\vec{c}$ or the relative address with respect to the first element of the matrix, D_i is the cardinal of the i-th attribute domain, and $\prod_{j=i+1}^{n-1} D_j$ is called its *weight* w_i. Obviously, the access index of the cell can be built from the offset, provided the attribute base is known, via integer division and modulus operations.

We now introduce the $KBM2L$ whose basic element is the *item*. An item is made up of adjacent elements in memory for which the DSS proposes the same action. The items represent *grains* of knowledge or sets of cases with the same optimal policy, i.e., decision contexts. If we use another base, we have the same knowledge but we change the granularity and perhaps, the memory requirements to store the final list of items. Our aim is to get a base that minimises the number of items, bringing up the grains of knowledge. This also provides a means of explanation, finding relationships between groups of attributes and the DSS proposal.

Hence, the contents of a $KBM2L$ are items represented as $< (offset, policy)|$. It reflects (1) that the offsets of the items are strictly increasing and (2) it summarises a set of adjacent cells with the same policy and different to the proposal of the next item. See [4] for further details on the formal conditions of consistency of a $KBM2L$, and how its internal structure is.

In our DSS, the $KBM2L$ is completed as long as the diagram is evaluated. The initial list has always only one item: $< (MaxOffset, unKB)|$, where $unKB$ means the absence of knowledge. Our software developed for the construction of the KB via a $KBM2L$ employs 18 rules for the management of the decision table and implements three algorithms for synthesis, learning and explanation of knowledge. In [4] we detail step-by-step how a $KBM2L$ is before and after applying the rules that add a new case $< (x, d)|$ to the list.

For δ attributes, the method for constructing the $KBM2L$ consists of reading the table inputs with the original initial order $(0, 1, ..., \delta - 1)$ in a structure without information. Note that the order of the inputs or cases is not important and, in general, the whole table may not be known, if it is very large. We try to improve the current base moving to another base. The information is then *copied* to the corresponding new $KBM2L$ structure. If this new list is more optimal than the old one (i.e., if it requires a shorter list), it is kept and the

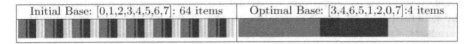

Fig. 1. *KBM2L* spectrum or sets of cases which the same optimal decision policy. Both lists have the same information (256 cases) but the optimal (right-hand) requires less memory space

process iterates to improve it again. Take into account that the information copy procedure between *KBM2L* structures in different bases may require up to *MaxOffset* + 1 elements to be copied and it is necessary to compare lists. But we can use some heuristic like taking only a sample of the copy to decide whether the base can be rejected. It reduces the computational burden because we do not have to look at the whole copy, which is not an easy task for such massive tables.

In trying to improve the current base, we should find bases that allow the items to be joined, that place equal items adjacently. The change of base affects the union/fragmentation of the items. And this is the key as we can see in Fig. 1.

Let us define two clearly different parts of an index from the point of view of an item. Let I_{inf} and I_{sup} be the vectors of indexes associated with the extreme cases of an item of the list. The first part is the *fixed* part of the index: its components that are evaluated on concrete values and that are common to all the cases of the item. The second part, which is complementary to the first, is the *variable* part: the cases do not share these values and therefore the attributes are irrelevant for the policy associated with the item. See [4] for some examples. These concepts open up automatic explanation possibilities.

Once we have built the *KBM2L* and we know how to manage its items, the list must be optimised. I.e., we now ask which is the order of the attributes that minimises the number of items stored as a *KBM2L* for a given matrix. The problem of finding the base with minimum storage space is one of combinatorial optimisation. In tables of δ attributes, we must consider $\delta!$ possible solutions, i.e., all the possible permutations of δ attributes. Finding the optimal base is a *NP*-hard problem that in addition must solve, at each step of the algorithm, an exponential problem: to copy the information from one *KBM2L* to another in a different base. In [4] we propose the use of modern global optimisation techniques like genetic algorithms (global search for $\delta \geq 20$) to solve the problem. Each individual is a base with δ genes. Crossover, mutation and selection operations allow the population to evolve. Also, we add heuristics to guide the search for the optimum: (1) partial information copy procedure by using samples; (2) move through the space of permutations towards elements of fixed or random Hamming distance for local search; (3) give more opportunity or probability of movement to the corresponding fixed part of the small items (those which represent few cases about certain policy) towards the zone of the variable part; etc. This process of base generation and test is guided because it learns how to generate better lists, preventing item fragmentation and promoting unions. The generation of information relative to the search space that can guide the optimisation process bears some resemblance to ant colony modern optimisation methods for discrete problems [2].

In short, the complexity of the optimal base search algorithm lies in the analysis of the fragmented item index and in the information transfer or copy between $KBM2Ls$ associated with the change of base.

3   Neonatal Jaundice Results

The base for the initial $KBM2L$ is $B_0 = \{$CBrb2, Emo, CBrb1, Soc, ...$\}$. We only specify the most relevant attributes out of the whole set of eighteen. The $CBrb1$ and $CBrb2$ attributes are bilirubin concentrations, Emo is the emotional cost and Soc is the social cost of the patient admission. The $KBM2L$ for this base has 12 grains of knowledge covering the whole set of 59,719,680 combinations, see Sect. 1. We use a two-column table to present this list, see below. The right-hand column includes the proposal of the system (as the influence diagram has two decisions, there is a proposal for each one). The left-hand column shows the attributes associated with each proposal. Only the fixed part (the attributes without changes for their cases) of each item is shown.

<((CBrb2:Normal,Emo:Low,CBrb1:Normal,...),	(Th2:TherapyNo,Th1:TherapyNo))|
<((CBrb2:Normal,Emo:Low,CBrb1:High,...),	(Th2:ObservationDischarge,Th1:Phototh6h))|
<((CBrb2:Normal,Emo:Medium,CBrb1:Normal,...),	(Th2:TherapyNo,Th1:TherapyNo))|
<((CBrb2:Normal,Emo:Medium,CBrb1:High,...),	(Th2:ObservationDischarge,Th1:Phototh6h))|
<((CBrb2:Normal,Emo:High,CBrb1:Normal,...),	(Th2:TherapyNo,Th1:TherapyNo))|
<((CBrb2:Normal,Emo:High,CBrb1:High,...),	(Th2:ObservationDischarge,Th1:Phototh6h))|
<((CBrb2:High,Emo:Low,CBrb1:Normal,...),	(Th2:TherapyNo,Th1:TherapyNo))|
<((CBrb2:High,Emo:Low,CBrb1:High,...),	(Th2:Phototh6hBloodExchangePhototh6h, Th1:Phototh6h))|
<((CBrb2:High,Emo:Medium,CBrb1:Normal,...),	(Th2:TherapyNo,Th1:TherapyNo))|
<((CBrb2:High,Emo:Medium,CBrb1:High,...),	(Th2:Phototh6hBloodExchangePhototh6h, Th1:Phototh6h))|
<((CBrb2:High,Emo:High,CBrb1:Normal,...),	(Th2:TherapyNo,Th1:TherapyNo))|
<((CBrb2:High,Emo:High,CBrb1:High,...),	(Th2:Phototh6hBloodExchangePhototh6h, Th1:Phototh6h))|

Note how lucky we have been with the initial base with only 12 items. However, this will often not be the case. For instance, $B = \{$CBrb1, Emo, Soc, CHgb1, CHgb2, Age1, Age2, CBrb2, ...$\}$ (Hgb: hemoglobin) yields 1,296 items.

The optimisation phase shows that the initial base is not optimal and by changing the order of the attributes we could get a shorter list and refine the knowledge about the decisive attributes. After 306 changes of base, the list has only four items, a quite significant improvement. The optimal base is $B_{final} = \{$CBrb1, CBrb2, Emo, Soc, ...$\}$, with a list shown below. This list can be read as four rules indicating the optimal global policy as a function of the key attributes, the fixed part of the item.

<((CBrb2:*[1],CBrb1:*,...),	(Th2:TherapyNo,Th1:TherapyNo))|
<((CBrb2:*,CBrb1:Normal),	(Th2:TherapyNo,Th1:Observation and Discharge))|
<((CBrb2:Normal,CBrb1:High,...),	(Th2:Observation and Discharge,Th1:Phototh6h))|
<((CBrb2:High,CBrb1:High,...),	(Th2:Phototh6hBloodExchangePhototh6h,Th1:Phototh24h))|

* means not available

Doctors can ask the DSS for any patient history in the jaundice protocol. They now know how the system explains its proposals and which rules are taken into account when making inferences. Thus, after the patient admission, if $CBbr1$ is normal, the baby is observed and discharged. If $Cbrb1$ level is high, the initial therapy is a Phototherapy of 6 hours long and then, if $Cbrb2$ level is normal, the baby is observed and discharged. Otherwise, if $Cbrb2$ level is high, doctors make a large session of Phototherapy with a blood exchange transfusion.

4 Conclusions

The preferences and the structure of dependencies and independencies represented in a decision model produce patterns of regularity in the proposals of the DSS. The granularity of the decision tables not only depends on the problem, but also on the internal organisation of the tables. A reorganisation may lead to a grouping of cases in contexts of identical proposals. A good organisation reduces the memory required to store the tables and brings out qualitative information about the variables: only some of them are really relevant in the contexts. Therefore, we discover relationships among the attributes using them to explain the DSS proposals. This is the case for the IctNeo system. The attainment of explicit decision-making rules and a means of observing the influence of parameter variation on these rules imply incidentally a practical procedure for performing sensitivity analysis.

The computational burden is not costly whenever we employ some resorts. For instance, we divide the evaluation process by instantiation of evidence [3], choosing some attributes to get a manageable size for the decision tables and producing the smallest impact on the propagation of uncertainty. IctNeo *learnt* from nine decision tables derived from the instantiation of two attributes.

The procedure presented in this paper is also applicable to data coming from mathematical programs, data bases or data acquisition systems. We are currently researching into further detail the rules to manage the list items, the operations among lists with different bases, suitable crossover operations for the genetic algorithm, possible connections with multivariate analysis, etc.

Acknowledgments

Research supported by Project CAM 07T/0027/2000.

References

1. Bielza, C., Gómez, M., Ríos-Insua, S., Fernández del Pozo, J. A. (2000) Structural, Elicitation and Computational Issues Faced when Solving Complex Decision Making Problems with Influence Diagrams, *Computers & Operations Research* 27, 7-8, 725-740. 89
2. Dorigo M., Di Caro, G., Gambardella, L. M. (1999) Ant Algorithms for Discrete Optimization, *Artificial Life*, 5, 2, 137-172. 92

3. Ezawa, K. (1998) Evidence Propagation and Value of Evidence on Influence Diagrams, *Operations Research* 46, 1, 73-83. 93
4. Fernández del Pozo, J. A., Bielza, C., Gómez, M. (2001) Knowledge Synthesis Optimising the Combinatorial Storage of Multidimensional Matrices, Working Paper, Technical Univ. of Madrid, *to be presented at ESI XIX*. 90, 91
5. Shachter, R. D. (1986) Evaluating influence diagrams, *Operations Research* 34, 6, 871-882. 89

Quasi-Fourier Modeling
for Individual and Count Outcomes

Michael Friger[1], Yelena Novack[1], and Ulrich Ranft[2]

[1] Epidemiology Department, Ben-Gurion University of the Negev
Beer-Sheba, Israel
{friger,novack}@bgumail.bgu.ac.il
[2] Medical Institute of Environmental Hygiene, H. Heine University,
Duesseldorf, Germany
ranft@uni-duesseldorf.de

Abstract. This article develops a model based on time-series analysis for investigating health outcome, such as disease or death, in relation to levels of air pollution. The model is built under assumption that any health outcome belongs to multivariate hierarchical system and depends on meteorology, pollution, geophysical and socio-cultural variables in it. The possible connections in this system are considered and mathematically formalized by means of trigonometric and polynomial functions. The model is tested by two simulations: (1) with count outcomes taken from Philadelphia daily mortality records for the period from 1974 to 1980; (2) with the individual outcomes taken from the peak flow measurements in 48 adults with vulnerable respiratory system in Leipzig, Germany, October 1990 - April 1991.

1 Introduction

In the last several decades air pollution is of great public-health concern throughout the world. A number of analyses have been recently published on associations of levels of urban pollution with variations in daily mortality and morbidity [1]. Depending on objectives and ways of understanding the problem, many different and sophisticated models have been proposed. Given the complexity of the problem, however, each model has its restriction and, therefore, no approach is accepted entirely so far. In this article we propose a new modeling approach, aimed to study the association of pollution with health, based on time-series techniques and system analysis, which contains an essential improvement of the model described in [2]. The proposed model makes believe to be a natural reflection of the reality and, therefore, a more reliable instrument for investigating the association of our interest. We show two simulations of the proposed approach for two different types of health outcome, count (death rates) and individual (health condition of a patient).

J. Crespo, V. Maojo, and F. Martin (Eds.): ISMDA 2001, LNCS 2199, pp. 95–100, 2001.

2   Sources of Data

As an example for count health outcome, we are going to use Philadelphia total daily mortality minus cancer mortality for 1974-1980. They were kindly made available for us by Prof. Johnathan Samet. Daily average temperature and dew point are meteorological variables (in degrees of Fahrenheit), pollutants (sulfur dioxide SO_2) are in parts per billion and total suspended particulate (TSP) is in micrograms per cubic meter.

As an example of individual health outcome, we take the data of the group of 48 adults with respiratory problems. This dataset comprises of daily peak expiration flow measurements (in l/min), daily measurements of two main pollutants (SO_2 in mg/m^3 and suspended particles in mg/m^3) and the daily meteorological measurements (temperature and humidity). The measurements were carried out during the period of seven months, starting from October 1990 till April 1991, in Leipzig, Germany.

3   Methods

3.1 Constructing the Model

Consider the concept of "health" as an outcome of our major interest. In our case, "health" is characterized by death rate in a given population or a patient's health state. We assume that variable "health" is part of the hierarchical system that includes meteorology, pollution and other variables (Figure 1).

Figure 1 derives from few assumptions we believe are in the base of the variable relationship. These assumptions are: (1) seasonal variation as a function of time-of-year (periodical geophysical affect G) has an effect on meteorology (M) and pollution (P) as well as health (H); (2) meteorological variables influence pollution and health; (3) pollutants affects health; (4) variations over week days can affect both pollutants and health.

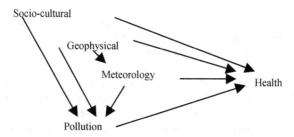

Fig. 1. Diagram for Relations among Health, Meteorology and Pollution

By all these assumptions we decompose the structural model proposed into 7 following paths: *(1) G→H; (2) S→H; (3) M→H; (4) G→M→H; (5) G→M→P→H; (6) S→P→H; (7) P→H*. (One can find a more detailed description in [2]).

Finally, we obtain the following function for the health outcome:

$$H_t = F_1^G(G_t,t) + F_2^S(S_t,t) + F_3^M(M_t,t) + F_4^G(G_t,t) \bullet F_4^{GM}(M_t,t) +$$
$$+ F_5^G(G_t,t) \bullet F_5^{GM}(M_t,t) \bullet F_5^{GMP}(P_t,t) + F_6^S(S_t) \bullet F_6^{SP}(P_S,t) + F_7^P(P_t,t),$$

$$(1)$$

where H_t is our dependent variable (health outcome); G_t, S_t, M_t, P_t are the vectors of geophysical, socio-cultural, meteorological and pollution variables respectively; t is the time variable; F_1^G, F_2^S, F_3^M, F_7^P are the functions which express the "direct" effects of geophysical, socio-cultural, meteorological and pollution factors on the dependent variable; F_4^G designates the "indirect" effects (via meteorology) of a geophysical factor on the dependent variable; F_4^{GM} stands for the "indirect" effects of meteorological factor on the dependent variable (after removing the influence of geophysical factor on meteorology); F_5^G is the "indirect" effects (via meteorology and pollution) of the geophysical factor on the dependent variable; F_5^{GM} is the "indirect" effects of meteorological factor (via pollution) on the dependent variable (after removing the influence of geophysical factor on meteorology); F_5^{GMP} is the "indirect" effect of pollution factor on the dependent variable (after removing the influence of geophysical and geophysical factors on pollution); F_6^S is the "indirect" effect of socio-cultural factor (via pollution) on the dependent variable; F_6^{SP} expresses the "indirect" effects of pollution factor on the dependent variable (after removing the influence of socio-cultural factors on pollution); symbol • stands for superposition of the functions.

The next step of the model construction is determining the type of the all the above functions of type F_*^{**}, which enter the model.

Let's consider now the functions that are related to G (geophysical factors). We put forward an a priori assumption that the periodic seasonal changes are, in fact, the reflection of geophysical processes which affects weather, pollution, and health outcome. Weather, in its turn, also affects pollution and health outcome. Hence it follows that the pollution-health outcome relationship is two-ways affected (directly and indirectly). By the "indirect effect" we mean that interaction between meteorology and its seasonal changes have effect on other variables, for example, pollution. Therefore, pairs of sinusoidal and co-sinusoidal functions with different periods could present all the functions related to G. Periodical changes of S (socio-cultural factors) are deduced as 6 terms of dummy variables for each day of the week. Other functions can be presented by polynomial and/or logarithmic functions. One of possible formalizations of the approach described can be a system of regression equations.

Let M_j $(j=1,...,r_m)$ and P_k $(k=1,..,r_k)$ be a meteorological and pollution variables respectively. Thus we obtain the following system of five equations (2-6):

$$
\begin{aligned}
Y_t = {}& q_0 + q^0 + \sum_{j=1}^{r_m} q_j M_j + \sum_{k=1}^{r_p} q_k P_k + \\
& + \sum_{i=1}^{g} \left(a_i \cos\left(\frac{it \cdot 2\pi}{365} \right) + b_i \sin\left(\frac{it \cdot 2\pi}{365} \right) \right) + \\
& + \sum_{j=1}^{r_m} \sum_{i=1}^{g} \left(a_{ij} M_j^* \cos\left(\frac{it \cdot 2\pi}{365} \right) + b_{ij} M_j^* \sin\left(\frac{it \cdot 2\pi}{365} \right) \right) + \\
& + \sum_{k=1}^{r_p} \sum_{j=1}^{r_m} \sum_{i=1}^{g} \left(a_{ij}^k M_j^* P_k^* \cos\left(\frac{it \cdot 2\pi}{365} \right) + b_{ij}^k M_j^* P_k^* \sin\left(\frac{it \cdot 2\pi}{365} \right) \right) + \sum_{s=1}^{6} c_{sk} P_k D_s
\end{aligned}
\tag{2}
$$

$$\hat{M}_j = \sum_{i=1}^{g} \left(c_{ij} \cos\left(\frac{it \cdot 2\pi}{365}\right) + d_{ij} \sin\left(\frac{it \cdot 2\pi}{365}\right) \right) \tag{3}$$

$$M_j^* = M_j - \hat{M}_j \quad (j = 1, \dots, r_m) \tag{4}$$

$$\hat{P}_k = \sum_{j=1}^{r_m} \sum_{i=1}^{g} \left(c_{ij}^k M_j^* \cos\left(\frac{it \cdot 2\pi}{365}\right) + d_{ij}^k M_j^* \sin\left(\frac{it \cdot 2\pi}{365}\right) \right) \tag{5}$$

$$P_k^* = P_k - \hat{P}_k \quad (k = 1, \dots, r_p) \tag{6}$$

where $2\pi/365$ is an yearly cycle; $i=1,2,...,g$ are the various sub-periods of a year (in our case, month, season, half a year and a year); D_s are the dummy variables (one for each day of the week), which represent a periodic component of the socio-cultural factor; $c_{ij}, d_{ij}, c_{ij}^k, d_{ij}^k, q_i, a_i, b_i, a_{ij}, b_{ij}, a_{ij}^k, b_{ij}^k$ are the constants obtained by appropriate type of multiple regression.

The model's goodness of fit is determined by adjusted R^2 for the individual health outcomes and deviance for the count data (Poisson distributed).

3.2 Interpreting the Model

The obtained model seems more problematic for interpretation then the standard linear models, where this process is trivial and based on the values of standardized regression coefficients and adjusted contribution of each variable in the model.

Numerous functional patterns of the independent variables (which we deal with in the given case) set us thinking about multi-layer interpretation strategy. Here is one of possible ways of interpreting the model.

We divide of the independent variables set in main factors and co-factors (covariates), depending on the study objectives. Thus, if the relationship of urban pollution and health is the subject of study, we define the pollutant variables $p_1, p_2 \dots, p_k$ as main factors and the rest of independent variables we treat as co-factors. Now, we transform the final equation of the model as the following:

$$Y_t = F_1(x_1(t), x_2(t), \dots, x_n(t), t) \cdot p_1 + F_2(x_1(t), x_2(t), \dots, x_n(t), t) \cdot p_2 + \dots$$
$$+ F_k(x_1(t), x_2(t), \dots, x_n(t), t) \cdot p_k \tag{7}$$

where x_i are the co-factors and t is time.

Then, we redefine the functions $F_i(x_1(t), x_2(t), \dots, x_n(t), t)$ as functions of time variable t, i.e. $F_i(x_1(t), x_2(t), \dots, x_n(t), t) = \Phi_i(t)$ for i=1,2,...,k.

As a final point, we obtain the following equation:

$$Y_t = \Phi_1(t) \cdot p_1 + \Phi_2(t) \cdot p_2 + \dots + \Phi_k(t) \cdot p_k \tag{8}$$

We'll call function $\Phi_i(t)$ "profile of variable p_i" and use calculus tools for their analysis (studying minimal and maximal points, intervals of increasing and decreasing and so on). This kind of information enables us to analyze the contribution and behavior of each of the main factors.

4   Results

4.1 Simulation of the Proposed Model on Count Data Set

Table 1 presents the results of how linear regression is used in the model with "total mortality minus cancer mortality" as a dependent variable. The table shows contributions of all significant terms to the explained variance by groups of M, S, G and P factors.

Table 1: Contributions of all factors to the explained variance of Mortality in Philadelphia, 1974-1982[1]

	Variable	Beta (Path Coefficient) (1)	R (2)	Contribution to Expl. Var. (1x2)
Geophysical	Cos–1 year	1.267	0.362	0.459
	Sin–1 year	0.250	0.197	0.050
	Sin–6 mon	-0.123	0.103	-0.012
				sum=0.497
Meterologi-cal	Dew	0.135	-0.321	-0.043
	Dew*Cos-1 year	0.421	0.296	0.125
	Dew*Sin-6 mon	0.162	0.009	0.002
	Temp*Cos-year	-1.216	0.310	-0.377
				sum=-0.293
Pollution	SO_2	0.045	0.125	0.006
	SO_2*Cos-4 mon	-0.088	-0.107	0.010
	SO_2*Day2	0.035	0.038	0.001
	TSP*Cos-3 mon	-0.071	-0.070	0.005
	TSP*Day1	0.108	0.115	0.012
				sum=0.034
Trend	Day	-0.130	-0.162	0.021

[1]For 13 terms: R^2=0.261; R^2_{adj}=0.257; Deviance=3114.97; Deviance/N=1.24

Table 2: Results of Deviance and Explained Variance in the Proposed Model and the Standard Model for the Period 1974-1980 and Each Year

	1974	1975	1976	1977	1978	1979	1980
Proposed Model Deviance Deviance/N Adjusted R^2	330.38 0.989 0.278	422.14 1.163 0.351	411.42 1.127 0.350	449.06 1.23 0.114	387.74 1.07 0.433	349.66 0.961 0.145	418.88 1.144 0.390
Standard Model Deviance Deviance/N Adjusted R^2	364.76 1.122 0.171	523.70 1.443 0.195	497.90 1.379 0.198	465.88 1.276 0.084	497.34 1.374 0.269	365.04 1.008 0.107	525.68 1.440 0.227

("Standard Model" denotes the linear regression model with four main variables: dew, temperature and the two pollutants)

Table 2 shows comparison between two modeling approaches (proposed and standard one). The lower the value of "Deviance/N" the better the fit of the data to the model. The model, taking into consideration the possible cyclic effect, likely has a better fitness estimation, both in terms of "Deviance/N" and explained variance.

4.2 Simulation of the Proposed Model on Individual Data Set

We used the hierarchical system from the previous example assuming an effect of the factors, which influence the mortality index, on the health condition of a patient. The same kinds of variables and their interactions are used, but the choice of possible cycles is different. The model was built for every person. For more than 60% of all individual models, proportion of explained variance in Quasi-Fourier Model is greater than 0.5, unlike that 18.7% explained by Standard Regression Model (contained M and P factors only). In Table 3 we put the three main factors with maximal contribution to the explained variance in the 48 individual models.

Table 3 Three factors with a greatest contribution to the patients' models

Types of the factors	First (n,%)	Second (n,%)	Third (n,%)
Periodic	38 (79.2%)	34 (70.8%)	23 (47.9%)
Periodic*Meteorological	7 (14.6%)	6 (12.5%)	14 (29.2%)
Periodic*Pollution	2 (4.2%)	7 (14.6%)	10 (20.8%)
Other (non-periodic)	1 (2.1%)	1 (2.1%)	1 (2.1%)

Table 3 demonstrates that for vast majority of the models the periodic factors and that connected with them contribute at most to explained variance. As one can see, the non-periodic variables, which are of the individual models, barely appear in the models.

5   Conclusions

The model we propose in the given paper is better to some extent then that published so far. This improvement concerns measurements of regular goodness of fit and takes place mainly from considering the direct and indirect effects of the environmental factors analyzed. Secondly, our study points out that pollution has a relatively small contribution to explained variance, even if we take into account the joint direct and indirect effect of pollution (Table 1 and 3).

References

1. Health Effects Institute. Particulate Air Pollution and Daily Mortality: Replication and Validation of the Selected Studies. Andover, Mass. Health Effects Institute, August (1995).
2. Goldsmith, J.R,, Friger, M.D. and Abramson, M.: Associations Between Health and Air Pollution an Time-Series Analyses Arch. Environ. Health (1996): Vol.51: 358-367.

An Anatomical and Functional Model for the Study of Cortical Functions

A. J. García de Linares[1] and L. de la Peña Fernández[2]

[1] R&D Department. Novasoft Sanidad. Málaga. Spain.
aglinares@novasoft.es
[2] Radiology Departament. School of Medicine.
University of Málaga. Spain
lpf@uma.es

Abstract. The increasing number of investigations focusing on the structural and functional organization of the brain makes necessary a better analysis of the results and the construction of tools that facilitate the integration of all this knowledge. We present an anatomical and functional cerebral model using the Visible Human dataset. The anatomical structures were labeled and assigned a unique color. In a parallel way, a database was created for including hierarchical anatomical information and the meta-analysis result from the human brain-mapping literature.

1   Introduction

Models of the anatomy of the human body are of increasing importance for scientists, engineers and physicians. The applications of these models vary widely from medical education and diagnostics to simulation of physical fields. To create anatomical models generally information extracted from medical images is used and advanced strategies of image processing are employed [6,7].

Since the Visible Human data set was created (© National Library of Medicine, Bethesda, Maryland, USA) [1,9] has become a staple to many applications used for teaching anatomy, models of surgical planning, and as a visual basis for surgical simulation and other virtual reality [6,12].

The explosive growth in brain imaging technologies has been matched by an extraordinary increase in the number of investigations focusing on the structural and functional organization of the brain. Human brain structure is so complex and variable across subjects that many research fields are required to manipulate, analyze and communicate brain data. Central to these tasks is the construction of comprehensive brain atlases [8,12], databases of 3-dimensional brain maps [2], templates and models to describe how the brain and its component parts are organized

Brain atlases provide a structural framework in which individual brain maps can be integrated. Most brain atlases are based on a detailed representation of a single sub-

J. Crespo, V. Maojo, and F. Martin (Eds.): ISMDA 2001, LNCS 2199, pp. 101-107, 2001.

ject's anatomy in a standardized 3D coordinate system, or stereotaxic space. The chosen data set acts as a template on which other brain maps (such as functional images) can be overlaid. The anatomical data provides the additional detail necessary to accurately localize activation sites, as well as providing other structural perspectives such as chemoarchitecture. Digital mapping of structural and functional image data into a common 3D coordinate space is a prerequisite for many types of brain imaging research, as it supplies a quantitative spatial reference system in which brain data from multiple subjects and modalities can be compared and correlated [5, 10, 11].

The purpose of this project is the creation of an anatomical and functional model of the human brain using the Visible Male brain dataset and with linked information about human functional mapping.

2   Material and Methods

This project has the following main tasks: (1) Volume creation, (2) Database creation, (3) Meta-analysis of functional papers and (4) Working Environment.

2.1   Volume Creation

We have used the Visible Human dataset (National Library of Medicine, Bethesda, Maryland, USA) for constructing the anatomical model. A total of 163 axial anatomical images concerning the male head were downloaded from then NLM-FTP site, each slice with a resolution of 2048 pixels by 1216 pixels, and each pixel defined by 24 bits of color (resulting about 7.5 megabytes of data/slice), at 1.0 mm intervals [9]. The images were preprocessed by removing background imagery such as the ruler and color bar, and the blue gelatin where the cadaver was embedded. Each cross-sectional image was also "cleaned" by application of an opening operation to all pixels which were within 10 pixels of the removed background [6, 7]. This opening operation removed small areas of gelatin which adhered to the skin after thresholding. Another preprocessing step is the detection and correction of differences in the color reproduction of the photos. The detection is performed using their color palette. The correction is done by transformations of the RGB values.

The pixel size in the "XY" plane was reduced to 1 mm in order to match the pixel spacing in the "Z" plane which is 1 mm. This made possible to obtain cubic voxels with 1 mm x 1 mm x 1 mm size. The slices were normalized into the Talairach space, anatomically defined by the bicommissural line, setting the central points of the anterior and posterior commissures manually [10,11]. The resulting volume dataset use x-y-z coordinates resolved to 1x1x1 mm volume elements within a standardized stereotaxic space. An array, indexed by x-y-z coordinates, that spans 87 mm (x), 133 mm (y) and 127 mm (z), provides high-speed access to data.

The images were segmented using interactive tracing, slice-to-slice propagation and editing of defined regions. At the same time, additional color-map entries were created, providing a unique color entry for each distinct anatomical structure. The defined anatomical regions were filled with the specific color assigned for that structure. Hemispheres, lobes, gyri and nuclei have been outlined and labeled. Gray matter, white matter and CSF regions have also been defined. For cerebral cortex, all Brodmann areas have been traced (Fig. 1).

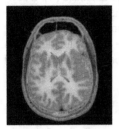 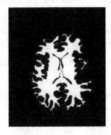 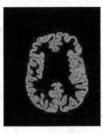 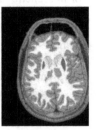

Fig. 1. From left to right. (A) Postprocessed anatomical slice. (B) White matter template. (C) Gray matter template. (D) Example of mixed labeled information in the same slice

2.2   Database

In order to provide an indexing structure useful for our knowledge base of brain structures and functions, we have designed a database with a comprehensive hierarchical nomenclature for structures of the human brain based on the Neuronames database [3].

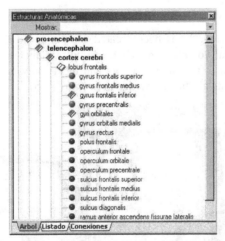

Fig. 2. The Nomina Anatomica window. Note the hierarchical structure used

The hierarchical organization (Fig.2), consistent with *Nomina Anatomica,* includes an exhaustive, nested set of mutually exclusive volumetric structures that represents the entire brain at each level of the Hierarchy and, a list of the superficial features that can be seen. We have included 790 structures (159 superficial features and 631 volumetric structures). The database was completed with additional information like the color used in the anatomical volume or the connection rules.

2.3   Meta-analysis

For the functional meta-analysis data we have used the Brainmap database [4], a software environment for the meta-analysis of the human functional brain-mapping literature that include 225 papers, 771 experiments and 7683 locations.

We have analyzed the results from 75 cortical activation studies, and included into the database. All these information was linked with the anatomical structures data and the volumetric data.

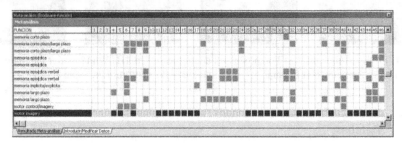

Fig. 3. Example of the meta-analysis information window showing information about some cognitive tasks (rows) and the activated Brodmann areas in red

2.4   Working Environment

A software program (Fig.4) has been created containing all the necessary tools for viewing the anatomical volume (OpenGL), editing the labeled structures, editing the contents of the database (anatomical names and meta-analysis results), and the most important task, integrate all the knowledge network (Fig. 5).

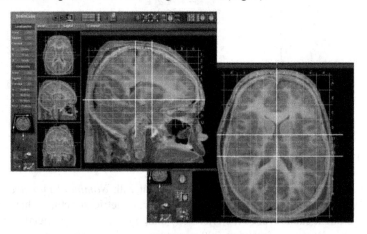

Fig. 4. Program window for the cerebral atlas

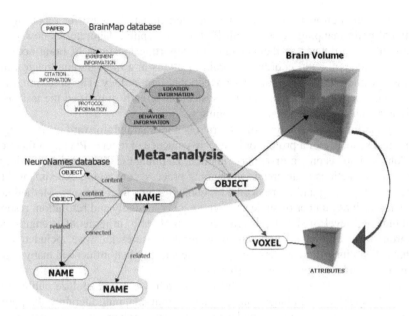

Fig. 5. Structure of the knowledge network

All the software programs have been programmed using Delphi 5.0 (INPRISE Inc) under Windows 2000 Professional (®Microsoft) and a Pentium III PC computer with 128Mb RAM and 19 Gb Hard disk. Sybase was chosen as the core component of our database.

3   Results and Discussion

A cerebral model has been created making possible to establish the spatial positions of the cerebral structures, the functions related with, as well as the existing spatial relationships. The spatial resolution allow the use of this tool as a cerebral atlas. The spatial normalization based on the Talairach space allow the correlation with other brain atlases or the use in brain studies.

Several digital atlases have been developed using photographic images of cryoplaned frozen specimens. Photographed material, while providing superior anatomic detail, has limitations. For accurate correlations, data must be placed in a plane equivalent to that of the image of interest. Acquisition of images in series directly from the consistently positioned cryoplaned blockface also avoids the need for serial image registration prior to reconstruction. Serial images can be reconstructed to a 3D anatomic volume that is amenable to various resampling and positioning schemes.

While not an atlas per se, the Visible Human imagery has sufficient quality and accessibility to make it a test platform for developing methods and standards [9]. The data has served as the foundation for developing related atlases of regions of the cerebral cortex, high-quality brain models and visualizations [8,12].

Bicommissural coordinates have become an international standard for reporting PET functional brain mapping. Virtually all PET brain-mapping laboratories now use bicommissural coordinates as their method for reporting locations of brain activation [5]. Using bicommissural coordinates brain locations in a tomographic image can be addressed without the ambiguities of conventional terminology. The precision, objectivity, and wide use of this coordinates system has greatly simplified the task of developing a database of human brain mapping.

Mapping the functional anatomy of the brain is not as straightforward as mapping the amino-acid sequence of a protein or base pair sequence of a gene. Placing a functional area "on the map" is only a first approximation. Defining the functional properties and functional interactions of an area is an ongoing process; converging experiments bring deeper understanding and more detailed models, but not final answers. Methodological details such as number of subjects used, imaging modality and resolution, response magnitude and level of statistical significance (preferably in terms of strength above background noise), and all pertinent behavioral measures must be included in the database. Enabling efficient meta-analysis is the strategy that influenced many aspects of the design and implementation of BrainMap [4].

The Brainmap database provide the ability to search, view, and analyze published, in press, and unpublished findings from the human brain-mapping literature. Its purpose is to promote the user's ability to understand and meta-analyze the functional anatomy of the human brain through rapid, exhaustive access to image-derived research on human functional neuroanatomy. In principle, functional brain imaging results should be amenable to systematic comparison across experiments and labs, provided the experiments being compared share similar base-line control conditions.

4   Conclusions

In spite of being based in just one brain this cerebral model could be a valuable tool for teaching, training, planning and for getting a better understanding of the cortical functions. At the present stage of the project the morpho-functional atlas has been used as a presurgical planning tool with excellent results.

References

1. Ackerman, M.I.: Viewpoint: The Visible Human Project. Journal Biocommunication, Vol. 18, No. 2, p. 14. (1991)
2. Bloom, F. E.: Databases of brain information. In Toga, A. W. (Ed.): *Three-Dimensional Neuroimaging*, Raven Press, New York, 1990, ch. 13, 273-306.
3. Bowden, Douglas M. & Martin, Richard F. NeuroNames Brain Hierarchy, *NeuroImage* 2:63-83, 1995.
4. Fox, P. T., Mikiten S., Davis, G., and Lancaster, J. L. *BrainMap: A database of human functional brainmapping. in Functional Neuroimaging: Technical Foundations* (eds. Thatcher, R. W., Hallett, M., Zeffiro, T., and John, E. R.), ch. 9, 95-105, (Academic Press Inc., Orlando, FL: 1994).

5. Friston K J, Passingham R E, Nutt J G, Heather J D, Sawle G V, Frackowiak R S
    J. (1989) Localization in PET images: direct fitting of the intercommissural (AC-
    PC) line. Journal of Cerebral Blood Flow and Metabolism 9:690-695.
6. Sachse, F., Werner, C., Mueller, M., Meyer-Waarden, K.: Preprocessing of the
    Visible Man Dataset for the Generation of Macroscopic Anatomical Models.
    Proc. First Users Conference of the National Library of Medicine's Visible Hu-
    man Project (1996)
7. Sachse, F., Werner, C., Mueller, M., Meyer-Waarden, K.: Segmentation and
    Tissue-Classification of the Visible Man Dataset Using the Computertomographic
    Scans and the Thin-Section Photos. Proc. First Users Conference of the National
    Library of Medicine's Visible Human Project. 1996
8. Tiede U., et al. A computerized three-dimensional atlas of the human skull and
    brain. in Am. J. Neuroradiology, 14, no. 3, 551-559, (1993).
9. Spitzer V, Ackerman MJ, Schersinger AL, Whitlock D, The Visible Human
    Male: a technical report. J AM Med Inform Assoc 1996; 3:118-130.
10. Talairach et al. (1967) Atlas d'anatomie stéréotaxique du télencéphale. Masson,
    Paris, 1967.
11. Talairach J and Tournoux P. Co-planar stereotaxic atlas of the human brain.
    Thieme Medical Publishers, Inc. New York, 1988.
12. Toh M, Falk RB, Main JS, Interactive Brain Atlas Using the Visible Human Proj-
    ect Data: Development Methods and Techniques, Radiographics, 1996; 16:1201-
    1206.

Predicting the Level of Metabolic Control Using Collaborative Filtering

Matthias Grabert[1], Reinhard W. Holl[2], Ulrike Krause[1],
Ingo Melzer[1], and Franz Schweiggert[1]

[1]Department of Applied Information Processing (SAI)
Helmholtzstr. 18, University of Ulm, D-89069 Ulm, Germany
{grabert,krause,melzer,swg}@mathematik.uni-ulm.de
http://www.mathematik.uni-ulm.de/sai
[2]Central Institute for Biomedical Engineering
Albert-Einstein-Allee 47, University of Ulm, D-89069 Ulm, Germany
reinhard.holl@zibmt.uni-ulm.de

Abstract. Collaborative Filtering is a well-approved method for prediction of consumer behaviour in marketing strategies. We adapt and evaluate this method for prognosis of the longterm metabolic control level in diabetic patients. The underlying data for the prediction were extracted from a central diabetic data pool (DPVSCIENT) [1],[2], containing longtime documentation of about 60% of all young patients with type-1 diabetes in Germany. Prediction results were successfully checked against random values and evaluated calculating sensitivity, specifity and total performance of a prognosis test. Best results were: sensitivity = 76%, specifity = 92% and total performance = 84%. This novel approach in diabetology demonstrates tracking for metabolic control and allows to predict favorable or unfavorable results, providing an objective basis to target intervention in individual patients.

Keywords: Diabetes, collaborative filtering, HbA_{1c} prediction, level of metabolic control

1 Introduction

1.1 Diabetes Mellitus

Diabetes mellitus is a chronic disease, more and more in focus of the public due to increasing incidence rates [3]. Successful longterm diabetes therapy in type-1 diabetes (insulin dependant diabetes) tries to keep the balance between a low level of metabolic control (HbA_{1c}-value) and as few hypoglycemic episodes as possible for the patient. A high HbA_{1c}-value correlates with a high probabilty of chronic complications such as impairment of eye and kidney or amputation of feet [4]. Therefore, the level of metabolic control is a key parameter of diabetes therapy. In this paper, we develop a prediction method for the average HbA_{1c}-value of the nth year after onset of diabetes using a data mining technology called "collaborative filtering" (or "social filtering" or "recommender systems") and test it for $n=6$.

J. Crespo, V. Maojo, and F. Martin (Eds.): ISMDA 2001, LNCS 2199, pp. 108–112, 2001.
© Springer-Verlag Berlin Heidelberg 2001

1.2   Collaborative Filtering

Collaborative filter techniques have been developed in the context of the World Wide Web since the early 1990s [5][6] and were also applied to one-to-one marketing. The main algorithm bases on the assumption that an unknown behaviour, preference, taste or characteristic of a person can be estimated using the similarity of this person to other persons. For example, a preference for or a rejection of a new product, can be predicted for a specific consumer, knowing his or her preference or rejection of other products [7]. The decision will be calculated taking into account recorded decisions of other clients for the very product, who have a similar purchase behaviour like the specific person.

Applied to diabetes, we try to predict the level of metabolic control in the 6th year of diabetes course for one patient. The estimation uses values of highly correlated patients, according to age, diabetes duration and former level of metabolic control.

2   Methods

The underlying data pool is DPVSCIENT [1], containing diabetes documentation of about 12,000 patients in Germany (at the end of the year 2000), mainly with type-1 diabetes. 652 patients with diabetes documentation of at least 6 successive years since onset could be found in the database. For each patient and each year, the average HbA_{1c}-value was calculated (total number of HbA1c-values: 5872; average number of HbA_{1c}-values per patient per year: 1.5). 88 patients were randomly selected into a prediction group (cf-group), and the remaining 564 patients formed the data-group. The following algorithm was then applied to predict the average HbA1c-value for the 6th year of diabetes course for a specific person P_0:

1. Select similar patients for P_0 from the data-group: year of birth should be at most 2 years earlier or later than P_0's year of birth; the same restriction applies for the onset of diabetes. This is assuring that P_0 and patients from the data-group have received a similar diabetes therapy.
2. Discard P_0 if not 10 or more *similar* patients were found in the data-group.
3. Calculate the Pearson correlation coefficient for P_0 and each *similar* patient P_k (according to step 1) from the data-group, using P_k's average HbA_{1c}-value $hb_{Pk,i}$ for each year $i=0,...,4$ of diabetes course and the overall average $\overline{hb_{Pk}}$ for all 5 years for patient P_k [8][9]:

$$w(P_0, P_k) = \frac{\sum_{i=0}^{4}(hb_{P0,i} - \overline{hb_{P0}})(hb_{Pk,i} - \overline{hb_{Pk}})}{\sqrt{\sum_{i=0}^{4}(hb_{P0,i} - \overline{hb_{P0}})^2 \sum_{i=0}^{4}(hb_{Pk,i} - \overline{hb_{Pk}})^2}}$$

4. Consider only patients Pk were w(P0, Pk) >a (a was modified during the test series).
5. Discard P0 if there remain less than 3 patients in the data-group after step 4.
6. Calculate a weight $K_{P0,a}$:

$$K_{P0,a} = \frac{1}{\sum\limits_{k:w(P0,Pk)>a} |w(P_0, P_k)|}$$

7. Then calculate the prediction for the 6th year after onset of diabetes ($i=5$) for patient P_0:

$$hb_{P0,5} = \overline{hb_{P0}} + K_{P0,a} \cdot \sum\limits_{k:w(P0,Pk)>a} w(P_0, P_k)(hb_{Pk,5} - \overline{hb}_{Pk})$$

3   Assessment of the Results

3.1   Definition of a Validation Test

We assume the prediction is *true*,

*   if $hb_{P0,5}$ differs only 0.5 or less from the true value $hbtrue_{P0,5}$ for patient P_0 in the 6th year of diabetes course
*   *or* the tendancy of the prognosis is right
    (i.e. ($hb_{P0,5} - hb_{P0,4}$) >0   and   ($hbtrue_{P0,5} - hb_{P0,4}$)>0)

Else, the prediction is *false*.

The HbA$_{1c}$ development for the patient is defined *positive,* if he or she has a lower average HbA$_{1c}$ value in the 6th year than in the 5th year. Else, it is defined *negative*.

Accordingly, the *test result* is *true positive (TP)*, if the HbA$_{1c}$ development is positive and the prediction is true. The test result is *true negative (TN)* , if the development is negative and the prediction is true.

3.2   Standard Evaluation

Mean and standard deviation for the best result (choice of a) were calculated and results were compared to randomly generated HbA$_{1c}$ values [10].

4   Results

4.1   Results for the Test

Table 1 gives the numbers for the test series. The value for a was increased from 0.1 to 0.9 during the series. Not all patients from the cf-group could be evaluated (see: *Methods*, step 2 and 5).

Table 1 Test series for CF prediction, ranked by total performance; TP% and TN% = percentage of true positive/negative tests; **Tperf % = Total Performance = (TP%+TN%)/2**

TP%	TN%	TPerf%	a	evaluated patients
75.5	91.7	83.6	0.7	73
75.0	88.9	81.9	0.9	25
82.5	71.4	77.0	0.8	61
85.5	67.9	76.7	0.5	83
83.9	62.1	73.0	0.2	85
87.3	58.6	72.9	0.4	84
85.5	58.6	72.0	0.3	84
80.7	62.1	71.4	0.1	86

4.2   Standard Evaluation of the Results

For the best cf-test series $(a=0.7)$, the mean absolute deviation of $hb_{P0,5}$ from $hbtrue_{P0,5}$ was *mean = 0.82* with *standard deviation = 0.78*. Range was [0.02; 5.20].

Random generated HbA_{1c}-values for 73 patients were computed, then the numbers where fed into the cf-algorithm $(a=0.7)$: *mean = 2.28, standard deviation = 1.38* and *range = [0.06; 6.45]*. This was significantly worse than in original HbA_{1c}-values.

A random prediction for the HbA_{1c}-value in the 6th year (random value was chosen from [4.5; 13.5]) was performed 100 times for 73 patients: *total mean=2,71, total standard deviation= 1.81* (best random series: *mean=2.04, standard deviation = 1.34)*

All random tests performed much worse than the cf-algorithm.

5   Conclusion

With the help of collaborative filtering, the level or the tendancy of metabolic control can be predicted in about 80% of the cases. Higher values for the correlation coefficient deliver better prediction results, as expected. Tight preconditions for the Pearson correlation coefficient restrict the numbers of evaluated patients too much (e.g., $a = 0.9$). Best results were achieved with $a=0.7$. From a clinical standpoint, this method, which has not been previously applied in diabetology, allows to predict favorable or unfavorable courses with respect to metabolic control in diabetes. If these findings are confirmed in independent groups of patients, this prediction may provide a basis to objectively decide on intensification of therapy (changes in insulin regimen, patient re-education etc). This would allow to target limited ressources available more efficiently, presumably improving the long-term outcome.

References

1. Grabert M., Schweiggert F., Holl R. W. and the German Pediatric Quality Control Group on Diabetes, 10 Years Successful Implementation Of a Diabetes Documentation System, Supporting External Benchmarking and Nation-wide Scientific Investigations. Diabetes, Nutrition & Metabolism Vol 13. N.4 (2000):pp.225

2. Hecker W, Grabert M, Holl RW, *Quality of paediatric IDDM care in Germany: A multicentre analysis.* German Paediatric Diabetology Group. J Pediatr Endocrinol Metab. 1999 Jan-Feb;12 (1):31-8

3. EURODIAB ACE study group, *Variation and trends in incidence of childhood diabetes in Europe.* Lancet 2000 11. März (9207), pp. 873- 876

4. Diabetes Control and Complications Trial Research Group, The effect of intensive treatment of diabetes on the development and progression of long-term complications of insulin-dependet diabetes mellitus. N. Engl. J. Med. 329: 977-986, 1993

5. Resnick P., Neophytos I., Mitesh S., Bergstrom P., Riedl J., GroupLens, *An Open Architecture for Collaborative Filtering of Netnews.* Proc. of CSCW '94: Conference on Computer Supported Cooperative Work (Chapel Hill, 1994), pp175-186, Addison-Wesley

6. Runte M., *Personalisierung im Internet – Individualisierte Angebote mit Collaborative Filtering,* Ph.D. thesis 2000, Christian-Albrechts-University of Kiel, Faculty of Economics and Social Sciences

7. Schafer, J.B., Konstan, J.A., and Riedl, J. (1999), *Recommender Systems in E-Commerce.* In ACM Conference on Electronic Commerce (EC-99), pages 158-166

8. Breese, J., Heckerman, D. and Kadie, C. (1998), *Empirical Analysis of Predictive Algorithms for Collaborative Filtering.* Proceedings of the Fourteenth Annual Conference on Uncertainty in Artificial Intelligence (UAI-98). San Francisco, CA: Morgan Kaufmann, 43-52.

9. Herlocker J.L., Konstan J.A., Borchers A., Riedl J. (1999), *An Algorithmic Framework for Performing Collaborative Filtering,* Proceedings of the 1999 Conference on Research and Development in Information Retrieval, August 1999

10. Balabanovic M., Shoham Y., Fab: *Content-Based, Collaborative Recommendation,* Communication of the ACM Vol.40 No. 3.(1997): pp. 66-72

Web-Enabled Knowledge-Based
Analysis of Genetic Data

Peter Juvan[1], Blaž Zupan[1,3], Janez Demšar[1], Ivan Bratko[1,2],
John A. Halter[4], Adam Kuspa[5,6], and Gad Shaulsky[6]

[1] Faculty of Computer and Information Science, University of Ljubljana, Sloveni
[2] Jožef Stefan Institute, Ljubljana, Slovenia
[3] Office of Information Technology and Department of Family and Community
Medicine
[4] Division of Neuroscience
[5] Department of Biochemistry and Molecular Biology
[6] Department of Molecular and Human Genetics
Baylor College of Medicine, Houston, TX, USA

Abstract. We present a web-based implementation of GenePath, an intelligent assistant tool for data analysis in functional genomics. GenePath considers mutant data and uses expert-defined patterns to find gene-to-gene or gene-to-outcome relations. It presents the results of analysis as genetic networks, wherein a set of genes has various influence on one another and on a biological outcome. In the paper, we particularly focus on its web-based interface and explanation mechanisms.

1   Introduction

Genetic research is one of the most effective approaches to the elucidation of biological processes. State-of-the-art technology has enabled the genomic sequencing of several simple organisms as well as complex organisms including human. While obtaining a genome sequence is an important milestone, it marks only the beginning of the effort needed to understand and use this knowledge. The hardest step awaits us in the field of functional genomics [6], which is concerned with the "development and application of global (genome-wide or system-wide) experimental approaches to assess gene function" [3].

Analysis of mutant data, a core task in functional genomics, has so far been performed manually. With advancing technology that enables higher rates of experimentation and data gathering, new computer-based approaches are required to support data analysis in functional genomics. We have developed a program called GenePath that provides intelligent assistance for analysis of genetic data. In discovery of gene functions, GenePath mimics expert geneticist by using the reasoning patterns geneticists would else employ manually. GenePath capitalizes on computer's processing power to systematically examine the data, thus automatizing potentially tiresome and error-prone process.

J. Crespo, V. Maojo, and F. Martin (Eds.): ISMDA 2001, LNCS 2199, pp. 113-119, 2001.

GenePath is implemented in Prolog [1] and for its reasoning uses elements of selected approaches from artificial intelligence. While its environment in Prolog was sufficient for prototyping and preliminary testing, participating geneticists strongly indicated that a more standard interface is needed. This pushed us towards the development of web-based interface (http://magix.fri.uni-lj.si/genepath), where Prolog-based core is seamlessly integrated within server-based application.

Basic elements of GenePath's core have been described in [8]. We here present the basics of its reasoning process, and then focus on its web-based implementation and methods that aim to explain its findings.

2   GenePath's Reasoning System

An input to GenePath is a set of genetic experiments, where each describes which genes were mutated and how and gives a qualitatively observed outcome of experiment. For example, consider a set of experiments on *Dictyostelium discoideum*, a soil ameba that is the subject of study in the laboratories of the authors from Baylor College of Medicine. *Dictyostelium* is particularly interesting for its social behavior and development cycle from single independent cells to a multicellular slug like form [7, 5, 4]. A sub process of *Dictyostelium*'s development is cell aggregation, which has been observed in experiments from Table 1.

Table 1. Genetic experiments: aggregation of *Dictyostelium*

Exp ID	Genotype	Aggregation
1	wild-type	+
2	yakA:: -	-
3	pufA:: -	++
4	yakA:: -, pufA:: -	++

Notice that in the first experiment from Table 1 no mutations were made and under normal conditions *Dictyostelium* aggregates. Under the same conditions, but with loss-of-function mutation of gene yakA (experiment 2), the aggregation does not take place. Additionally mutating pufA, aggregation is restored and actually takes place faster compared to wild-type *Dictyostelium* (experiment 4).

When geneticists analyze such data, they most often use a set of informal, unwritten but intuitive rules to derive relations between genes and outcome. For instance, an example of a simple rule is "*IF mutation of gene A changes the outcome P (compared to the wild type) THEN gene A is influencing the outcome P*". Using this rule, it can be concluded from Table 1 that both genes yakA and pufA influence the aggregation. An example of a more complex rule is "*IF mutation of gene A changes the outcome P (compared to the wild type) and adding the mutation of gene B reverses the outcome P THEN gene B acts after gene A in a path for the outcome P*". Using this rule and experiments 2 and 4 from Table 1, it can be concluded that pufA acts after yakA in the path for aggregation.

GenePath currently includes about 10 such rules, which are also referred to as patterns. It uses them to abduce the following gene-to-gene or gene-to-outcome relations:

o *parallel*: both `GeneA` and `GeneB` influence `Phenotype`, but are on separate (parallel) paths;

o *epistatic*: `GeneB` is epistatic to `GeneA` in a path for `Phenotype` with a given `Influence` (both genes are therefore on the same path and `GeneB` acts after `GeneA`);

o *influences*: `GeneA` either excites or inhibits (`Influence`) the `Phenotype`;

o *not influences*: `GeneA` does not influence the `Phenotype`.

As a final result of data analysis, GenePath derives genetic networks by satisfying abduced network constraints [8]. The network consists of nodes (genes and an outcome), and arcs that correspond to direct influences of genes on other genes and outcome. GenePath can derive models that include two types of influence: *excitation* (→) and *inhibition* (—|). As additional input, GenePath can also consider known parts of the network – a prior knowledge specified by the geneticist.

3   A Web-Based Interface to GenePath

To make GenePath available to a wider audience, and in particular to experts and students in functional genomics, we have developed an interactive graphical user interface. The primary requirement was to design the interface that could be used on a wide variety of platforms. To avoid maintenance of different platform-specific versions, we have developed a web interface incorporating a server-based application that exports its user interface through a web browser. The resulting benefits are platform independence and low processing requirements on the client's side. No specific client-side installation procedure is required. A potential drawback is slower response time, especially at periods of intensive usage from several users, and at some points awkward user interface (compared to potential capabilities of stand-alone application), which is limited by HTML capabilities.

Our server-based application uses Active Server Pages (ASP) technology and Microsoft's IIS 5.0 web service. GenePath's abductive inference engine is implemented in SICStus Prolog (http://www.sics.se), and the communication between the engine and the interface is realized through SICStus's Visual Basic interface. Clickable images of genetic networks are generated using graph visualization software GraphViz (http://www.graphviz.org).

The user interface is quite intuitive and does not require special explanation. It follows a linear structure from the selection of a project, through definition of genetic data and background knowledge, all the way to the presentation of derived genetic networks and provision of explanation as to how the specific relations where found.

3.1 Data Entry

Data entry consists of specification of genes, outcomes, genetic experiments and background knowledge. The interface is straightforward, and supports savings and uploads to and from the client's system. Fig. 1 shows an entry screen for mutant data of *Dictyostelium*, where aggregation is observed as the outcome.

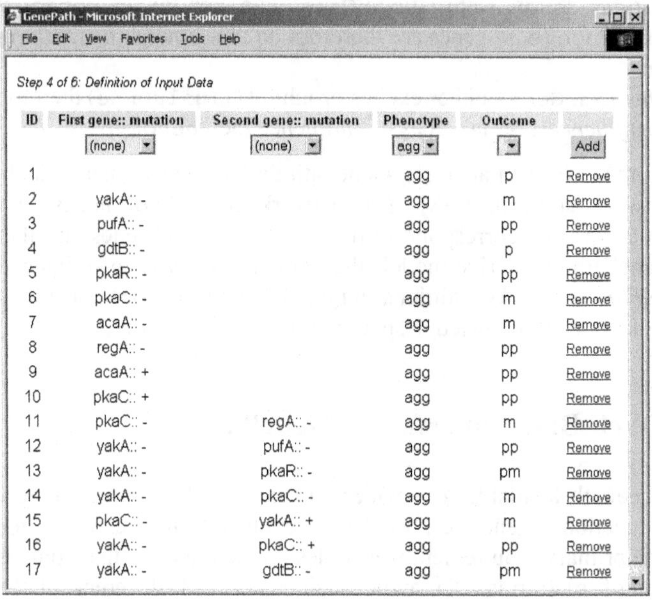
GenePath - Microsoft Internet Explorer

File Edit View Favorites Tools Help

Step 4 of 6: Definition of Input Data

ID	First gene:: mutation	Second gene:: mutation	Phenotype	Outcome	
	(none)	(none)	agg		Add
1			agg	p	Remove
2	yakA:: -		agg	m	Remove
3	pufA:: -		agg	pp	Remove
4	gdtB:: -		agg	p	Remove
5	pkaR:: -		agg	pp	Remove
6	pkaC:: -		agg	m	Remove
7	acaA:: -		agg	m	Remove
8	regA:: -		agg	pp	Remove
9	acaA:: +		agg	pp	Remove
10	pkaC:: +		agg	pp	Remove
11	pkaC:: -	regA:: -	agg	m	Remove
12	yakA:: -	pufA:: -	agg	pp	Remove
13	yakA:: -	pkaR:: -	agg	pm	Remove
14	yakA:: -	pkaC:: -	agg	m	Remove
15	pkaC:: -	yakA:: +	agg	m	Remove
16	yakA:: -	pkaC:: +	agg	pp	Remove
17	yakA:: -	gdtB:: -	agg	pm	Remove

Fig. 1. A screen for definition and revision of genetic data

3.2 Presentation of Genetic Network and Constraints

For the data from Fig.1 GenePath finds a number of network constraints and three direct relations: yakA → pkaC, regA —| pkaC, and yakA —| pufA. Together with background knowledge (not shown here), the resulting genetic network is shown in Fig.2. The user can request the display of any type of constraints found by GenePath (*precedes* relations are displayed in the shown screenshot), or can click on any gene or edge of the network to display relevant experiments and constraints.

3.3 Explanation

The essential capability of GenePath's interface is the ability to provide explanation on abduced constraints. By clicking on the related evidence field of a specific constraint, the explanation is shown in a separate window. This includes the description of the pattern that was used to derive the constraint, and the experiments (or relations from background knowledge) that were involved.

For instance, Fig. 3 shows an explanation of the last constraint from Fig. 2: pufA is epistatic to yakA in a path for aggregation with a negative influence (inhibition). GenePath tells us that pufA was found to act after yakA in a path for aggregation because mutating these two genes separately leads to different outcomes, but mutating both genes at the same time leads to the same outcome as mutating only pufA. Therefore, it concludes that pufA blocks the influence of yakA; this is possible only if pufA is in the same path but after yakA.

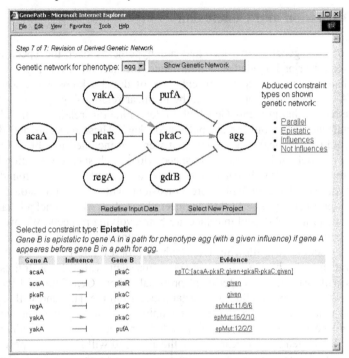

Fig. 2. Derived genetic network for cell aggregation and abduced constraints of type *precedes*

ID	First gene mutation	Second gene mutation	Phenotype	Outcome
2	yakA:: -		agg	m
3	pufA:: -		agg	pp
12	yakA:: -	pufA:: -	agg	pp

Constraint type EPISTATIC, pattern **epMut**

epMut: assuming a linear pathway, IF two different mutations (A and B) result in two different phenotypes AND the phenotype of the double gene mutation is the same as one of the single gene mutations (B), THEN that single gene mutation (B) is epistatic AND gene B is considered to act after gene A.

pufA acts after *yakA* because the outcomes of the single gene mutations in experiments 3 and 2, respectively, are different from each other and the outcome of the double gene mutation in experiment 12 is the same as for the single gene mutation in *pufA* (experiment 3).

Close Window

Fig. 3. Constraint explanation of the last constraint in Fig. 2: yakA —| pufA

Notice that GenePath's provision of explanations is possible because of its knowledge-based approach. The patterns that it uses for abduction of network constraints also define the language in which explanations are communicated. Since it was the domain experts that defined the patterns, GenePath's reasoning and explanation is bound to be transparent and comprehensible by biologists.

4   Discussion and Conclusion

GenePath derives genetic networks that are hypotheses over the specified set of experiments and prior knowledge. For instance, the network from Fig. 2 is slightly different than expected from the current state of domain knowledge, where genes yakA, pufA and pkaC are considered to be in linear relationship (yakA —| pufA —| pkaC). The reason that prevents GenePath to determine this relation is the absence of experimental data that would relate pufA and pkaC. These experimental data were obtained from biochemical experiments that were not included in table 1 [4, 5]. The advantage of GenePath is the ease and speed with which such observation is found. Furthermore, for the data shown in this paper, the expert biologists found that the constraints derived by GenePath were consistent with their knowledge, and that additional experiments can be further engineered based on what GenePath has found.

GenePath and its web-based interface are both evolving projects. We are currently extending their functionality by considering a combination of abductive inference and qualitative reasoning [8], allowing GenePath to propose and rank a set of potential networks rather than show a single network consistent with the constraints. Further extensions will also include experiment proposal, where GenePath will indicate for which genes the relations could not be established from the data, and will suggest the experiments that would resolve the resulting ambiguities in the genetic network.

The approach we are developing is intended for functional genomics community, particularly for students and researchers in the area, and will for that purpose be freely available on the Internet. Interested reader is welcome to check and use GenePath at `http://magix.fri.uni-lj.si/genepath`. The web site also provides for a number of test cases, including the one under the name "Project 3a: Dictyostelium Development (Aggregation Only)" described in this paper.

References

1. Bratko, I.: *Prolog Programming for Artificial Intelligence*. 3rd edition. Addison-Wesley (2001)
2. Flach, P.: Simply Logical: Intelligent Reasoning by Example. John Wiley & Sons (1994)
3. Hieter, P., Boguski, M.: Related Articles Functional genomics: it's all how you read it. *Science* (1997) 278(5338):601-2
4. Souza, G. M., da Silva, A. M., Kuspa, A.: Starvation promotes dictyostelium development by relieving PufA inhibition of PKA translation through the YakA kinase pathway. *Development* (1999) 126(14):3263-3274
5. Souza, G. M., Lu, S., Kuspa, A.: YakA, a protein kinase, required for the transition from growth to development in Dictyostelium. *Development* (1998) 125(12):2291-2302

6. Zhang, M. Q.: Large-scale gene expression data analysis: a new challenge to computational biologists. *Genome Res* (1999) 9:681-688
7. Zimmer, C.: The slime alternative. *Discover* (May 1998) 86-93
8. Zupan, B., Bratko, I., Demšar, J., Beck, J. R., Kuspa, A., Shaulsky, G.: Abductive Inference of Genetic Networks. *Proc. Artificial Intelligence in Medicine Europe*. Cascais, Portugal (2001)

Fuzzy Sets Applied to Image Processing and Quantification of Interstitial Fibrosis and Glomerular Size in Computer Assisted Microscopy

Elzbieta Kaczmarek [1], Aldona Wozniak [2], and Wieslawa Salwa-Zurawska[2]

[1] Chair and Department of Informatics and Statistics,
Karol Marcinkowski University of Medical Sciences,
60-529 Poznan, Dabrowskiego 79

[2] Chair and Department of Patomorphology,
Karol Marcinkowski University of Medical Sciences,
60-355 Poznan, Przybyszewskiego 49
elka@usoms.poznan.pl

Abstract. The aim of the paper is to present the application of fuzzy sets to image processing and analysis of renal biopsies in light and confocal microscopy. Fuzzy segmentation was applied to processing of grey scale images. Colour images were processed by fuzzy-like approach. Segmented glomerular profiles and interstitial fibrosis were then quantitatively assessed. The mean glomerular volume and the degree of fibrosis were estimated in light microscopy. The volume of glomerular mesangium was assessed with a confocal microscope. Concluding, fuzzy processing makes morphometric studies of renal biopsies more practical for clinical diagnosis of diseases.

1   Introduction

Interstitial fibrosis and morphological changes in renal glomeruli are the structural effects of many diseases. In normal cases, in light microscopy, we can observe a network of thin blue fibres around renal glomeruli and interstitium distributed in red interstitial tissue. In process of pathological changes related with the formation of excessive fibrous tissue, some areas of the interstitial tissue become blue. A reliable and objective method to quantify the extent of interstitial fibrosis and, at least, the mean size of renal glomeruli is needed for both clinical practice and experimental studies. Previous works focussed on 3D visualisation and quantification of renal capillaries [2], [3], [4]. This paper presents the design of image processing application for quantifying interstitial fibrosis and glomerular size in the same tissue section. The fuzzy logic algorithms were used for segmentation of renal glomeruli from epifluorescent images observed in confocal laser scanning microscopy.

J. Crespo, V. Maojo, and F. Martin (Eds.): ISMDA 2001, LNCS 2199, pp. 120–125, 2001.
© Springer-Verlag Berlin Heidelberg 2001

2   Material Preparation

Kidney biopsies were subjects of quantitative light microscopy studies. Material for light microscopy was routinely PAS stained and then Masson's trichrome staining was performed. Material for confocal microscopy was first perfusion fixed in neutral buffered formalin overnight then washed several times in phosphatate buffered salline and sectioned on a vibratome into 200 microm sections. Each section was inserted into a biopsy cassete, and then stained with eosin. Then, the sections were transferred to glass slides and mounted in immersion oil with refractive index of 1.596 [3].

3   Image Acquisition

Kidney images were registered with a computer-assisted light microscope. Each colour image of 760x570 pixels (24 bits per pixel) was recorded and stored by using image analysis system MicroImage v.4.0 (Olympus).

A sequence of optical sections thorough the entire glomerular volume was acquired with a confocal laser scanning microscope with an oil-immersion objective (40x, NA1.3). Illumination was 488nm from an argon laser. Each epifluorescent image of 256x256 pixels and 256 grey levels was obtained by averaging eight image inputs recorded in one second each [2], [3], [4].

4   Fuzzy Logic for Image Processing of Kidney

In this study, fuzzy sets built for input image pixels represent intervals that are the intensity features. The membership function specifies the membership grade, which the colour of a pixel belongs to. The membership grade is defined as a value in the range [0, 1] where '0' denotes no membership and '1' denotes a full membership.

In the input image, each entry may be corrupted by a noise. A fuzzy mean process for filtering is generated by the weighted average procedure. Pixels of the noise-corrupted image located in the sample matrices are summed to get the weighted average. The fuzzy mean process results in a value for the pixel being filtered. Then, a final decision process selects the value closest to the fuzzy estimator. This is the filtered pixel value.

4.1   Fuzzy Sets for Processing of Grey Scale Kidney Images

Let X be the original grey scale input image with L grey levels. A fuzzy set built for the image pixels represented an interval of the grey scale, for instance *'dark', 'median', 'bright.'*

Let now F denotes a filtering function on the input image X. The weight associated with each pixel were decided by referring to the membership function of associated intensity feature, for instance *'dark', $DK=[DK_{begin}, DK_{end}]$.* If all pixels in the sample matrix had a zero membership grade according to their grey levels, then $F(x)$ was set to zero, x was the pixel value.

Analogously, we generated a fuzzy mean process for bright by referring to the membership function of associated intensity feature *'bright''*, $BR=[BR_{begin}, BR_{end}]$,

and a fuzzy mean process for median associated with the intensity feature *'median'*, $MD=[MD_{begin}, MD_{end}]$. Then, each pixel value x was processed in the following way:

```
procedure Fuzzy (DK, MD, BR, x, F(x))
  {DK=[DK_begin, DK_end], MD=[MD_begin, MD_end], BR=[BR_begin, BR_end]};
  for x ≤ BR_begin and x ≥ DK_end do I(x):=1 else I(x):=0; {The
  decision process of the filtering procedure};
  begin
      If abs(F(x_DK)-I(x)) < abs(F(X_MD)-I(x))
  then F(x):= F(x_DK);
      If abs(F(x_BR)-I(x))< abs(F(x)-I(x))
  then F(x):= F(x_BR);
  end.
```

Thus, the filter is basically a mean filter operating with coefficients $F(x)$.

Brightness normalisation was performed on the basis of histogram extremes of an image that was chosen as a reference image. Then, analysed structures were segmented on the basis of the defined three classes of pixels:

'background' – grey levels corresponding with the general scene against which the structures were viewed,
'interior' – grey levels as inside the analysed structures,
'outer neighbourhood' - grey levels as in the nearest neighbourhood surrounding analysed structures.

On the basis of the defined classes of pixels, membership functions related with the reference histogram were then determined. Minimal frequencies of a reference histogram reflected crossing points of membership functions, whereas maximal frequencies of the histogram were equal 1 and corresponded to the membership function. The degree of pixel membership was defined by IF-THEN fuzzy rules. For instance:

IF   pixel x_1 belongs to *'background'*   AND   pixel x_2 belongs to *'outer neighbourhood'* THEN set pixel x_2 as *'black'*;
IF pixel x_1 belongs to *'outer neighbourhood'* AND pixel x_2 belongs to *'interior'* THEN set the pixel x_2 as *'white'*.

The use of the method for processing of epifluorescent images of renal glomeruli acquired with a confocal microscope allowed to segment renal capillaries and mesangium (Fig. 1).

4.2   Fuzzy Sets for Segmentation of Interstitial Fibrosis

Colour images of interstitial tissue were first smoothed before detection the fibrosis areas. The averaging approach within a 3x3 sample matrix of pixels was used to remove noisy pixels. The average colour of the central pixel within the sample matrix was determined taking into account the colours of its eight neighbouring pixels in RGB colour space as follows:

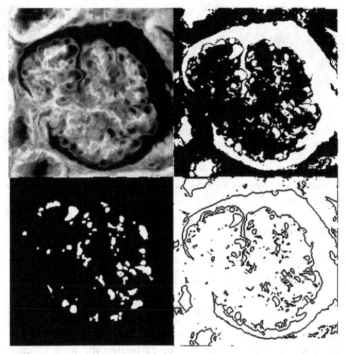

Fig. 1. A confocal image of a renal glomerulus (top left), binary version of the pre-processed image (top right), segmented capillary profiles (bottom left), edges of the segmented glomerulus and capillaries (bottom right)

[45; 75] for red, [105; 155] for green and [140; 180] for blue coordinates. The remaining colours represented the normal part of the tissue (in red tones). The colour of each pixel's was compared with colours of eight, 3x3 matrices of neighbouring pixels (namely, two 3x3 neighbourhoods in four directions). For each of the neighbourhoods, the average colour in RGB colour space was first found.

Then, colour contrast between two pixels was defined as the square of the Euclidean distance between the colour vectors $v_1=(R_1, G_1, B_1)$ and $v_2=(R_2, G_2, B_2)$ as shown in Eq. (1).

$$\text{Contrast } (v_1, v_2) = (R_2 - R_1)^2 + (G_2 - G_1)^2 + (B_2 - B_1)^2. \qquad (1)$$

The contrast between the two colour vectors: [45, 105, 140] and [75, 155, 180] resulted 5000 (Eq. 1), and defined the threshold for blue tones, t_{blue}.

Colour contrast between a pixel and the average colour of each of its eight neighbourhoods were then calculated and compared with the threshold t_{blue}.

If a contrast (Eq.1) at one direction exceeded the threshold t_{blue} then the pixel was decided to belong to the red tone area else to blue tone spots. In this way edges between red and blue areas were detected (Fig. 2).

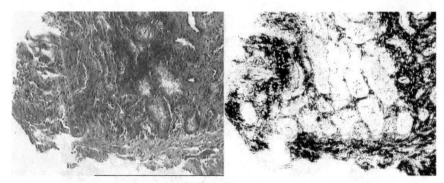

Fig. 2. A light microscopy image of the interstitial tissue (left), binary version of the segmented fibrosis (in black) (right)

5   Implementation

The segmented glomerular profiles $glom_i$ allowed the estimation of the mean glomerular volume $\bar{v}$ in random section analysis [2], [7], as shown in Eg. 2

$$\bar{v} = \sum Area\ (glom_i) / n. \tag{2}$$

where n is the number of detected glomerular profiles.

Analysing series of confocal images, we calculated the total volume V of each glomerulus [2], [7], as a single particle volume (Eq. 3.)

$$V = z \sum Area\ (\ glom_i\ ) \tag{3}$$

where z is the step of optical sections acquired with a confocal microscope and $glom_i$ is the glomerular profile on section i $(i=1, ... , k;\ k$ is the number of confocal images representing consecutive profiles of the entire glomerulus).

Analogously, we assessed the volume of mesangium in confocal images. The degree of fibrosis was assessed as shown in Eq. 4.

$$\%fibrosis = 100 \bullet \sum Area\ (\ blue\ )\ /Area\ (\ red\ ) \tag{4}$$

where *blue* denotes the part of the tissue in blue tones while *red* in red tones.

Techniques presented in this paper were implemented for preliminary comparative light microscopy studies of 15 cases with minimal change disease 'mcd' and 15 cases with focal segmental glomerulosclerosis 'fsgs' in children. The mean glomerular volume in 'mcd' was $13.1 \pm 4.4 \times 10^5$ microm^3 while $14.9 \pm 7.9 \times 10^5$ microm^3 in "fsgs". The degree of fibrosis was $20.6\% \pm 6.2\%$ in 'mcd' while $48.7\% \pm 10.7\%$ in 'fsgs'. A network of blue fibres around glomeruli and interstitum in 'mcd' cases constituted, on average, 20.6% of the tissue. In 'fsgs' cases the results were 2.3 times higher than in 'mcd' cases and showed how much the fibrosis expanded in interstitial tissue in process of the disease.

Studies of normal rat renal glomeruli developed in confocal microscopy indicated that the glomerular volume ranged from 16.3 to 27.8×10^5 microm^3 and confirmed previous results [2], while the volume of mesangium was on average 14.3×10^5 microm^3.

6   Final Comments

Fuzzy sets have recently attracted much attention in medical imaging and were also used for segmentation of kidney boundaries in MR images [1]. Major problems in processing of kidney images studied in microscopy were related with the use of several rank and/or median filters [3]. Since weighted fuzzy mean filters show lower computational complexity, than the standard median filter [5], therefore, the weighted average approach and fuzzy logic were implemented in this study.

Studies on membranous glomerulonephritis [6] showed that the percentage of fibrosis varied from 10.3% in stage I of the disease to 34.2% in stage V. In our study, the area of detected blue rings around glomeruli was included in the determined %fibrosis and increased the results. However, comparing the results of "mcd" cases with 'fsgs' cases, we can assess the progress of pathological changes with the same systematic error of measurements. Our further work will be focussed on the elimination of the 'glomerular ring' bias.

References

1.   Jendrysik F., Eichweld H., Graumann R.: Fuzzy Segmentation Method Applied to the Extraction of Kidney Boundaries in Medical Images. Proc. EUFIT'97, Aachen, Spetember 8-11, 1997: 2360-2364
2.   Kaczmarek E: Quantification of three-dimensional vascular patterns in renal glomeruli. Acta Stereol. 1998 Vol. 15/2: 147-152
3.   Kaczmarek E., Becker R. L.: Three-Dimensional Modeling of Renal Glomerular Capillary Networks. Analytical and Quantitative Cytology and Histology. Vol. 19, (1997): 93-101
4.   Kaczmarek E: Visualization and modelling of renal capillaries from confocal images. Med. Biol. Eng. Comput. 1999 Vol. 37: 273-277
5.   Lee C.-Y., Kuo Y.-H., Yu P.-T.: Weighted fuzzy mean filter for image processing. Fuzzy Sets and Systems. 1997 Vol. 89: 157-180
6.   Paparaskevakou H. Et al.: Membranous glomerulonephritis: A morphometric study. Pathology, Research & Practice. 2000 Vol. 196(3): 141-144
7.   Russ J.C., Computer Assisted Microscopy. The Measurement and Analysis of Images. Plenum, New York, third edition, 1992

Cancer Epidemiology of Small Communities: Using a Novel Approach to Detecting Clusters

E. Kordysh[1], A. Bolotin[1], M. Barchana[2], and R. Chen[3]

[1]Ben-Gurion University of the Negev, P.O.B. 653, Beersheba 84 105, Israel
{kordish,arkadyv}@bgumail.bgu.ac.il
[2]Israel Cancer Registry, Jerusalem, Israel
micha.barchana@moh.health.gov.il
[3]Impulse Dynamics, Haifa, Israel
rinach@internet-zahav.net.il

Abstract. Cancer cluster detection in small communities is an important but complicated field of cancer epidemiology, due to large statistical errors of both types associated with the detection. In this paper, authors show the use of a new approach to this problem. This approach is based on three complementary techniques. One is aimed at detection of the cluster, and two others are applied after cluster detection in order to confirm or reject the cluster. Included is application of the approach in small agricultural-industrial communities of the South of Israel. The approach reduces both types of statistical errors, increases the chance to detect a true clustering and enables a first step in the identification of the cause of a cluster detected.

Keywords: Cluster analysis for medical applications, Temporal pattern analysis, Cancer epidemiology, Small agricultural-industrial communities.

1 Introduction

For the last years, detection of cancer clusters in local communities has been grown up to a stand-alone problem, which professional meetings and special journal issues are devoted to [see, for example, Ref. 4 and 12]. A fact that numerous epidemiological investigations report relatively high rates of site-specific cancer among agricultural workers speaks in favor of the significance of this problem [1, 3, 9, 10, 12, 13, 15, and 16]. Moreover, a pretty high incidence rate of lympho-proliferative cancers among residents of a rural farming community reported also increase the problem actuality [14].

As a matter of fact, all Israel agricultural-industrial communities (AIC) have apparent chemical exposures, thus providing a good base for epidemiological studies. Previous studies of the use of pesticide in AIC show that both occupational and environmental exposures can occur when residential neighborhoods are in close proximity to sprayed areas. Furthermore, Blair et al. [2], consider research results of agricultural factors as

J. Crespo, V. Maojo, and F. Martin (Eds.): ISMDA 2001, LNCS 2199, pp. 126–132, 2001.

a clue to understanding the etiology of cancer in the general population (which may be exposed to agricultural chemicals distributed in the forms of food, water and air pollutants).

Our study was planned and carried out in view of these findings, and in response to the belief expressed by the communities' members that cancer rates were in general high in some of the AIC in South Israel.

Due to the fact that both types of statistical errors are bound to inflate, it is important to consider the possibility that a detected cluster is false, i.e., related to a rare occurrence rather than to an exposure. Chen R. et al. proposed to apply several complementary techniques in order to detect and to interpret clusters in small communities [4-8]. These techniques made the method we used in our study.

2   Materials

The residents of 45 AIC were included in the study. These communities were established in the period from 1937 to 1957. The distribution of population by age (divided by 5-years intervals: 0-4, 5-9, etc.) and gender for each year over 1972-1996 period was acquired from two organizational bodies of AIC.

Cancer incidence data in AIC over 1972-1996 years were obtained from Israel Cancer Registry and AIC clinics. Observed cancer cases in AIC were stratified by age, gender and by site (by ICD9). As baseline rates we used the gender-age and site-specific incidence rates of the Jewish population in Israel in each of the 25 years of observation.

3   Methods

The analysis comprises the following techniques: (1) cluster detection, (2) cluster confirmation (3) possible interpretations of the cluster. The detection and confirmation are based on tests of significance; each of them is applied to a distinct part of the data. The first test, CUSCORE-test, is a procedure of sequential type [7]. If the test gives a significant result, we consider it as a cluster and apply the special confirmatory test to the first 5 cases following the detected cluster. The cluster interpretation is based on the temporal pattern of the cases [5, 6].

3.1 The q-Interval

The q-interval is the probability for no case within the time interval observed between consecutive cases in the data set [5]. For example, if the 9-th case occurred on November 15 1969, and the 10-th case occurred on January 15 1971, q_{10} is the null probability for no case within the 14-month period (between Nov. 15, 1969 and Jan. 15, 1971). This probability is evaluated under the assumption that the distribution of the time interval between consecutive cases is exponential [5]. Namely,

$$q_i = \exp(-RI_i) \quad , \tag{1}$$

where RI_i is the expected number of cases in the relevant period.

Although q_i is evaluated as a probability, it is actually a random variable, since its value is determined by a random time interval. Its distribution is uniform over 0-1 and its expected value is 0.5 [5].

When the cases are more frequent than that expected (as it happens within a cluster), the q-values are likely to be larger than 0.5. Accordingly, a sequence of large q-intervals (larger than 0.5) indicates clustering.

The efficiency of the CUSCORE-test for the q-interval is not adequate when the dataset is large. Therefore, a modified q-interval is used for data sets that are larger than 23.

The modified q-interval (which we will call $q(3)$-interval) is defined as a probability to observe less than 3 cases over the time interval in which 3 cases were registered. The value of every $q(3)$-interval is calculated by the gamma distribution. Since the exponential distribution is a special case of the gamma distribution, the q-interval effectively is the $q(1)$-interval.

3.2 The CUSCORE-Test of Significance

The CUSCORE test [7] is aimed at detection of temporal clustering of some events embedded within the data set. Each interval is defined as either short or long, according to the expected number of events within it. It is defined as short if the RI is equal to or smaller than an appropriate critical value k. The critical value k of the CUSCORE-test of significance is determined with accordance to the data size and $q(1)$- or $q(3)$-interval.

Table 1. Critical interval (k) between cases for given number of events (S)

S	q(1)	k
5	0.451	0.797
6	0.493	0.707
7	0.554	0.590
8	0.579	0.546
9	0.606	0.501
10	0.623	0.474
11	0.638	0.450
12	0.649	0.433
13	0.659	0.417
14	0.667	0.405
15	0.674	0.394
16	0.681	0.384
17	0.687	0.376
18	0.692	0.368
19	0.696	0.362
20	0.701	0.355
21	0.705	0.350
22	0.708	0.345
23	0.712	0.340

The test is based on a cumulative score. Initially, the score equals 0 and it increases by 1 with every case if the interval is short and decreases by 1 in opposite situation. However, the score is never smaller than 0. When a long interval appears and the score after the previous case is 0, the test is recycled, namely the score value remains 0 (not −1). The test is significant (i.e. cluster is found) if the score equals 5 for any of the S analyzed cases.

Using Markov-chain approach, the critical values k were calculated for significance levels 0.05 (using n = 5) [7]. Tables 1 presents the $q(1)$ and critical values k for 5÷23 cases (S). Table 2 presents the $q(3)$ and the associated k for $S = 24÷60$.

Table 2. Critical interval (k) until the 3rd case for given number of events (S)

S	q(3)	k
24	0.579	2.364
27	0.606	2.263
30	0.623	2.201
33	0.638	2.145
36	0.649	2.104
39	0.659	2.065
42	0.667	2.036
45	0.674	2.009
48	0.681	1.984
51	0.687	1.963
54	0.692	1.943
57	0.696	1.928
60	0.701	1.909

3.3 The Confirmatory Technique

Two confirmatory procedures have been put forward, based on the RI corresponding to the first 5 cases observed after the cluster is detected [6]. One technique is based on the mean; the other is based on the median RI value. According to the results of the test one of the following is concluded: (1) The cluster is if the statistic (mean or median RI) is smaller than the corresponding critical reference value t_1. (2) The cluster is rejected if the statistic is above t_2. (3) The judgment about the cluster is reserved if the statistic value is between t_1 and t_2. The median confirmatory technique is used when less than 6 cases are expected between the cluster detection and the end of the study. The mean technique is functional if the expected number of cases is larger than 5. The reference values for both methods were aimed at confirming only 25% of the false clusters and 97.5% of the true clusters when the rate is twice the baseline rate. Accordingly, for the median technique $t_1=0.4455$ and $t_2=0.9600$; for the mean technique $t_1=0.6737$ and $t_2=1.0242$ [6].

3.4 The Temporal Pattern of the Cases

The q-intervals reflect the temporal incidence rates of the cases. This temporal pattern may be used for cause interpretation of the detected cluster [5, 8].

3.5 How the Techniques Work Altogether: An Example from Our Study

Here we present an example where $q(3)$ is in use. Table 3 presents 35 cases of all cancer sites in males of AIC No. 6. The date of each third case is shown in this table.
RI_1 is the number of cases expected between 1/1/72 (the start date) and the date of the
3rd case, RI_2 is the number of cases expected between the 3rd and the 6th cases.

The critical value k for 35 cases is 2.145. Therefore, the score is in-
creased/decreased by 1 if the observed RI_i is smaller/larger than 2.145. All RI_i where
$i \leq 5$ are smaller than k, hence a cluster is detected on the date of 15th case (31/12/82).
Here the mean confirmatory technique is applied to the time interval from the cluster
detection date (31/12/82) to the date of 20th case (31/8/84-not shown in the table). The
RI for this period (from 31/12/82 to 31/8/84) is 1.2647; thus the mean RI is 0.2529.
As *this mean* is smaller than t_1=0.6373, the cluster is confirmed. The $q(3)$ values,
clearly support these results as except of the last one, each of them is larger than 0.5,.

The procedure for evaluation of $q(1)$ is demonstrated in "Method".

Table 3. Data of all sites cancer in males of AIC No. 6

i	Case No.	Case date	RI	$q(3)$	CUSCORE
1	3	31/1/74	0.7334	0.962	1
2	6	31/01/78	1.9389	0.693	2
3	9	31/03/80	1.1738	0.886	3
4	12	31/01/82	1.2240	0.874	4
5	15	31/12/82	0.6406	0.973	5
6	18	01/05/84	1.0685	0.907	
7	21	31/05/85	0.8039	0.952	
8	24	30/06/87	1.7618	0.741	
9	27	31/12/89	2.2031	0.622	
10	30	30/06/91	1.2928	0.859	
11	33	30/06/93	1.7361	0.748	
12	36	>31/10/96	>3.006	<0.422	

4   Results

We found clusters in 14 AICs (over all 45 we analyzed). In 7 of 14 AICs an exposure
to local cancer risk factor(s) has a solid basis as a reason leading to true cluster, because the results display the only cluster confirmed. Table 3 shows up the analysis
outcome for this case. The clusters detected in 4 AICs are not confirmed because they
were found at the end of observation period. Therefore further follow up is required in
order to make decision to reject or confirm those clusters.

Datasets of 3 AICs are composed of two periods: alarming interval (time when the
cuscore is growing up to 5) and time when observed cases are going down (they are
lower than expected ones). Such a phenomenon can happen when all sensitive individuals (especially in a closed community) have already responded to the local cancer
risk factor(s), or when the local cancer risk factor(s) has ceased to exist. We can call
this observable fact "past clustering".

5   Conclusions

Using the analysis, we managed to find certain important scenarios about increased cancer risk in AIC. These scenarios are: 1) confirmed cluster; 2) detected cluster that requires further observation, 3) "past" clustering. In all 3 scenarios, it is logical to assume that exposure to local cancer risk factor(s) is a reason of cancer clustering.

We can highly recommend to use the approach every time when one needs to detect clusters of any kind (not only cancer ones) in small quasi-close communities.

References

1. Blair A, Zahm SH. Agricultural exposures and cancer. Environ Health Perspect, 1995, 103 (Suppl 8): 205-8
2. Blair A, Zahm SH, Pearce NE, Heineman EF, Fraumeni JF Jr. Clues to cancer etiology from studies of farmers. Scand J Work Environ Health, 1992, 18:4, 209-15
3. Cerhan JR, Cantor KR, Williamson K, Lynch CF, Torner JC, Burmeister LF. Cancer mortality among Iowa farmers:recent results, time trends , and lifestyle factors. Cancer Causes Control, 1998,9:3,311-9.
4. Chen R. Exploratory analysis as a sequel to suspected increased rate of cancer in a small residential or workplace community. Statistics in Medicine, 1996,15:807-816
5. Chen R. The cumulative q-interval as a starting point in disease cluster investigation. Statistics in Medicine, 1999,18:3299-3307
6. Chen R, Connely RR and Mantel N. Analysing post alarm data in a monitoring system, in order to accept or reject the alarm. Statistics in Medicine, 1993,12:1807-1812
7. Chen R. Goldbourt U. Analysis of data associated with seemingly temporal clustering of a rare disease. Methods of Information in Medicine, 1998, 37:26-31
8. Chen R, Iscovich J, Goldbourt U. Clustering of leukemia cases in a city in Israel. Statistics in Medicine, 1997, 16:1873-1887
9. Fleming LE, Bean JA, Rudolph M, Hamilton K.Mortality in a cohort of licensed pesticide applicators in Florida. Occup Environ Med, 1999 Jan, 56:1, 14-21
10. Ji BT , Silverman DT, Stewart PA et al. Occupational Exposure to Pesticdes and pancreatic cancer. Am J Ind Med, 2001,39: 92-99
11. National Conference of Clustering of Health Cases. Am J Epidemiol 1990, Sp(suppl), 1-202, vol 132
12. Ritter L, Wigle DT, Semenciw RM, Wilkins K, Riedel D, Mao Y. Mortality study of Canadian male farm operators: cancer mortality and agricultural practices in Saskatchewan. Med Lav, 1990 , 81 (6): 499-505
13. Simpson J, Roman E, Law G, Pannett B. Women's occupation and cancer preliminary analysis of cancer registrations in England and Wales, 1971-1990. Am J Ind Med, 1999,36:1,172-85
14. Waterhouse D, Carman WJ, Schottenfeld D. et al. Cancer incidence in the rural community of Tecumseh, Michigan: A pattern of increased lymphopoietic neoplasms. Cancer, 1996 , 77 (4):763-70

15. Wiklund K, Dich J. Cancer risks among male farmers in Sweden. Eur J Cancer Prev, 1995, 4:1 81-90
16. Zhong Y, Rafnsson V. Cancer incidence among Icelandic pesticide users. Int J Epidemiol, 1996, 25(6): 1117-24

Hybrid Pattern Recognition Algorithms with the Statistical Model Applied to the Computer-Aided Medical Diagnosis

Marek Kurzynski, Edward Puchala, and Jerzy Sas

Wroclaw University of Technology,
Faculty of Electronics, Division of Systems and Computer Networks,
Wyb. Wyspianskiego 27, 50-370 Wroclaw, Poland
kumar@zssk.pwr.wroc.pl

Abstract. The present paper is devoted to the pattern recognition procedures that simultaneously use the information contained in the empirical data (learning set) and the set of expert rules with unprecisely formulated weights understood as conditional probabilities. Adopting the probabilistic model the combined and unified recognition algorithms are derived. In the first approach algorithm is based simply on the both set of data, in the second however, one set of data is transformed into the second one. Proposed algorithms were applied practically to the diagnosis of acute renal failure in children. Obtained results have proved its effectiveness in the computer medical decision-making.

1   Introduction

The design of the classifier in statistical pattern recognition generally depends on what kind of information is available about the probability distribution of classes and features. If this information is complete, then the Bayes decision scheme can be used. If such information is unknown or incompletely defined, a possible approach is to design a system, which will acquire the pertinent information from the actually available data for constructing a decision rule. Usually it is assumed that available information on the probability characteristics is contained in a learning set consisting of a sequence of observed features of patterns and their correct classification. In such a case many learning procedures are known within empirical Bayes decision theory, which lead to the different sample-based pattern recognition algorithms (e.g. [1]).

Another approach, interesting from both theoretical and practical point of view, supposes that appropriate information is contained in expert knowledge. A typical knowledge representation consists of rules of the form IF A THEN B with the weight (uncertainty measure) α. These rules are obtained from the expert as his/her conditional beliefs: if A is known with certainty then the expert's belief into B is α. In this case numerous inference procedures are proposed and very well investigated for different formal interpretations of the weight α [2-4].

J. Crespo, V. Maojo, and F. Martin (Eds.): ISMDA 2001, LNCS 2199, pp. 133-139, 2001.

Since till now there is lack of methods which combine features of these two approaches: sample-based recognition and knowledge-based methods, hence in this paper we shall focus our attention on decision algorithms for the case in which both the learning set and expert rules are available. Additionally, adopting the probabilistic interpretation of weight coefficients, we suppose that expert rules are not provided with exact value of α (i.e. conditional probability), but only an interval is specified (by its upper and lower bounds), into which this probability belongs. In one of the discussed concept first the learning set is transformed into the set of "artificial" expert rules, and then - having the homogenous form of information - we calculate approximated values of *a posteriori* probabilities, which can be used in the Bayes decision scheme.

This paper is a sequel to the author's earlier publications [5,6] and it yields an extension of the results included therein.

2   Preliminaries and the Problem Statement

Let us consider the pattern recognition problem with probabilistic model. This means that vector of features describing recognized pattern $x \in X \subseteq R^d$ and its class number $j \in M = \{1,2,...,M\}$ are observed values of a couple of random variables X and J, respectively. Its probability distribution is given by *a priori* probabilities of classes $p_j = P(J = j)$, $j \in M$, and class-conditional probability density functions (CPDFs) of X $f_j(x) = f(x/j)$, $x \in X$, $j \in M$. Pattern recognition algorithm ψ maps the feature space X to the set of class numbers M, viz.

$$\Psi : X \rightarrow M. \tag{1}$$

If probabilities (1) and CPDFs (2) are known, i.e. in the case of complete probabilistic information, the optimal (Bayes) recognition algorithm Ψ^* minimizing the probability of misclassification Pe makes decision according to the following rule:

$$\Psi^*(x) = i \quad \text{if} \quad p_i(x) = \max_{k \in M} p_k(x), \tag{2}$$

where *a posteriori* probabilities $p_j(x)$ can be calculated from the Bayes formula.

Let us now consider the original and interesting from practical point of view concept of recognition. We assume that *a priori* probabilities and CPDFs are not known, whereas the only information on the probability distribution of J and X is contained in the two qualitatively different kinds of data:

Learning set

$$S = \{(x_1, j_1), (x_2, j_2), ..., (x_L, j_L)\}, \quad x_i \in X, \quad j_i \in M, \tag{3}$$

where x_i denotes the feature vector of the *i*-th learning pattern and j_i is its correct classification. Additionally, let S_i denotes the set of learning patterns from the *i*-th class.

Expert rules

$$R = \{R_1, R_2, ..., R_M\}, \tag{4}$$

where

$$R_i = \left\{ r_i^{(1)}, r_i^{(2)}, ..., r_i^{(N_i)} \right\}, \quad i \in M, \quad \Sigma N_i = N \tag{5}$$

denotes the set of rules connected with the i-th class. The rule $r_i^{(k)}$ has the following general form:

IF $w_i^{(k)}(x)$ THEN $\boldsymbol{J} = j$ WITH probability greater than $\underline{p}_i^{(k)}$ and less than $\overline{p}_i^{(k)}$

where $w_i^{(k)}(x)$ denotes a predicate depending on the values of the features x. We will continue to adopt the following equivalent form of the rule $r_i^{(k)}$:

$$\underline{p}_i^{(k)} \le p_i(x) \le \overline{p}_i^{(k)} \quad \text{for} \quad x \in \mathsf{D}_i^{(k)}, \tag{6}$$

where

$$\mathsf{D}_i^{(k)} = \{x \in \mathsf{X} : w_i^{(k)} = \text{true}\} \tag{7}$$

will be called rule-defined region.

Now our purpose is to construct the recognition algorithm

$$\Psi(S, R, x) = \Psi_{SR}(x) = i, \tag{8}$$

which using information contained in the learning set S and the set of expert rules R recognizes a pattern on the basis of its features x.

3 Pattern Recognition Algorithms

In the sample-based classification, i.e. when the only learning set S is given, one obvious and conceptually simple method is to estimate *a priori* probabilities and CPDFs and then to use these estimators to calculate *a posteriori* probabilities (let say $p_i^{(S)}(x)$), i.e. discriminant functions of the optimal (Bayes) classifier (2).

On the other hand, using this concept in the case when only the set of rules R is given, we obtain the so-called GAP (the **G**reatest **A**pproximated *a posteriori* **P**robability) rule-based algorithm, which originally was introduced in [5]:

$$\Psi_R(x) = i \quad \text{if} \quad p_i^{(R)}(x) = \max_{k \in M} p_k^{(R)}(x), \tag{9}$$

where $p_i^{(R)}(x)$ denotes approximated *a posteriori* probability of i-th class calculated from the set R (details of estimation procedure can be found in [6]). In the sequel, we shall suppose that both sets S and R are given. Now, in order to find the algorithm (8) we propose the following concepts:

Mixed algorithm

In this approach we have:

$$\Psi_{SR}(x) = i \quad \text{if} \quad p_i^{(SR)}(x) = \max_{k \in M} p_k^{(SR)}(x), \tag{10}$$

where $p_i^{(SR)}(x) = \beta \, p_k^{(S)}(x) + (1 - \beta) \, p_k^{(R)}$ and mixing coefficient $\beta \in [0,1]$ can be calculated experimentally.

Unified algorithms

Now, in order to find (8) we will transform one set of data into the second set and next, having the homogenous form of information, we can simply use either the GAP algorithm (for transformation $S \rightarrow R$) or recognition algorithm with learning (e.g. empirical Bayes or NN - nearest neighbour decision rule [1]) for transformation $R \rightarrow S$. Our proposition of procedures for „the unification of information" is as follows:

Algorithm $S \rightarrow R$

Idea of this algorithm consists in interval estimate of *a posteriori* probability [7] on the base of learning set for each rule-defined region and next the confidence limits of this interval are treated as upper and lower bounds of *a posteriori* probability in a new „artificial" rule. Namely:

1. Adopt initial conditions: the number of „artificial" rules for decision i - L_i, rule-defined regions - $D_i^{(k)}$ ($k = 1,2,...,L_i$),

2. Calculate: $\underline{p}_i^{'(k)} = \dfrac{m}{n} - u_\alpha \sqrt{\dfrac{\dfrac{m}{n}(1 - \dfrac{m}{n})}{n}}$, $\overline{p}_i^{'(k)} = \dfrac{m}{n} + u_\alpha \sqrt{\dfrac{\dfrac{m}{n}(1 - \dfrac{m}{n})}{n}}$,

where n and m denote the number of all learning patterns and the number of learning patterns from the ith class belonging to $D_i^{'(k)}$, respectively. u_α is a critical value of standardized Gaussian distribution for given level of confidence α.

3. Repeat steps 1 and 2 for all $i \in M$.

Algorithm $R \rightarrow S$

1. Adopt initial conditions: the number of „learning" patterns per rule - m,

2. For rule $r_i^{(k)}$ generate m couples (x,i), where x is uniformly distributed in $D_i^{(k)}$ random number and $i \in M$ is natural number generated as follows:

$$i = \begin{cases} j & \text{with probability } (\overline{p}_i^{(k)} + \underline{p}_i^{(k)})/2, \\ k(\neq j) & \text{with probability } [1 - (\overline{p}_i^{(k)} + \underline{p}_i^{(k)})/2]/(M - 1) \end{cases}$$

3. Repeat the step 2 for all rules $r_i^{(k)} \in R_i, i \in M$.

All the decision algorithms that are depicted in this chapter have been experimentally tested as far as the decision quality is concerned. Measure for the decision quality is the frequency of correct diagnoses for real data that are concerned with diagnosis of acute renal failure in children. The purpose of our research and associated tests was not only the comparative analysis of the presented algorithms but also answering the question whether mixed and unified algorithms (i.e. algorithms using both sets of data) would yield a better decision quality as compared to rule-based (GAP) and sample-based (EB-empirical Bayes [1]) algorithms. The next chapter describes the performed tests and their outcome.

4   Computer-Aided Diagnosis of Acute Renal Failure (ARF)

The diagnosis of ARF as a pattern recognition task includes the following ten classes (etiologic types of ARF): toxicosis, nephrotic syndrome, sepsis, acute glomerulonephritis, uremic-haemolytic syndrome, circulatory failure, renal vain thrombosis, andrenogenital syndrome, postrenal failure, others (prerenal or intrarenal) [8]. The vector of features x contains the values of 53 items of clinical data (general, past and/or concurrent diseases, anamnesis, physical examinations, laboratory examinations, gasometric examinations, morphology of the blood, serum, serum ionogram, urine).

In the Department of Pediatric Nephrology of Wrocław Medical Academy the set of 380 case records of children suffering from ARF were collected, which constitute the learning set (3). Each case record contains administrative data, values of clinical features and a firm diagnosis. Most of the diagnoses were made during the period of hospitalization according to the generally accepted criteria. 25 children had died and the anatomopathologic findings provided a definite diagnosis.

Furthermore, the knowledge base for the diagnostic problem in question contains 165 rules (4) which connect the observed values of clinical data with etiologic type of ARF. For example: **IF** {skin=icteric} **AND** {trombocytes=increased} **AND** {reticulocytes=increased} **THEN** uremic-haemolytic syndrome **PROBABILITY** 0.5-0.6.

In order to study the performance of the proposed recognition concepts and evaluate their usefulness to the computer-aided establishing of the etiology of ARF, the computer experiments were made. The outcome is shown in Table 1. It includes the frequency of correct diagnoses for the investigated algorithms.

Table 1. Results of empirical tests

No	Algorithm	Accuracy [%]
1	GAP algorithm with the set R	83,2
2	EB algorithm with the set S	91,6
3	Mixed algorithm (10) with β=0.25	86,3
4	Mixed algorithm (10) with β=0.4	87,1
5	Mixed algorithm (10) with β=0.5	88,5
6	Mixed algorithm (10) with β=0.6	90,3
7	Mixed algorithm (10) with β=0.75	92,8
8	GAP algorithm with sets R+S (α=0.01 in the unification procedure)	85,2
9	GAP algorithm with sets R+S (α=0.025 in the unification procedure)	85,8
10	GAP algorithm with sets R+S (α=0.05 in the unification procedure)	86,4
11	GAP algorithm with sets R+S (α=0.1 in the unification procedure)	84,3
12	EB algorithm with sets R+S (m=1 in the unification procedure)	93,8
13	EB algorithm with sets R+S (m=2 in the unification procedure)	95,6
14	EB algorithm with sets R+S (m=5 in the unification procedure)	96,4
15	EB algorithm with sets R+S (m=10 in the unification procedure)	95,1

5   Conclusion

In this paper we have focused our attention on the recognition technique via empirical data (learning set) and the expert rules (knowledge representation). Taking the probabilistic model of classification, we discuss different concepts of pattern recognition algorithms. Their classification functions, based on the Bayes decision scheme, are obtained as approximated values of class *a posteriori* probabilities. This means, that the both sets of data are treated as a source of information about the probability distribution of appropriate random variables.

Presented algorithms have been experimentally tested on the real data. All the experiments show that algorithms which use the both sets of data are much more effective as far as the correct decision frequency is concerned than algorithms which include only one set of data. This testifies that the proposed conceptions are correct, and demonstrates effectiveness of the proposed algorithms in such computer-aided medical diagnosis problems in which both the learning set and expert rules are available.

References

1. Devroye L., Gyorfi L., Lugosi G.: A Probabilistic Theory of Pattern Recognition. Springer Verlag (1996)
2. Pearl J.: Probabilistic Reasoning in Intelligent Systems. Morgan Kaufman Publishers, Inc., San Francisco (1992)

3. Dubois D., Lang J.: Possibilistic Logic, In: Handbook of Logic in Artificial Intelligence and Logic Programming. Oxford Univ. Press (1994) 439-513
4. Neapolitan R.: Probabilistic Reasoning in Expert Systems. Wiley, New York (1990)
5. Kurzynski M., Sas J., Blinowska A.: Rule-Based Medical Decision-Making with Learning. Proc. 12th World IFAC Congress, Vol. 4, Sydney (1993) 319–322
6. Kurzynski M., Sas J.: Rule-Based Classification Procedures Related to the Unprecisely Formulated Expert Rules. Proc. SIBIGRAPI Conference, Rio de Janeiro (1998) 241-245
7. Sachs L.: Applied Statistics. A Handbook of Techniques. Springer Verlag, New York, Berlin, Tokyo (1984)
8. James A. J.: Renal Diseases in Childhood. The C.V.Mosby Co., Saint Louis (1976)

Computer-Aided Diagnosis:
Application of Wavelet Transform to the Detection of
Clustered Microcalcifications in Digital Mammograms

María J. Lado[1], Arturo J. Méndez[1], Pablo G. Tahoces[2],
Miguel Souto[3], and Juan J. Vidal[3]

[1] Department of Computer Science, University of Vigo,
Campus Lagoas-Marcosende, 36200 Vigo, Spain
{mrpepa, mrarthur}@uvigo.es
[2] Department of Electronics and Computer Science, University of Santiago de
Compostela, Campus Sur, 15782 Santiago de Compostela, Spain
mrpablo@usc.es
[3] Department of Radiology, University of Santiago de Compostela,
San Francisco 1, 15782 Santiago de Compostela, Spain
mrmiguel@usc.es

Abstract. Computer methodologies are being developed to assist radiologists, as second readers, in the interpretation of mammograms. This could represent further amelioration by increasing diagnostic accuracy in the screening programs. We have developed a computerized scheme to detect clustered microcalcifications in digital mammograms, using 100 mammograms that were randomly selected from the mammographic screening program, currently undergoing at the Galicia Community (Spain). After the digitization process, the breast border was initially determined. A wavelet-based algorithm was employed to detect the clusters of microcalcifications. The sensitivity achieved was 79% at a false positive detection rate of 1.83.

1 Introduction

Although breast cancer is still one of the main causes of death in women [1], it is recognized that an early detection and treatment can reduce the mortality rates produced by this disease. An independent double reading improves breast cancer detection rates [2], but the additional cost that double reading implies is considered to be beyond the possibilities of many departments and health service administrations [3]. Several researchers have pointed out the possibility to employ computer-aided diagnosis (CAD) schemes to aid radiologists, in the interpretation of mammograms [4], During the last decade CAD has been largely developed to improve the diagnostic accuracy in both the detection and classification of masses [5, 6] and clustered microcalcifications [7, 8], signs that may indicate the presence of breast cancer.

J. Crespo, V. Maojo, and F. Martin (Eds.): ISMDA 2001, LNCS 2199, pp. 140-145, 2001.
© Springer-Verlag Berlin Heidelberg 2001

Many investigators have reported automated algorithms to detect microcalcifications in mammograms. Veldkamp and Karssemeijer [7] have developed a computer-aided diagnostic method based on the use of Bayesian techniques and application of a Markov random field model. Others employed filter based methods or wavelet transform techniques to detect the microcalcifications [9, 10]. Finally, we have also proposed, as a further step in our CAD schemes [11], that wavelet transform techniques could be used for the detection of clustered microcalcifications. In fact, we have developed a method based on the wavelet transform applied to the complete mammogram, employing digital mammograms digitized at a pixel size of 87.5 µm and 1024 gray levels previously developed at our Laboratory, and consequently published [12], with the same image database. In this work, we have digitized the mammograms at a pixel size of 87.5 µm and 4096 gray level values.

2   Materials and Methods

1.1   Acquisition of Digital Mammograms and Database Characterization

Fifty-five mammograms containing 95 clusters o microcalcifications were digitized at a resolution of 2000x2500 pixels, and 4096 gray level values (12 bits precision) employing a Lumiscan 85 laser scanner (Lumisys Inc., Sunnyvale, CA). Images were directly stored via SCSI interface on a magnetic disk array Sun StorEDGE A5100, and a Sun Ultra 80 Workstation (Sun Microsystems, Inc., Mountain View, CA), was used for all the calculations.

All the lesions were ranked by two experienced radiologists by consensus in a four-level decision scale, *level 1*, corresponding to obvious cases (24), *level 2*, for relatively obvious cases (36), *level 3*, corresponding to subtle cases (24), and *level 4*, for very subtle cases (11).

Contrast value and size for each microcalcification were computed to characterize the database. A mean size of 29.61±23.63 pixels was obtained. The mean contrast computed was 0.03325±0.0196.

1.2   Detection of Clusters of Microcalcifications

The general scheme to detect clusters of microcalcifications is a five-step process, that involves: a) detection of the breast border, b) application of one-dimensional wavelet transform, c) application of local gray level threshold, d) clustering procedure, and e) reduction of false positives.

Detection of the breast border: to detect the breast border, an algorithm that computes the gradient of gray levels was applied. First, a thresholded version of the entire mammogram was calculated, obtained to avoid artefacts that produced distortion when the border was calculated. Next, five points were automatically selected as reference points to divide the breast into three regions. To calculate these points, an analysis of the relative position of the breast and the film border was performed. These five reference points delimited three regions over the breast. Then, a tracking algorithm, based on the relationship between gray level values of neighbour pixels, was applied over the three regions in a similar way, varying only on the starting point and the direction of application of the algorithm [13].

Application of wavelet transform: when the breast border was calculated, wavelet transform techniques were applied. Previous studies [12] have demonstrated that one-dimensional wavelet transform provides similar results in detecting microcalcifications to those of the two-dimensional wavelet transform, and saves computation time. Because of this, one-dimensional wavelet transform techniques were implemented. Each image was divided into vertical lines, and wavelet transform was applied over each line constituting the image. Lines were recomposed employing the high frequency components of the wavelet sub-images that enhanced the microcalcifications, previously determined [12]. The result was an image with the high frequency components enhanced, while the low frequency background structure was removed. Over the reconstructed image obtained for each mammogram, a global threshold was applied, and a binary image giving all the possible points of microcalcifications was created. This threshold value was based on the values of the wavelet coefficients; to obtain it, several maxima values of the wavelet coefficients were calculated for each line constituting the image. The pixel positions corresponding to values of wavelet coefficients that were greater that an imposed constraint value, were considered as points of microcalcifications and translated to the binary image.

Application of local gray level threshold: a local gray level threshold, based on the difference between the gray level value of each detected signal and the gray level value of a region of the original mammogram, centered on the signal, was applied over the points of the binary image translated to the original one [12]. In this way, the seed points of microcalcifications were calculated, and a region growing algorithm was applied. Average gray level value of each seed point and the eight pixels spatially connected to it was calculated, as well as the standard deviation. A new spatially connected pixel was considered. If the difference between the gray level value of the new pixel and the average gray level value previously calculated was lower or equal than the standard deviation, the pixel was included into the microcalcification, and a new average and gray level value were calculated. The procedure continued until there were no more spatially connected pixels verifying the required condition. A contrast test was then applied over the detected signals to reduce the number of false detections.

Clustering procedure: several definitions of cluster of microcalcifications have been given. We have chosen the definition given by Kopans, that describes a cluster as five or more signals within region of 1 cm^2 of area [14]. To group the detected microcalcifications, and according to the definition of Kopans, we have considered a window of 1 cm^2 of area, initially situated at the lower left-hand corner of the image [12]. The number of signals present in the area limited by this window was counted: if there were 5 or more signals, they were considered to form a cluster of microcalcifications. Otherwise, they were considered as false positives and rejected. The window was then moved 0.5 cm in the vertical direction, and the process was repeated. When the window reached the upper limit of the image, it was moved 0.5 cm in the horizontal direction. The process continued until all the image was examined. Since there were regions of the mammogram that were analyzed more than once, microcalcifications located in these regions could belong to different clusters at the same time. To avoid these overlapping problems, clusters with at least one common microcalcification were considered to be the same cluster.

Reduction of false positives: the final step in the detection process was the reduction of false positives by employing discriminant analysis. This was performed by applying the SPSS software package for Windows [15] to some input properties of the detected clusters, previously calculated.

3   Results

The 55 mammograms of our study were analyzed to detect possible clusters of micro-calcifications employing the automated detection scheme described above. Figure 1 shows an example of an original image containing a cluster of microcalcifications, and the results of the detection procedure.

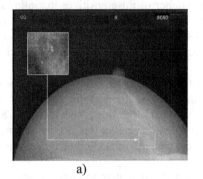 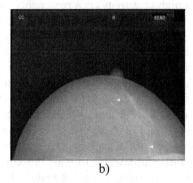

a)   b)

Fig. 1. a) An original mammogram containing a cluster of microcalcifications, and b) Results of the detection process (indicated by white arrows): the cluster detected, and the presence of a false positive

The system achieved a sensitivity of 79% with a mean number of 1.83 false positives per image.

4   Discussion

Computerized detection of microcalcifications has been at the frontispiece of investigation over the last years. Research on interpretation and analysis of mammograms has shown that detectability of microcalcifications depends on the subtlety of the original signals, but also on the limited contrast sensitivity of film screen system, on the image noise, or the presence of artifacts. However, it is clear that a computer scheme will be clinically useful only when it provides a detection rate higher or equal than when either the human observer or the computer work alone.

In this work we are investigating on an automatic wavelet-based algorithm for the detection of clusters of microcalcifications on digital mammograms. We have applied one-dimensional wavelet transform over each vertical line constituting the image, in order to enhance the microcalcifications. This is a less-time consuming process, because the wavelet transform is only computed in one direction, and it is not limited to either square or rectangular regions, because it performs over each line of the image and, as a result, it can be applied over irregular areas, such as the mammographic region.

In a previous study [12], we have developed a similar method to detect clustered microcalcifications in digital mammograms, employing a 10 bit precision scanner for the digitisation process. We have obtained a sensitivity of 76.43% at a false positive of 1.57 per image. In this work, our sensitivity has increased up to 79%, as well as the mean number of false detections: 1.83 per image. This is due to the fact that the algorithm has not been neither optimised nor modified for the new parameters that necessarily include the increase in gray level values, produced by the digitisation process at 12 bits precision. Even although the sensitivity needs to be improved, we do not believe that this implies that the detection system is not beneficial for breast cancer detection: one of the requirements for a computer detection scheme to be helpful, apart from a high sensitivity, is a reasonably low number of false positives that allows the radiologists to analyze mammograms easily. The mean number of false positives per image yielded by our system will not confuse the radiologist by suggesting normal areas as suspicious. Thus, the use of our detection scheme could lead to a reduction in the number of biopsies to be performed.

Other techniques employing wavelet transform are applied over ROIs (Regions Of Interest). Zhang et al. [16] employed weighted wavelet transform algorithms over ROIs of 12.8x12.8 mm^2, obtaining a sensitivity of 83% with a specificity of 80%. Yoshida et al. [13] have also developed a technique based on wavelet transform, obtaining a 95% of sensitivity and 1.5 false detections per image, but they combined wavelet transform with a filtering procedure.

Our results suggest that the system developed is competent to complement the interpretation of radiologists in their daily practice, and also to improve their diagnostic performance. Future work will address to the issue of optimising the parameters for the high resolution system, in order to improve the sensitivity and to reduce the number of false detections.

Acknowledgments

The authors are grateful to Roberto Patiño for his technical assistance in the edition of this manuscript. This work has been partially supported by Secretaría de Estado de Universidades, Investigación y Desarrollo (ref. 1FD97-0147).

References

1. Landis, S. H., Murray, T., Bolden, S., Wingo, P.A.: Cancer statistics 1998. CA Cancer Journal for Clinicians 48 (1998) 6-29
2. Thurfjell, E. L., Lernevall, K. A., Taube, A. A. S.: Benefit of an independent double reading in a population-based mammographic screening program. Radiology 191 (1994) 241-244

3. Tonita, J.M., Hillis, J.P., Lim, C.H.: Medical radiologic technologist review: Effects on a population-based breast cancer screening program. Radiology 211 (1999) 529-533
4. Tahoces, P.G., Correa, J., Souto, M., Gómez, L., Vidal, J.J.: Computer-assisted diagnosis: The classification of mammographic breast parenchymal patterns. Physic in Medicine and Biology 40 (1995) 103-117
5. Yin, F. F., Giger, M. L., Doi, K., Vyborny, C. J., Schmidt, R. A., 1994, Computerized detection of masses in digital mammograms: Automated alignment of breast images and its effect on bilateral subtraction technique. Medical Physics 21, 445-452
6. Méndez, A.J., Tahoces, P.G., Lado, M.J., Souto, M., Vidal, J.J.: Computer-aided diagnosis: Automatic detection of malignant masses in digitized mammograms. Medical Physics 25 (1998) 957-964
7. Veldkamp, W., Karssemeijer, N.: Accurate segmentation and contrast measurement of microcalcifications in mammograms: A phantom study. Medical Physics 25 (1998) 1102-1110
8. Gavrielides, M.A., Lo, J.Y., Vargas-Voracek, R.,Floyd, C.E.: Segmentation of suspicious clustered microcalcifications in mammograms. Medical Physics 27 (2000) 13-22
9. Chan, H.P., Doi, K., Vyborny, C.J., Schmidt, R.A., Metz, C.E., Lam, K.L., Ogura, T., Wu, Y., MacMahon, H., Improvement in radiologists' detection of clustered microcalcifications on mammograms. The potential of computer-aided diagnosis. Investigative Radiology 25, (1990) 110
10. Yoshida, H., Doi, K., Nishikawa, R.M., Giger, M.L., Schmidt, R.A.: An improved computer-assisted diagnostic scheme using wavelet transform for detecting clustered microcalcifications in digital mammograms. Academic Radiology 3 (1996) 621-627
11. Souto, M., Correa, J., Tahoces, P.G., Carrascal, F., Méndez, A.J., Lado, M.J., Carreira, J.M., Vidal, J.J.: A limited PACS dedicated to a research environment. Nine years' experience in Santiago de Compostela. Medical Informatics, 21 (1996) 123-132
12. Lado, M.J., Tahoces, P.G., Méndez, A.J., Souto, M., Vidal, J.J.: A wavelet-based algorithm for detecting clustered microcalcifications in digital mammograms. Medical Physics 26 (1999) 1294-1305
13. Méndez, A.J., Tahoces, P.G., Lado, M.J., Souto, M., Correa, J., Vidal, J.J.: Automatic detection of breast border and nipple in digital mammograms. Computer Methods and Programs in Biomedicine 49 (1996) 253-262
14. Kopans, D.B: Breast Imaging. Lippincott-Raven, Philadelphia (1998)
15. Norussis, M.J.: SPSS for Windows. Professional Statistics. SPSS, Chicago (1992)
16. Zhang, W., Yoshida, H., Nishikawa, R.M., Doi, K.: Optimally weighted wavelet transform based on supervised training for detection of microcalcifications in digital mammograms. Medical Physics 25 (1998) 949-956

A Methodology for Constructing Expert Systems for Medical Diagnosis*

L. M. Laita[1], G. González-Páez[1], E. Roanes-Lozano[2], V. Maojo[1],
L. de Ledesma[1], and L. Laita[3]

[1] Universidad Politécnica de Madrid, Dept. Artificial Intelligence,
Campus de Montegancedo, Boadilla del Monte, 28660-Madrid, Spain
`laita@fi.upm.es`
`g_gonzalezp@yahoo.es`
`{maojo,ledesma}@fi.upm.es`
[2] Universidad Complutense de Madrid, Dept. Algebra,
Edificio "La Almudena", c/ Rector Royo Villanova s/n, 28040-Madrid, Spain
`eroanes@eucmos.sim.ucm.es`
[3] CEU Madrid, Nursing School,
Campus de Montepríncipe, 28660-Madrid, Spain

Abstract. We propose a methodology, based on Computer Algebra and implemented in CoCoA language, for constructing rule based expert systems, that can be applied to the diagnosis of some illnesses. For the sake of clarity, our proposal uses a simplified description of depression, assuming that our aim is the proposal of a general methodology rather than the study of this particular illness.

1 Introduction

We propose a method of construction of rule based expert systems (denoted as RBES) for diagnosis of some illnesses. Depression is used as illustration, even though, for the sake of simplicity, only a very small amount of information on depression is used.

RBES have usually three components: a "knowledge base", an "inference engine" and an "user interface".

Our particular **knowledge base** encodes information about depression, in form of propositional logic formulae (called "production rules") of the form:

$$\circ x[i] \wedge \circ x[j] \wedge ... \wedge \circ x[k] \to \circ y[l]$$

where "∘" represents the symbol "¬" (meaning "no") or no symbol at all; "∧" and "→" stand for "and" and "implies", respectively. In some formulae below the symbol "∨", which stands for "or" is also used.

Our **inference engine** proceeds as follows: first, logical formulae are automatically translated into polynomials and second, "Gröbner bases" and "normal

---

* Partially supported by projects TIC2000-1368-C03-01 and TIC2000-1368-C03-03 (Ministry of Science and Technology, Spain).

J. Crespo, V. Maojo, and F. Martin (Eds.): ISMDA 2001, LNCS 2199, pp. 146–152, 2001.

Table 1. Predisposing factors

Rules	$x[3] \land x[4]$	$x[3] \land \neg x[4]$	$\neg x[3] \land x[4]$	$\neg x[3] \land \neg x[4]$
$x[1] \land x[2]$	$y[1]$	$y[1]$	$y[2]$	$y[2]$
$\neg x[1] \land x[2]$	$y[1]$	$y[1]$	$y[3]$	$y[3]$
$x[1] \land \neg x[2]$	$y[2]$	$y[2]$	$y[3]$	$y[4]$
$\neg x[1] \land \neg x[2]$	$y[2]$	$y[3]$	$y[4]$	$y[4]$

forms" are applied to these polynomials using CoCoA [1]. The background theory is original of a group of researchers to which the authors belong.

The **user interface** provides an Internet implementation of the "HARD" (*Humeur, Anxieté, Ralentissement, Danger*) diagram of Ferreri and Rufin [5] developed by one of the authors of this paper [3].

2   The Knowledge Base

The knowledge base is constructed by weighting the factors (only some predisposing, triggering and symptomatic factors will be considered) that lead to a diagnosis of depression.

2.1   Predisposing Factors

We only consider as predisposing factors: familiar antecedents, hormonal alterations, personality and external influences (translated by the variables $x[1]$, $x[2]$, $x[3]$ and $x[4]$, respectively). Any of these variables preceded by the symbol "$\neg$" represent the non-existence of the corresponding factor.

The information about predisposing factors is set into a table (Table 1), that summarizes the 16 conjunctions of four different elements taken from the set of the variables above and their negations. An intensity, called "intensity 1" is assigned to each of these conjunctions: $y[1]$, $y[2]$, $y[3]$ and $y[4]$ mean: high, medium, low and non-existing "intensity 1", respectively.

Such an assigning gives rise to 16 implications between each of the mentioned 16 conjunctions and its corresponding intensity. They can be logically simplified to 9 production rules (in this case), of which one is transcribed as illustration:

$$R5 : x[1] \land \neg x[2] \land \neg x[3] \land x[4] \rightarrow y[3]$$

$R5$ translates the statement: "IF familiar antecedents = yes AND hormonal alterations = no AND personality problems = no AND external influences = yes, THEN intensity 1 (of predisposing factors for depression) = low".

2.2   Triggering Factors

We only consider as triggering factors: family separations and/or deaths (denoted $x[5]$) and personal failure (denoted $x[6]$). The non existence of these factors is denoted $\neg x[5]$ and $\neg x[6]$, respectively.

In the antecedent of each production rule corresponding to triggering factors, a variable of the set "intensity 1" (e.g $y[1]$) must appear in order to reflect that triggering factors do not enter into action if there are not predisposing factors.

The "intensity 2" levels of triggering factors are represented by $z[i]$ ($i = 1, .., 4$) meaning, respectively, high, medium, low and non-existing. A table, similar to Table 1, gives rise, after logical simplification, to eleven production rules, R10 to R20, of which R12 is transcribed as illustration:

$$R12 : y[2] \wedge x[5] \wedge \neg x[6] \rightarrow z[2]$$

$R12$ translates the statement "IF intensity 1 (of predisposing factors) = medium AND separations and/or deaths = yes AND personal failure = no, THEN intensity 2 (of triggering factors) = medium".

2.3   Symptoms

We only consider as symptoms: isolation ($x[7]$), sadness ($x[8]$), lack of auto-esteem ($x[9]$) and suicide thoughts ($x[10]$).

An "intensity 3" is assigned to each of the 16 conjunctions of symptoms and/or their negations. $w[1]$ ($i = 1, .., 4$), mean, respectively, high, medium, low and non-existing "intensity 3". They are resumed in eleven production rules, R21 to R31, of which R24 is transcribed:

$$R24 : \neg x[7] \wedge x[8] \wedge \neg x[9] \wedge \neg x[10] \rightarrow w[3]$$

$R24$ translates the statement: "IF isolation = no AND sadness = yes AND lack of auto-esteem = no AND suicide thoughts = no, THEN intensity 3 (of symptoms) = low".

2.4   Diagnosis

Twenty four production rules, R12 to R55, of which R39 is transcribed as illustration, correspond to diagnosis. $v[1]$, $v[2]$, $v[3]$ and $v[4]$ respectively denote severe, moderate, low and non-existent depression.

$$R39 : w[2] \wedge (y[1] \vee y[2]) \wedge (z[2] \vee z[3] \vee z[4]) \rightarrow v[2]$$

$R39$ translates the statement "IF intensity 3 = medium AND (intensity 1 = high OR medium) AND (intensity 2 = medium OR low OR non-existent), THEN diagnosis = moderate depression".

3   The Inference Engine

The basic concepts and results on which the inference engine is based is summarized next [2,4,6].

3.1   Basic Logical and Mathematical Concepts

A logical formula A_0 is a "consequence" of the formulae $A_1, A_2, ..., A_m$ (that represent the rules and facts of the knowledge base of our expert system) iff whenever A_1, A_2, ..., A_m are true, then A_0 is true.

Rules and facts of the RBES are translated into polynomials by assigning a polynomial to each basic logical formula, as follows:

$$\neg x_1 \rightsquigarrow 1 + x_1$$
$$x_1 \vee x_2 \rightsquigarrow x_1 x_2 + x_1 + x_2$$
$$x_1 \wedge x_2 \rightsquigarrow x_1 x_2$$
$$x_1 \rightarrow x_2 \rightsquigarrow x_1 x_2 + x_1 + 1$$

Intuitively, polynomials with addition and multiplication form a "polynomial ring". Certain good-behaviour subsets of polynomial rings are called "ideals". The ideal generated by a finite set of polynomials is the set of sums of products of elements of the ring by generators.

The main result is that *A formula A_0 is a consequence of the formulae $A_1, A_2, ..., A_m$, that represent production rules and potential facts of a RBES (potential facts are in this paper the variables $x[i]$ ($i = 1, .., 10$) and their negations), if and only if the polynomial translation of the negation of A_0 belongs to the ideal generated by both the set of polynomials that translate the negations of $A_1, A_2, ..., A_m$ and the set formed by the polynomials $x_1^2 - x_1, x_2^2 - x_2, ..., x_n^2 - x_n$.*

This can be intuitively denoted as

$$NEG(A_0) \in J + N + I$$

where J is the ideal generated by the polynomial translations of the negations of the production rules. I is the ideal generated by $x_1^2 - x_1, x_2^2 - x_2, ..., x_n^2 - x_n$ (the effect of introducing the ideal I is that the exponents of all variables of all polynomials are reduced to 1).

Potential facts are taken subdivided into "maximal consistent subsets". This means that these subsets do contain each potential fact or its negation but not both simultaneously. N represents the ideal generated by the polynomial translation of (the negation of) the facts in a maximal consistent set of facts.

3.2   Implementation of the Expert System

As said above, the expert system is implemented in CoCoA (v. 3.0)[1]. The polynomial ring A with coefficients in Z_2 (that is, allowing coefficients 0 and 1) and 26 variables; and the ideal I are declared first.

---

[1] CoCoA, a system for doing Computations in Commutative Algebra. Authors: A. Capani, G. Niesi, L. Robbiano. Available via anonymous ftp from: cocoa.dima.unige.it

```
A::=Z/(2)[x[1..10],y[1..4],z[1..4],w[1..4],v[1..4]];
USE A;

I:=Ideal(x[1]^2-x[1],...,x[10]^2-x[10],y[1]^2-y[1],...,
        y[4]^2-y[4],z[1]^2-z[1],...,z[4]^2-z[4],w[1]^2-w[1],...,
        w[4]^2-w[4],v[1]^2-v[1],...,v[4]^2-v[4]);
```

The polynomial translation of the basic formulae (see §3.1) is:

```
NEG(M):=NF(1+M,I);
OR1(M,N):=NF(M+N+M*N,I);
AND1(M,N):=NF(M*N,I);
IMP(M,N):=NF(1+M+M*N,I);
```

Rules R1 to R55 are entered in prefix form. For instance:

```
R5:=NF(IMP(AND1(AND1(AND1(AND1(x[1],NEG(x[2])),NEG(x[3])),
        x[4]),y[3])),I);
```

All potential facts are entered afterwards.

```
F1:=x[1]; ... F10N:=NEG(x[10]);
```

Ideal generated by the negations of all the rules:

```
J = Ideal(NEG(R1) ,..., NEG(R54));
```

In order to find diagnoses consider, as illustration, the following ideals generated by maximal consistent sets of facts.

```
K:=Ideal(NEG(F1N),NEG(F2N),NEG(F3N),NEG(F4N),NEG(F5N),NEG(F6N),
        NEG(F7N),NEG(F8N),NEG(F9N),NEG(F10N));
L:=Ideal(NEG(F1N),NEG(F2),NEG(F3),NEG(F4N),NEG(F5),NEG(F6N),
        NEG(F7),NEG(F8),NEG(F9),NEG(F10N));
N:=Ideal(NEG(F1),NEG(F2N),NEG(F3),NEG(F4),NEG(F5N),NEG(F6),
        NEG(F7N),NEG(F8N),NEG(F9),NEG(F10N));
T:=Ideal(NEG(F1),NEG(F2),NEG(F3N),NEG(F4N),NEG(F5N),NEG(F6),
        NEG(F7N),NEG(F8),NEG(F9N),NEG(F10));
```

The severity of the diagnosis ($v[1]$, $v[2]$, $v[3]$ or $v[4]$) is determined using normal forms (denoted "NF"), that is a certain kind of polynomial reduction [7]. The output is 0 for exactly one of them (previously, a verification should take place; see [4] for details). For instance the answers of:

```
NF(NEG(v[1]),K+J+I);
NF(NEG(v[2]),K+J+I);
NF(NEG(v[3]),K+J+I);
NF(NEG(v[4]),K+J+I);
```

are, respectively: v[1]+1, v[2]+1, v[3]+1, 0. This means that for the facts in K, depression is non-existent.

Similarly, we obtain:

for ideal L: 0, v[2]+1, v[3]+1, v[4]+1
for ideal N: v[1]+1, v[2]+1, 0, v[4]+1
for ideal T: v[1]+1, 0, v[3]+1, v[4]+1

which means that, for the facts in L, N and T, depression is: severe, low and moderate, respectively.

4   Complete Approach and User Interface

As said in the introduction, a user Internet interface based on the HARD diagram has been developed. It calls a knowledge base far more complex than the one that illustrates this paper (but built using the methodology proposed here). It is freely available from the web page: **sidide.iespana.es/** (in Spanish).

5   Conclusions

A new methodology for diagnosis has been proposed. It consists of the following steps:

1) Assign propositional variables to factors, arrange the combinations of these variables (and their negations) in tables and assign in each table an intensity to each of these arrangements. This gives rise to the set of production rules (forming the knowledge base).
2) Introduce the ring A and the ideal I and enter the production rules and the potential facts into the CoCoA language.
3) Gröbner bases and normal forms are respectively used to check consistency and find diagnoses.

References

1. A. Capani and G. Niesi, *CoCoA User's Manual (v. 3.0b)* (Dept. of Mathematics University of Genova, Genova, 1996).   147
2. J. Chazarain, A. Riscos, J. A. Alonso and E. Briales, Multivalued Logic and Gröbner Bases with Applications to Modal Logic. *Journal of Symbolic Computation*, **11** (1991) 181-194.   149
3. G. González Páez, *Sistema Distribuido para el diagnóstico de la Depresión Utilizando CoCoA* (Ltd. Dissertation, Facultad de Informática, Universidad Politécnica de Madrid, 2001).   147
4. L. M. Laita, E. Roanes-Lozano, L. de Ledesma and J. A. Alonso, A Computer Algebra Approach to Verification and Deduction in Many-Valued Knowledge Systems. *Soft Computing* **3**-1 (1999) 7-19.   149, 150
5. P. Morand de Jouffrey, *La Depresión* (Acento Ed., Madrid, 1999).   147

6. E. Roanes-Lozano, L. M. Laita and E. Roanes-Macías, A Polynomial Model for Multivalued Logics with a Touch of Algebraic Geometry and Computer Algebra. *Mathematics and Computers in Simulation* **45**-1 (1998) 83-99. 149

7. W. W. Adams and P. Loustaunau, *An Introduction to Gröbner Bases*. Graduate Studies in Mathematics 3 (American Mathematical Society, Providence, RI, 1994). 150

An Expert System for Microbiological Data Validation and Surveillance

E. Lamma[1], P. Mello [2], A. Nanetti [3], G. Poli [4], F. Riguzzi [1], and S. Storari [1]

[1] Department of Engineering, University of Ferrara
Via Saragat 1, 44100 Ferrara, Italy
{elamma,friguzzi,sstorari}@ing.unife.it
[2] DEIS, University of Bologna,
Viale Risorgimento 2, 40136 Bologna, Italy
pmello@deis.unibo.it
[3] Clinical, Specialist and Experimental medicine department
Microbiology section, University of Bologna, Italy
ananetti@med.unibo.it
[4] DIANOEMA S.p.A.
Via de' Carracci 93, 40131 Bologna, Italy
gpoli@dianoema.it

Abstract. In this work, we describe a system for microbiological laboratory data validation and bacteria infections monitoring. In the following sections we report about the first results we have obtained with a prototype that adopts a knowledge-base approach for identifying critical situations and correspondingly issuing alarms. The knowledge base has been obtained from international standard guidelines for microbiological laboratory practice and from expert suggestions.

1 Introduction

The main goal of this work is to describe the design and the implementation of an Expert System for Microbiological Data Validation and Surveillance. For bacterial infections, stored data usually includes: information about the patient (sex, age, hospital unit where the patient has been admitted), the kind of material (specimen) to be analysed (e.g., blood, urine, saliva, pus, etc.) and its origin (the body part where the specimen was collected), the date when the specimen was collected (often substituted with the analysis request date) and, for every different bacterium identified, its species and its antibiogram. For each isolated bacterium, the antibiogram represents its resistance to a series of antibiotics [1] and it is usually represented by a vector of couples (antibiotics, resistance), where four types of resistance to antibiotics are possibly recorded: R when resistant, I when intermediate, S when susceptible, and null when unknown. The set of antibiotics to be tested can be defined by the user.

About microbiological data validation, the quality of antibiogram results is a critical point because clinicians use directly these results for therapy definition. Some

J. Crespo, V. Maojo, and F. Martin (Eds.): ISMDA 2001, LNCS 2199, pp. 153-160, 2001.

instruments execute intelligent controls on performed antibiotic test results but these controls are limited because they do not have information about specimen, patient characteristics and infection history. A system, capable of using all available information, may be a better support for laboratory personnel in the validation task. This system should also control the application of standard antibiotic testing guidelines: these guidelines, used by almost all microbiological laboratories, indicate antibiotic test execution methods and result interpretations. Examples of problems that this system should manage are: automatic correction of antibiotic results for particular species that present in vitro susceptibility but in vivo resistance, controls on the list of tested antibiotics, predictions of test results for a group of antibiotics using some representative antibiotics (ex. Tetracycline is representative for all tetracyclines), intelligent reporting.

The expert system presented in this work is able to provide automatic data validation performing a series of controls. Regarding bacteria infection monitoring, the system identifies critical situations for a single patient (e.g., unexpected antibiotic resistance of a bacterium) or for a hospital unit (e.g., contagion events) and alarms the microbiologist. The prototype adopts a knowledge-base approach to identify critical situations and correspondingly generate alarms. The knowledge base has been obtained from international standard guidelines for microbiological laboratory practice and from expert suggestions. Rules have been validated by laboratory experts and also by an automatic system that uses Data Mining techniques for automatic knowledge extraction [2].

In following sections, we describe the first results we have obtained in a testing trial on two-year real microbiological data.

2   Microbiological Surveillance Expert System

A Surveillance system may be realized using an Expert System programming approach. This Artificial Intelligence programming technique has been applied to the medical field since 1980. In an Expert System [3], also called Knowledge Based System (KBS), knowledge about the problem is translated into special data structures and rules. An inference engine applies these rules to the available data to perform some specific tasks.

Specifications and Features

Given a newly isolated bacterium and the related antibiogram, the system performs five main tasks: validates the culture results, reports the most suitable antibiotics list, issues alarms regarding the newly isolated bacterium, issues alarms regarding patient clinical situation and identifies potential epidemic events inside the hospital.

In the validation of culture results, the system finds antibiotics not tested but necessary, identifies impossible antibiotic results for particular species and tests common relations between antibiotic results.

In the intelligent reporting of antibiotics results, the system associates to each antibiotics a suitability, obtained considering some antibiotic characteristics: costs, infection site, bacteria specie and hospital ward.

In single analysis alarms, the system provides information regarding the bacteria (dangerous resistance, multiresistant bacteria, etc.).

In single patients alarms the system issues alarms considering the infection history of the patient. For example:

- **Polimicrobic population:** if two or more bacteria species where found in two different (consecutive) time points in the same sample material;
- **Resistance Acquisition:** if the newly identified bacteria has more antibiotic resistances than the last previous one of the same specie.

The system will also provide *information regarding the hospital ward* (contagion) and *epidemic breakout alarm*: the system architecture is ready but these controls are not implemented yet.

Knowledge elicitation

For knowledge elicitation we selected NCCLS [4], the international standard organization recognized by almost all laboratories as the reference in routinely work. NCCLS writes an annual compendium [5] containing testing guidelines for microbiological laboratories. NCCLS guidelines are basically composed, for each species, of: a table that specifies antibiotics to be tested, a table that specifies antibiotic test interpretation and a list of exceptions regarding particular antibiotic test results.

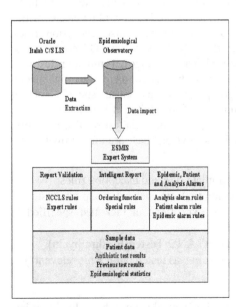

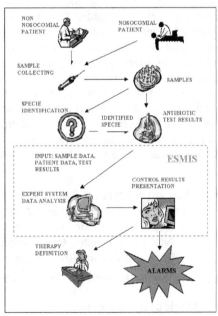

Fig.1 Databases and Data types   **Fig. 2** Control flow of the overall system

System Architecture

A laboratory information system called Italab C/S (developed by Dianoema S.p.A. an information technology company operating in the health care market) manages and stores all the information concerning patients, analysis requests and analysis results in an Oracle database and transfers in real-time microbiological data to a dedicated database called Epidemiological Observatory. Description of databases and data types are shown in figure 1. ESMIS will became part of the routinely laboratory result production process as described in figure 2. ESMIS introduces in the process the automatic validation step: in this step ESMIS presents the results of its controls to laboratory personnel that will decide to agree or disagree with them and to make, if necessary, changes on antibiotic test results. ESMIS also produces the final report and issues alarms regarding the patient clinical situation.

3   Implementation and First Prototype Description

We developed an ESMIS prototype using the Expert System Tool Kappa-PC 2.4 by Intellicorp [6] which offered a good cost/features degree and a simple and powerful programming language. Moreover, it works in interpreted and compiled mode and can perform both forward and backward chaining reasoning.

Knowledge Base

Since NCCLS compendium guidelines can change each year, ESMIS rules are designed as templates: rules are general and are dynamically instantiated referring to NCCLS table entries, so they can be updated with the last guidelines version by simply updating the table. Thus the problem of continuous knowledge update by qualified people is avoided since it is sufficient to update NCCLS table entries which are stored in an Oracle database. We have implemented also exception rules, representing particular cases not considered in NCCLS tables. Of course these exception rules need to be changed if the specific cases changes. Template rules work on a NCCLS table that specifies antibiotics to be tested on a specific species subdivided in: Main reporting antibiotic groups (basic, advanced, specific and for urinary tract infections), Antibiotic subgroups (antibiotics with similar characteristics) and Antibiotic equivalencies (antibiotics with the same bacteria test result). Examples of template and exception rules used in ESMIS knowledge base are the following:

- There are two types of Rack test rules: template rule and exception rules.
    - **Template rules** verify if at last one antibiotic from each subgroup was tested.
    - **Exception rules** are used to represent exceptions in rack test specified in NCCLS table notes. One example is:
        IF   **InfectionSite** = "Urinary Tract" AND **Tested**(Erythromycin)
        THEN   DisplayComment("Erythromycin was tested but it isn't relevant")

- Single analysis alarms
    -For implementing the Resistance Acquisition control we use the following rule:

Considering the patient infection history

IF   **SpeciesOfLastBacteria** = **BacteriaSpecies**(*IdentifiedBacteria*) **AND**
       ResistanceNumOfLastBacteria > **ResistanceNumOfNewBacteria**
THEN   **IssueAlarm**("Therapy is failed! Bacteria has increased the number of antibiotic resistances")

Graphical User Interface

In every medical software application, the system GUI is very important and needs particular attention. Laboratory personnel use ESMIS as a decision support system so the information provided must be simple, direct and self-explaining in order not to introduce a delay in the results production process. These objectives are obtained tuning the knowledge base and organizing the main window in a suitable manner.

4   Results of First ESMIS Testing Trial

Actually we have realized a prototype of ESMIS that contains knowledge regarding the *Staphylococcus* species and the *Enterobacteriaceae* species. The KB is composed of: 9 culture result validation template rules, 24 culture result validation exception rules for the *Staphylococcus* species, 29 culture result validation exception rules for the *Enterobacteriaceae* species, 8 single patient alarm rules and 6 single analysis alarms rules.

This prototype has been tested off-line on two-year culture results collected from the Clinical, Specialist and Experimental medicine department, Microbiology section of the University of Bologna (Italy). During these two years, another microbiological expert system was used for microbiological data validation. This system presents some problems: the knowledge base is "closed" and no change can be made on it, some controls were not implemented and must be manually executed by laboratory personnel and finally there are no clear descriptions about generated alarms.

ESMIS analysis results were compared with the previously adopted expert system. Even if data have been already validated, ESMIS was able to discover inconsistencies over data. Figure 3 shows ESMIS evaluation process results regarding a *Staffilococcus Aureus* bacterium:

REP.GRP.	ANTIBIOTIC	STRUM. RES.	ESMIS RES.	DER.	TO REPORT	RACK NOTE	VALID. NOTE	REPORT NOTE
C41	RIFAMPIN	S	S	no	no	--	--	N_REP1
B41	VACOMYCIN	S	S	no	*	--	--	--
B21	CLINDAMYCIN	R	R	no	*	--	--	--
B11	CLARITHROMYCIN	R	R	no	*	--	--	--
---	NETILMYCIN	S	>R<	no	*	N_RACK1	N_VALI1	--
A11	OXACILLIN	R	R	no	*	--	--	--
A21	PENICILLIN	R	R	no	*	--	--	--
B31	SULFA/TRIMETH	R	R	no	*	--	--	--
---	CLOXACILLIN	-	>R<	*	no	--	--	N_REP2
---	DICLOXACILLIN	-	>R<	*	no	--	--	N_REP3

Fig.3 Antibiogram results after ESMIS evaluation

For each alarm there is an associated note explaining the name of the rule applied and its description. Please notice that in Figure 3, an inconsistency arises between NETILMYCIN (belonging to the AMINOGLYCOSIDE antibiotic group) and OXACILLIN. The validation note about this inconsistency is N_VALI1:

```
VALIDATION NOTE: N_VALI1 --> 1: ( Vali_Stafi_23_5)
     If OXACILLIN test result is Resistance (R) then test results for
AMINOGLYCOSIDE should be Resistance too. The expected test result is R.
```

Beside data validation, further objectives achieved by ESMIS are:

1. **Flexibility:** ESMIS knowledge base is mainly composed by rules obtained by NCCLS international guidelines. These rules are not always recognized as correct and sometimes personalization are needed to adapt the control to the local environment. The expert has easily applied his personalization and has made ESMIS better tailored to the local situation.

2. **Clarity:** Now, only the description of issued alarms (customizable by the laboratory expert) is showed, allowing a simpler problem identification. For every validation step, the evolution of reasoning is also shown.

3. **Intelligent reporting:**   the intelligent reporting features of ESMIS was recognized by experts as one of the most important innovation. For each bacteria, only the antibiotic results of less dangerous antibiotics (to which the bacterium is susceptible) must be presented in the final report. The expert may customize the final report and guide therapy definition by creating appropriate reporting rules. The reporting note for RIFAMPIN antibiotic, presented in Fig.3, is N_REP1:

```
REPORTING NOTE:  N_REP1 --> 1: ( Ref_Stafi_29)
Antibiotics belonging to Group C and U should be presented in the
final report only if the infection location is Urinary tract.
```

4. **Contagion alarms:** ESMIS has found some possible contagion events by analyzing the culture results of some patients. The laboratory expert has analyzed these alarms and recognized that these events need further investigation.

5. **Patient infection surveillance:** for each patient, culture results are compared with the previous ones on the same patient and alarms regarding possible dangerous bacteria mutations and infection evolutions are issued.   Experts recognize that these alarms may be useful for supporting therapy control.

6. **Performance:** In real-time analysis simulation the first ESMIS prototype has evaluated each antibiogram in 33 second and this performance is compatible with the normal production process of analysis results.

5   Related Work

During the last few years, many surveillance systems have been developed in order to monitor microbiological analysis results and to early identify infection and epidemiological events. All these systems have peculiar features that make them not suitable for efficient and correct analysis of Italian data. Significant examples of these systems are WHONET 5 [7], GermWatcher [8] and TheraTrac 2 [9]. WHONET 5 is a database software for the management of microbiology laboratory test results.

GermWatcher is an expert system, which applies both local and international culture-based criteria for detecting potential nosocomial infections. TheraTrac 2 is a system for microbiological data validation and real-time alarming. It directly interacts with Vitek [10] an expert system for test results validation, that is integrated in particular analytical instruments. All systems use international standard guidelines in order to defining controls to be executed on laboratory test results. WHONET is an off-line tool useful for medium and long term data analysis but it is not suitable for real-time monitoring and alarm generation. GermWatcher works on-line but in order to work correctly needs a lot of data not available in Italy. TheraTrac 2 works on-line but is designed for USA hospital organization (focused on pharmacists) that is different from Italian hospital organization.

In the past, DEIS University of Bologna and Dianoema S.p.A. have designed and implemented an expert system for the validation of biochemical analysis [11].

6   Conclusions and Future Work

In this paper we have described a system for microbiological laboratory data validation and bacteria infections monitoring. We also described the first results we have obtained with a prototype that adopts a knowledge-base approach to identify critical situations and to correspondingly issue alarms. Expert system technology gives the following advantages to our system: knowledge base easy update (thanks to template rules), quality of service, clarity and flexibility. In [2] we have also experimented automatic knowledge validation and extraction of ESMIS rules by using Data Mining techniques.

In the future we plan to further develop our system by identifying the final tool for ESMIS implementation, by extending ESMIS knowledge base and by integrating the system with datamining techniques and time series analysis.

Acknowledgements

We are grateful to Leonardo Maestrami for his help in the ESMIS implementation and to MURST [12] (project 23204/DSPAR/99) that has partially supported this project.

References

1.   A.Balows, W.J.Hauser,Jr, K.L.Herrmann, H.D.Isenberg, H.J.Shadomy, *Manual of Clinical Microbiology*, 5°Ed, American Society for Microbiology, Washington, 1991
2.   E.Lamma, M.Manservigi, P.Mello, A.Nanetti, F.Riguzzi, S.Storari, *The Automatic Discovery of Alarm Rules for the Validation of Microbiological Data*, IDAMAP2001, London, UK
3.   M. Stefik, *Introduction to knowledge systems*, Morgan Kaufmann, 1995

4. National Committee for Clinical Laboratory Standards (NCCLS), www.nccls.org, Accessed 10 July 2001
5. NCCLS, Performance Standards for Antimicrobial Susceptibility Testing; Ninth Informational Supplement, M100-S9 Vol. 19 No. 1, January 1999
6. Intellicorp, Inc., http://www.intellicorp.com, Accessed 10 July 2001
7. World Health Organization, WHONET 5 – Microbiology Laboratory Database Software, WHO/CDS/CSR/DRS/99.1
8. M.G.Kahn, S.A.Steib, V.J.Fraser, W.C.Dunghan, *An Expert System for Culture-Based Infection control Surveillance*, Washington University, 1992
9. Theratrac, Biomerieux, http://www.theratrac.com, Accessed 10 July 2001
10. Vitek, Biomerieux, http://www.biomerieux.com, Accessed 10 July 2001
11. M.Boari, E.Lamma, P.Mello, S.Storari, S.Monesi, *An Expert System Approach for Clinical Analysis Result Validation*, ICAI 2000,Las Vegas, Nevada, USA
12. Ministero dell'università e della ricerca scientifica e tecnologica, www.murst.it, Accessed 30 June 2001

Hierarchical Clustering of Female Urinary Incontinence Data Having Noise and Outliers

Jorma Laurikkala and Martti Juhola

[1] Department of Computer and Information Sciences,
33014 University of Tampere, Finland
{jpl,mj}@cs.uta.fi

Abstract. We studied pre-processing of a female urinary incontinence data set by removing uninformative variables, outliers, and noise, to allow hierarchical clustering methods to find partitions that resemble the diagnostic classes. Outliers were identified with box plots and Mahalanobis distances, while noisy cases were detected with the repeated edited nearest neighbor rule. The cleaned data were analyzed with six clustering methods. The best results, as measured with Fowlkes and Mallows similarity measure, were achieved with complete linkage (0.90) and Ward's method (0.84). These methods managed to separate the two largest diagnostic classes, stress and mixed incontinence, from each other. Unfortunately, single linkage, average linkage, centroid, and median methods were not able to differentiate between these classes. The results are in accord with our earlier results indicating that supervised methods suit better for classification of this data than cluster analysis. However, outliers, noise, and clusters, which were identified, may be of interest to expert physicians.

1   Introduction

We extend our previous work [1,2] concerning the cluster analysis of the female urinary incontinence data. We have studied earlier [1] this data with the k-means clustering method and recently a number of hierarchical clustering methods were applied to the extended data set [2]. The results of the k-means cluster analysis showed that the data contained clusters dominated by the five most frequent diagnostic classes.

In the later work, analyses with supervised multivariate statistical methods and machine learning techniques [2,3] have shown that the data can be assigned accurately into the diagnostic classes on the basis of the diagnostic parameters. However, in [2] the hierarchical cluster analysis [4-6] could not establish partitions which would correspond to the five diagnostic classes. Only normal patients, i.e. the continent women, could be identified, while the rest of the data were placed into a huge cluster, dominated by the two largest diagnostic groups, and into small splinter groups.

Medical knowledge suggests that one reason for the poor performance of the clustering methods is the overlapping class boundaries. For example, there is a diagnostic

J. Crespo, V. Maojo, and F. Martin (Eds.): ISMDA 2001, LNCS 2199, pp. 161-167, 2001.
© Springer-Verlag Berlin Heidelberg 2001

class, mixed female urinary incontinence, for patients who have both stress symptoms and symptoms of urgency. Another difficulty is uninformative variables, outliers, and noise which often cause problems both for statistical and machine learning methods. As an unsupervised method, cluster analysis is especially sensitive for these problematic aspects of data, which are common in the real-world data sets. Therefore, if possible, the data is often pre-processed before applying cluster analysis [4-6].

We studied here whether data pre-processing would allow us to find data partitions that resemble more the diagnostic groups than partitions in our previous work. Especially, we were interested in how the two largest diagnostic groups, stress and mixed incontinence, could be separated from each other after pre-processing. Variable set was reduced by using the results in [2]. Since in [7] we found that there were suspicious cases in our data set, the data were reduced by removing outliers. In addition, noisy cases, which were identified with the repeated edited nearest neighbor method [8], were excluded from the data.

2   Materials and Methods

The female urinary incontinence data (N=529), which were collected in the Department of Obstetrics and Gynaecology of Kuopio University Hospital, Finland, consist of the stress, mixed, sensory urge and motor urge incontinence cases and of the continent women (Table 1). The missing values due to the retrospective data collection were filled in with the Expectation-Maximization method as in [2].

The original variable set had 16 variables and 11 of them were processed with the logistic regression analysis and clustering methods in [2]. Variables that are unrelated to the clusters are known to produce decrements in the ability of clustering methods to recover clusters [4,6]. In [2] logistic regression analysis identified 8 of the 11 independent variables as statistically significant ($p<0.05$) in relation to the diagnoses. For this reason, we used these variables, instead of the 11 variables, in this study.

Outliers [9] are observations which appear to be inconsistent with the remainder of the data. Human error often produces unintentional outliers. Outliers are also frequently generated as the result of the natural variation of population or process one cannot control [9]. There are two types of outliers. Univariate outliers are extreme data values of distribution of an individual variable (or attribute). Multivariate outliers are cases (or examples) which have unusual value combinations. Multivariate outliers have sometimes univariate outlier values. However, multivariate outliers are not necessarily outliers in univariate sense, because unusual combinations of normal values may cause a case to be a multivariate outlier.

Quinlan defines *noise* as mislabeled examples (class noise) or errors in the values of attributes (attribute noise) [10 pp. 92]. Outlier is a broader concept than noise, because it includes errors, as well as discordant data produced by the natural variation of population. Examples with class noise are outliers produced by sampling error, while attribute noise may or may not show in the data as outlying values.

Some clustering methods perform well in presence of outliers and noise, but often these data pose a problem to clustering methods [4,6]. For example, of the hierarchical methods, the single linkage method suffers from chaining. The method may fail to identify distinct clusters, if there are a few intermediate observations (noise) between them. Another example is the well-known *k*-means method which is extremely sensitive to outliers and noise, when random starting points are used.

Multivariate outliers and cases with the most univariate outlier values were identified within the diagnostic groups with an informal method that utilizes box plots and Mahalanobis distances [7]. Repeated Edited Nearest Neighbor rule (RENN) [11 pp. 267] was used to drop noise from the data. Wilson's ENN algorithm [8,11] removes cases whose class label differs from the class label of the majority of three nearest neighbors. RENN repeats the ENN algorithm until no cases are removed from data [11]. Heterogeneous value difference metric [12] was used as the distance measure.

Table 1 shows the frequencies of the original (T) and reduced data (S_1, S_2, and S_3). Also, frequencies of the outliers (O) and noisy cases (N) are shown. The first reduced data set S_1, was produced by removing 55 outlier cases (10.4%) from T. Total of 88 noisy cases (16.6%) were excluded from T to create the reduced data set S_2. The union of outliers and noisy cases (112, 21.2% of T) were dropped from T to produce the third reduced set S_3. In R 27.7% of the cases were both outliers and noisy.

Table 1. Frequencies of the diagnoses in the original (T) data set and reduced data sets S_1, S_2, and S_3 created by removing outliers (O), noise (N) and the union of outliers and noise ($R=O \cup N$) from T, respectively

Diagnosis	T	S_1	O	S_2	N	S_3	R
Stress	323	291	32	299	24	279	44
Mixed	140	123	17	112	28	109	31
Sensory urge	33	31	2	9	24	9	24
Motor urge	15	12	3	3	12	3	12
Normal	18	17	1	18	0	17	1
Sum	529	474	55	441	88	417	112

We applied hierarchical agglomerative clustering methods which start from the first partition P_n, which contains n single-member clusters, and generate a series of partitions $P_n, P_{n-1}, ..., P_1$ of the data by fusing clusters. The last partition P_1 consists of all n objects [4-6]. The analyses were performed with the statistical software package SPSS for Windows 10. Comparative research has shown that the performance of a clustering method depends on the data to be partitioned [4]. A number of clustering methods should be used to avoid overly optimistic or pessimistic inferences based on the results of a single method [4-6]. Therefore, the female urinary incontinence data were partitioned as in [2] using the single linkage, complete linkage, average linkage, centroid, median, and Ward's clustering methods.

3   Results

Data sets were standardized before applying cluster analyses with the squared Euclidean distance. The dendrograms (or trees) were cut at level of five to allow the comparison of the classes and partitions. Fowlkes and Mallows B_k measure [4,5,13] was used to assess the similarity between two partitions of data both having k clusters (B_k ? [0,1]). B_5 measures for the hierarchical clustering methods are shown in Table 2.

Table 2. Fowlkes and Mallows B_5 similarity measure values between the diagnostic classes and cluster partitions in the earlier work [2], the original (T) and reduced (S_1, S_2, and S_3) data sets

Method	[2]	T	S_1	S_2	S_3
Single linkage	0.68	0.70	0.72	0.75	0.77
Complete linkage	0.59	0.79	0.56	0.84	0.90
Average linkage	0.70	0.70	0.74	0.75	0.78
Centroid	0.70	0.69	0.74	0.76	0.77
Median	0.68	0.70	0.74	0.70	0.80
Ward	0.70	0.66	0.78	0.77	0.84
Mean	0.68	0.71	0.71	0.76	0.81

Dropping of the three uninformative variables increased similarity measures slightly for all methods, except for the centroid and Ward's methods, in comparison with our earlier results with 11 variables [2]. In comparison with the original data T, outlier removal increased similarity measures slightly for all methods, except complete linkage, whose B_5 value decreased unexpectedly from 0.79 to 0.56. On the other hand, excluding noisy cases increased similarities for all the methods.

Clear increase in similarity values, in comparison with the results of T, were obtained when both outliers and noisy cases were discarded. To validate this result, we created 10 reduced data sets by removing randomly 20% of cases from the original data. Then, the 10 data sets were clustered and B_5 values were calculated. Mean of these values was 0.69, range 0.46-0.76, and standard deviation 0.05.

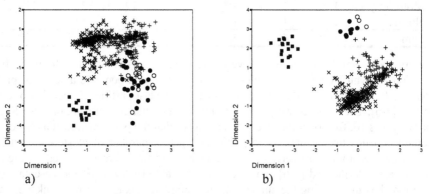

a)   b)

Fig. 1. Scatter plot of principal component analysis scores for a) original and b) reduced data. x = Stress, + = mixed, • = sensory urge, and o = motor urge incontinence. ? = normal

In addition to cluster analysis, we performed a linear principal component analysis with the standardized data, to provide two-dimensional views of the data sets. Fig. 1 a) shows the scatter plot of the first two eigenvalues, which accounted approximately for 54% of the total variance, for the original data. Fig. 1 b) presents a scatter plot for the reduced data set S_3. The first two eigenvalues accounted for 59% of the total variance.

4   Discussion

Data pre-processing of the female urinary incontinence data with variable, outlier, and noise removal allowed the hierarchical clustering methods to produce partitions that were more similar to the diagnostic groups than partitions found in our previous work [2]. Exclusion of uninformative variables improved the results slightly in comparison to the larger set of variables. Dropping of outliers and noisy cases gave slightly better results than the results obtained with the reduced variable set. Clear improvement was obtained with data set S_3 from which uninformative variables, outliers, and noisy cases were removed (Table 2).

However, the main problem, overlapping of the stress and mixed incontinence classes, was not solved decisively. Only complete linkage and Ward's method were able to clearly separate these groups from each other in the data set S_3. Other methods performed almost the same way as the single linkage method which assigned practically all of the stress and mixed incontinence cases into the same cluster.

Fig. 1 a) illustrates why the hierarchical clustering methods had difficulties in finding the diagnostic classes. The scatter plot shows that in the original data there is a large group, which contains the incontinent women, and a group for the normal patients. The larger group has two centers made of the stress and mixed urinary incontinence cases which overlap extensively. The scatter plot in Fig. 1 b) presents the data set S_3. As expected, the diagnostic groups are more distinct after cleaning of the data. Outlier removal has cleaned the data by dropping unusual cases within groups, while the RENN rule has removed noise. Although the decision borders were widened, there are still stress and mixed incontinence cases that occupy the same area. The normal cases have moved farther away from the other groups.

A large number of cases (21.2% of the original data) were removed to produce reduced set S_3, and, unfortunately, most of the sensory and motor urge cases were lost during the cleaning process. For this reason, we produced an additional reduced data set S_4 so that outliers were removed from all the classes, while noise was removed only from the two largest groups. The results were mostly only slightly lower than results obtained in the reduced set S_3 (mean of B_5 values was 0.78 and range 0.72-0.92). However, a large portion of the sensory and motor urge cases was often placed in the same cluster with the stress and mixed incontinence cases.

In [1] we applied k-means cluster analysis with initial values, while in [2] and the current study, hierarchical methods were used, because these methods are more objective than optimizing methods. In contrast to hierarchical clustering, optimizing methods try to produce a partition with a certain number of clusters, which is as good as possible, with respect to some numerical criterion. For comparison with the hierarchical cluster analyses, data sets S_3 and S_4 were analyzed with the k-means method using the means of diagnostic groups as the initial values. B_5 similarity values were 0.94 and 0.90, respectively. As expected, these values were higher than those of the hierarchical cluster methods, whose mean B_5 values with these data sets were 0.81 and 0.78, respectively.

It must be noted, that although the cluster analysis methods process data in an unsupervised manner, we had the class labels available for the data pre-processing methods. This is naturally a limitation. When class information is unavailable, other methods, such as graphical presentations of the data derived from the raw data may be useful aids for pre-processing of data [4-6]. Derived data may also be the actual input to the clustering. We applied in this work the linear principal component analysis only to visualize data.

The aim of cluster analysis in our earlier work [1,2] was to explore how the data could be classified using the diagnostic parameters alone. The results of the present study are better than previous results in [2]. However, the results are in accord with other earlier results in [2,3] where supervised statistical and machine learning methods outperformed both the hierarchical methods and k-means cluster analysis. For these reasons, we will use also in future supervised methods to build classifiers for computer-aided diagnosis of female urinary incontinence [3]. However, outliers and noise that were identified, as well as the clusters obtained from the cleaned data, may be of interest to the expert physicians. Future research should focus more on exploring the data. For example, identifying the optimal number of clusters or clustering within the diagnostic groups might give additional insight into the data.

References

1. Laurikkala, J., Juhola, M., Penttinen, J., Aukee P.: Parameter Evaluation of the Differential Diagnosis of Female Urinary Incontinence for the Construction of an Expert System. In: Pappas, C., Maglaveras, N., Scherrer J.-R., (eds.): Medical Informatics Europe'97. Studies in Health Technology and Informatics, Vol. 43. IOS Press, Amsterdam (1997) 671-675
2. Laurikkala, J., Juhola, M., Lammi, S., Penttinen, J., Aukee, P.: Analysis of the Imputed Female Urinary Incontinence Data for the Evaluation of Expert System Parameters. Comput. Biol. Med. 31 (2001) 239-257
3. Laurikkala, J., Juhola, M., Lammi, S., Viikki, K.: A Comparison of Genetic Algorithms and Different Classification Methods in the Diagnosis of Female Urinary Incontinence. Methods Inf. Med. 38 (1999) 125-131
4. Everitt, B.S.: Cluster Analysis. Wiley, London (1993)
5. Jain, J.K., Dubes, R.C.: Algorithms for Clustering Data. Prentice-Hall, New Jersey (1988)
6. Sharma, S.: Applied Multivariate Techniques. Wiley, New York (1996)
7. Laurikkala, J., Juhola, M., Kentala, E.: Informal Identification of Outliers in Medical Data. In: Lavrac, N., Miksch, S., Kavsek, B., (eds.): The Fifth Workshop on Intelligent Data Analysis in Medicine and Pharmacology (IDAMAP'2000), Berlin (2000) 20-24
8. Wilson, D.L.: Asymptotic Properties on Nearest Neighbor Rules Using Edited Data. IEEE Trans. Syst. Man. Cybern. 2 (1972) 408-421
9. Barnett, V., Lewis, T.: Outliers in Statistical Data. 2nd edn. Wiley, Norwich (1987)
10. Quinlan, J.R.: Induction of Decision Trees. Mach. Learn. 1 (1986) 81-106
11. Wilson, R.D., Martinez, T.R.: Reduction Techniques for Instance-based Learning Algorithms. Mach. Learn. 38 (2000) 257-286

12. Wilson, R.D., Martinez, T.R.: Improved Heterogeneous Distance Functions. J. Artif. Intell. Res. 6 (1997) 1-34
13. Fowlkes, E.B., Mallows, C.L.: A Method for Comparing Two Hierarchical Clusterings. J. Am. Stat. A. 78 (1983) 553-568

ACMD: A Practical Tool for Automatic Neural Net Based Learning

Roland Linder and Siegfried J. Pöppl

Institute for Medical Informatics, Medical University of Luebeck
Ratzeburger Allee 160, D-23538 Luebeck

Abstract. Although neural networks have many appealing properties, yet there is neither a systematic way how to set up the topology of a neural network nor how to determine its various learning parameters. Thus an expert is needed for fine tuning. If neural network applications should not be realisable only for publications but in real life, fine tuning must become unnecessary. We developed a tool called ACMD (Approximation and Classification of Medical Data) that is demonstrated to fulfil this demand. Moreover referring to six medical classification and approximation problems of the PROBEN1 benchmark collection this approach will be shown even to outperform fine tuned networks.

1   Introduction

For applications in medicine multilayer perceptrons (MLP) trained by the backpropagation algorithm [1] are most popular. Despite the general success of backpropagation in learning neural networks several deficiencies are still needed to be solved. Learning can be trapped into local minima, the training process does converge slowly, and there are difficulties in explaining the network's response. Since 1986 when Rumelhart et al. had "re-invented" backpropagation, various coping strategies have been published [2]. Some of these strategies will be presented in this paper, existing ones as well as newly developed approaches. But the most apparent disadvantage is that the convergence behaviour depends very much on the choice of the network topology and diverse parameters in the algorithm such as the learning rate and the momentum. Therefore the presence of an expert seems to be absolutely necessary when training backpropagation networks. The need for fine tuning may be the greatest obstacle for a wide-spread use of neural network techniques in medicine.

Attempts in designing at least the network structure automatically have been undertaken by various constructive algorithms [3] that can be roughly divided into dynamic node creation [4] and cascade correlation [5]. These algorithms build up the network dynamically. Assuming the future availability of hard-coded neural networks the automatic training of a fixed network architecture remains highly desirable.

Therefore we will present an approach called ACMD (Approximation and Classification of Medical Data) that mainly relies on an expanded version of a multi-neural-

J. Crespo, V. Maojo, and F. Martin (Eds.): ISMDA 2001, LNCS 2199, pp. 168-173, 2001.

network architecture by Anand et al. [6] in connection with *adaptive propagation* [7], an improvement of the backpropagation algorithm. This network can be trained without any fine tuning. Its performance will be demonstrated by solving five medical multiclass classification problems and one medical approximation problem. These problems are part of the established PROBEN1 benchmark collection from Prechelt [8]. Moreover we will prove the usefulness of an ensemble of multi-neural-networks.

2   Methods

For purposes of more clarity, strategies for improving the generalisation performance will be separately listed from those accelerating the convergence speed. Naturally overlapping can not be avoided. Due to the lack of space we will restrict to the most important strategies.

2.1   Strategies for Improving the Generalisation Performance

For the classification tasks we used a modular network architecture similar to that published by Anand et al. [6], reducing a k-class problem to a set of k two-class problems and training a neural network module for each two-class problem. Differently from Anand et al. the a-priori probabilities of each class were taken into account by feeding a further MLP with the outputs of the modules.

In order to avoid so-called *overfitting* we used *early stopping* terminating the learning phase after a predefined number of epochs (1000). Afterwards the test set performance was computed for that state of the network which had the minimum validation set error during the training process.

Most often in medicine there is only a small amount of data available. In order not to waste valuable data we suggest to make use of a network ensemble consisting of five multi-neural-networks as described above. So all training data have to be divided into five equally sized sets A to E. The first multi-neural-network will be trained by set A, B, C, and D. Set E will serve as a validation set. Training the second multi-neural-network, the training set consists of set A, B, C, and E, set D will be the validation set and so on. To get one common result for each class, the output activities of the five multi-neural-networks can be averaged. It is appropriate to neglect the minimum and maximum output value (in case that one of the multi-neural-networks fails). The mean value will be calculated only averaging the three remaining output activities.

As a quick alternative to slow standard backpropagation and its known derivates we developed an algorithm called *adaptive propagation* (APROP), useful not only to accelerate the convergence speed but also for improving the generalisation performance. APROP prefers adapting those weights that lead to successful neurons. The success of a neuron is defined by the amount and the distribution of its δ-errors. For a detailed description and benchmarking please refer to [7].

In medicine there are frequently different prior class probabilities. In order to take also small classes into account sufficiently, we suggest a modified error function (squared δ-errors of the output neurons with keeping their sign):

$$\delta_{output\ layer} = f'(activation\ function) \cdot sign(t - o) \cdot (t - o)^2 \qquad (1)$$

$\delta_{output\ layer}$ designates the error δ of an output neuron, t denotes the target output, and o the real output. The effectiveness of this modification was examined in [9].

In accordance with the *generalised back-propagation algorithm* by Ng et al. [10] we propose to square the derivation of the activation function so as to improve the convergence by preventing the error signal to be dropped to a very small value.

2.2   Strategies for Accelerating the Convergence Speed

It is well known that a fast convergence speed can be achieved by oversizing the network structure. However most researchers follow the spirit of Occam's razor and choose the smallest admissible size that will provide a solution, because in their opinion the simplest architecture is the best for generalisation. Notwithstanding several neural net empiricists have published papers showing that surprisingly good generalisation can in fact be achieved with oversized multilayer networks. From our experience oversizing the network architecture leads to a dramatic increase of convergence speed as well as to an improved generalisation performance (assuming early stopping). In the following a network will be chosen that comprises only one hidden layer (facilitating rule extraction later on) but 100 hidden neurons.

On the side, oversized networks guarantee a sufficient approximation capacity when learning different classification tasks of varying complexity using always the same number of hidden neurons (as we do, see Chapter 3).

The APROP algorithm is ideally suited for oversized networks. When compared to algorithms like RPROP, Vario-Eta, or Quasi-Newton techniques [7] APROP could save up to three-quarters of learning time needed by the other algorithms.

In order to save learning time, we suggest to stop training after a predefined number of oscillating epochs in the generalisation curve - e.g. ten epochs - or after a maximum number of epochs leading to no further decrease of the validation set error, say 100 epochs at a total amount of 1000 learning epochs.

3   Implementation and Benchmarks

ACMD was implemented as a prototype using the programming language MS Visual C++ 6.0 SP 4 and a Pentium III-1000 DP. Because C++ is not very comfortable in programming the graphical user interface, MS Visual Basic was used for creating the GUI, calling C++ DLLs that contain the actual neural network code. The compiler settings were optimised for speed, the multithreaded code was optimised by an extensive use of pointers, small dimensioned arrays, avoidance of if-statements or consecutive instructions that hamper pipelining. Also an approximation of the exponential function proposed by Schraudolph [11] has been proved to speed up calculation.

ACMD was realised as already suggested in Chapter 2. All experience was gained by evaluating signals from an electronic nose [9]. None of our suggestions was influenced by the benchmarks presented here. Otherwise our results might have been distorted. As the only pre-processing data were z-transformed. Carefully all weights were initialised randomly within an interval of [-0.01, +0.01]. As activation function for the hidden neurons a hyperbolic tangent was employed. Its advantage over the standard logistic sigmoid function is the symmetry of its outputs with respect to null. The standard logistic sigmoid function was used for the output neurons. There were no short-cut connections in order not to disturb the building up of an internal hierarchy. Learning was performed as batch learning. After the second epoch, a momentum term was utilised with a momentum factor μ set at 0.9. The global learning rate was set at 0.1. As pre-tests demonstrated there was no need to start several runs from different weight initialisation. Thus only two runs where done per benchmark: the first one used all data excluding the test data and employed a network ensemble. The second one used exactly the same learning set, validation set, and test set as demanded for the benchmark.

The performance was tested by solving five multiclass classification problems and one medical approximation problem of the standardised PROBEN1 benchmark collection from Prechelt [8]. These six of thirteen benchmarks are those that refer to real medical classification tasks:

cancer: Diagnosis of breast cancer.
diabetes: Diagnosis of diabetes of Pima Indians.
gene: Detection of intron / exon boundaries (slice junctions) in nucleotide sequences.
heartc: Prediction of heart disease.
thyroid: Diagnosis of thyroid hyper- or hypofunction.
heartac: Differently from *heartc* the benchmark *heartac* uses a single continuous output that represents the number of vessels that are reduced.

Table 1 gives an overview of the number of inputs, outputs, and examples available. The data sets contain binary inputs as well as continuous ones. For each dataset the total amount of examples was divided into three partitions: a learning set (50%), a validation set (25%), and a test set (25%). For each benchmark PROBEN1 contains three different permutations, which differ only in the ordering of examples, e.g. *cancer1*, *cancer2*, and *cancer3*.

Table 1. Properties of the benchmarks used

Benchmark	cancer	diabetes	gene	heartc	thyroid
Inputs	9	8	120	35	21
Outputs	2	2	3	2	3
Examples	699	768	3175	303	7200

As fine tuning for each problem, Prechelt used 12 different MLP topologies (comprising 2, 4, 8, 16, 24, 32, 2+2, 4+2, 4+4, 8+4, 8+8, and 16+8 hidden nodes), experimented with linear output nodes and those using the sigmoid activation function, and he proved shortcut connections to be effective or not. For each benchmark Prechelt chose the architecture achieving the smallest validation set error. For a detailed description of architecture and learning parameters please refer to [8]. As classification method *winner-takes-all* was used, i.e. the output with the highest activation designates the class. For the approximation tasks Prechelt defined a *squared error percentage* that is similar to the MSE.

4   Results

Using the proposed network ensemble the percentages of misclassifications and the squared error percentages were significantly smaller than those of the manually designed MLP by Prechelt (Wilcoxon signed ranks test over all 18 results, p=0.026). Without ensemble and thus using the same learning set, validation set, and test set as Prechelt did, our results were also significantly better than the results by Prechelt's fine tuned MLP (same significance value p=0.026), see Table 2.

Table 2. Comparison of the percentages of misclassification or the squared error percentages

Benchmark	Tuned by Prechelt	With ensemble	Without ensemble
cancer1	1.38	2.30	2.87
cancer2	4.77	4.02	4.02
cancer3	3.70	4.02	4.02
diabetes1	24.10	23.44	23.44
diabetes2	26.42	22.92	24.48
diabetes3	22.59	21.53	22.40
gene1	16.67	11.48	11.48
gene2	18.41	8.45	8.95
gene3	21.82	10.34	11.22
heartc1	20.82	17.33	17.33
heartc2	5.13	6.67	4.00
heartc3	15.40	12.00	14.67
thyroid1	2.38	1.83	6.00
thyroid2	1.86	1.67	1.67
thyroid3	2.09	2.39	2.28
heartac1	2.47	2.29	2.26
heartac2	4.41	3.04	3.06
heartac3	5.37	3.78	4.05

5   Conclusions

The aim was to develop an universal approach that makes fine tuning unnecessary. Contrary to expectation this approach could be shown not only to achieve the same generalisation performance as Prechelt did when manually designing his MLP, but even to outperform his results in a statistically significant way. Due to the small number of output neurons needed for the benchmarks used above, the multi-neural-network approach might be even more promising for classification tasks comprising more classes. In our opinion oversizing the networks combined with early stopping is the key for these encouraging results. Also Prechelt himself speculates that more than 32 hidden neurons (the maximum number he used) may produce superior results [8].

In future we will have to evaluate our results using further benchmarks and to analyse the effectiveness of each strategy in detail. Moreover we will add missing values strategies, feature selection, and some kind of knowledge extraction. When implemented all this in an intuitively applicable fashion, ACMD will be made accessible via the internet and hopefully the basis will be done for a wide-spread use of neural network technique in numerous medical fields.

References

1. Rumelhart, D. E., Hinton, G. E., & Williams, R. J.: Learning Representations by Back-Propagating Errors. Nature 323 (1986) 533-536
2. Orr, G. B., Müller, K.-R. (eds.): Neural Networks: Tricks of the Trade. Lecture Notes in Computer Science, Vol. 1524. Springer-Verlag, Berlin Heidelberg New York (1998)
3. Kwok, T.Y., Yeung, D.Y.: Constructive algorithms for structure learning in feed forward neural networks for regression problems. IEEE Trans. on Neural Networks 8(3) (1997) 630-645
4. Ash, T.: Dynamic node creation in backpropagation networks. Connection Science 1(4) (1989) 365-375
5. Fahlman, S.E., Lebiere, C.: The cascade-correlation learning architecture. In: Touretzky, D.S. (ed.): Advances in Neural Information Processing Systems 2, Morgan Kaufmann, CA (1990) 524-532
6. Anand, R., Mehrotra, K., Mohan, C.K., Ranka, S.: Efficient Classification for Multiclass Problems Using Modular Neural Networks. IEEE Trans. on Neural Networks. 6(1) (1995) 117-124
7. Linder, R., Wirtz, S., Pöppl, S.J.: Speeding up Backpropagation Learning by the APROP Algorithm. Second International ICSC Symposium on Neural Computation, Proceedings CD, Berlin (2000).
8. Prechelt, L.: Proben 1 – a set of neural network benchmark problems and benchmarking rules. Technical Report 21/94, Fakultät für Informatik, Universität Karlsruhe. Available via ftp.ira.uka.de in directory /pub/papers/techreports/1994 as file 1994-21.ps.Z. (1994)
9. Linder, R., Pöppl, S.J.: Backprop, RPROP, APROP: Searching for the best learning rule for an electronic nose. Neural Networks in Applications '99. In: Proc. of the Fourth International Workshop, Magdeburg, Germany, (1999) 69-74
10. Ng, S.C., Leung, S.H., Lik, A.: Fast Convergent Generalized Back-Propagation Algorithm with Constant Learning Rate. Neural Processing Letters 9 (1999) 13-23
11. Schraudolph, N.N.: A Fast, Compact Approximation of the Exponential Function. Neural Computation 11 (1999) 853-862

Development of a Mammographic Analysis System Using Computer Vision Techniques

J. Martí[1], P. Planiol[1], J. Freixenet[1], J. Español[2], and E. Golobardes[3]

[1] University of Girona. Computer Vision and Robotics Group - IIiA
Campus de Montilivi, 17071. Girona
{joanm,planiol,jordif}@eia.udg.es

[2] University Hospital of Girona "Dr. Josep Trueta". Department of Oncology
Avda. de França s/n, 17071 Girona
jespanyol@bsab.com

[3] Universitat Ramon Llull. Computer Science Department
Passeig Bonanova, 8 08022 Barcelona
elisabet@salleURL.edu

Abstract. This work presents an application intended to work as a second reader in Radiology Services for digital mammograms, which makes use of several Computer Vision algorithms. Although the presented prototype basically focuses on the detection and the characterization of microcalcifications, the system has the capability to grow up by adding new abnormalities (e.g. masses) or new classification patterns. Experimental results of the system's performance have been obtained through digital mammograms of the Regional Health Area of Girona.

1 Introduction

Breast cancer is one of the most extended among women in the western society. Although its behaviour depends on every country, the statistics shows that there are more than 700.000 new cases over the world per year, which about 20% turns into malign tumours. Breast cancer screening has been proved as a good practical tool for detecting and removing breast cancer prematurely, and it also increases the survival percentage in women aged 50 and older. This screening test program produces a lot of mammograms to be diagnosed by radiologist, increasing from 38% in 1987 to 60% in 1990 the percentage of women over 40 years old who had ever received at least one mammogram [1]. However, some controversy arises, especially with respect to the accuracy of screening mammography and the related costs of errors. Mammography accuracy is limited, both in sensitivity (some cancers are missed) and specificity (many non-cancer cases are referred for invasive procedures).

The problems of missed cancers (false negatives) and the high number of unnecessary follows-ups (false positives) both of them have been approached using computer aided diagnosis (CAD). CAD generally follows steps similar to the radiologist's procedure to read a mammogram: detection (where abnormalities can

J. Crespo, V. Maojo, and F. Martin (Eds.): ISMDA 2001, LNCS 2199, pp. 174–180, 2001.

be found), segmentation (identification of the boundaries of objects at those locations), feature extraction (measurement of the characteristics of the potential abnormalities), and finally, classification (differentiate benign from malignant cases) [1].

The results from a previous research work performed in the Regional Health Area of Girona [2] were used as the starting point in the development of the current prototype *Higiea*. In such a work, a total number of 216 mammograms were analyzed in order to build a statistical model to predict the cancer risk, taking into account only the shape of doubtful microcalcifications.

2   Image Analysis

There are different kinds of lesions in a mammogram that can be used as an early warning of the presence of a breast cancer. In the current version of the application, only information related to the shape of the microcalcifications is used. The procedure for issuing a diagnosis, follows these four steps: detection of seed pixels, segmentation, feature extraction, and classification. Attending the experimental nature of this prototype, every step includes more than one possibility for achieving the final results; therefore, different algorithms have been set out for detecting the seed pixels, segmenting the microcalcificacions, or extracting features. Its daily use in a mammographic unit will report further results about their behaviour.

The detection of seed pixels in the microcalcification can be manual or automatic, and often is integrated in the segmentation step. *Higiea* allows the user to manually detect the seed pixels, or use an automatic criterion based on the average grey level of the region [3] to select them.

As for the segmentation concerns, three different algorithms have been included: a region-growing one [3], based on mathematical morphology [4], or based on the wavelet transform [5].

The region-growing algorithm starts from the seed pixels, selected in the previous step. A region growing process is started on every seed pixel $p(i,j)$ by adding its 4-connected neighbours, provided that they belong to the region if the following condition is accomplished:

$$(1 + \tau)(F_{max} + F_{min})/2 \geq p(i,j) \geq (1 - \tau)(F_{max} + F_{min})/2 \qquad (1)$$

where F_{max} and F_{min} are the current maximum and minimum pixel values of the region being grown, and τ is the growth tolerance (where its value is between 0 and 1).

The segmentation stage uses different techniques: mathematical morphology to extract the pixels, and Markov Random Fields to label the pixels.

We used the Top-Hat morphology operator, defined as the subtraction of the opening operator $\gamma_B(f)$ to the identity operator f:

$$TH(f) = f - \gamma_B(f) \qquad (2)$$

Table 1. Feature set used to characterize the microcalcifications

Feature Variable Description
Area The number of pixels in the microcalcification.
Number of Holes The number of holes in the microcalcification.
Feret Elongation A measure of the shape of the microcalcification: $\frac{FeretMaxDiameter}{FeretMinDiameter}$
Roughness A measure of the roughness: $\frac{Perimeter}{ConvexPerimeter}$
Elongation Similar to the Feret Elongation: $\frac{Lenght}{Breath}$
Compactness A measure of the roundness, it's equal to: $\frac{Perimeter^2}{4\pi Area}$
Principal Axis The angle between the horitzontal and the principal symmetry axis of the microcalcification: $-0.5 * \arctan \frac{2*Moment_{1,1}}{Moment_{2,0} - Moment_{0,2}}$

The opening operator eliminates the elements of the image with more luminance that are smaller than the structural element; therefore, when it is substracted from the identity image, the elements that have been eliminated are extracted. To be able to extract the microcalcifications, the structural element must be bigger than the biggest microcalcification. Mossi and Albiol [4] propose to select a square or a circle with the appropriate size as a structural element.

Once the segmented image has been obtained, we can extract a set of features from every microcalcification individually as well as from the whole cluster, which will be used in the classification step. Although there are several works that propose a wide range of features, *Higiɛα* uses a set of shape-based features for the microcalcifications:

The classification step will label the mammography as benign or malignant using the features $(X_1, \ldots, X_k)$ extracted in the previous step. A statistical model based on the logistic regression model normit/probit obtained from the microcalcification features is used to assign the probability p_i, according to the equation:

$$\phi^{-1} = \beta_0 + \beta_1 X_{1i} + \ldots + \beta_k X_{ki} \qquad (i = 1, \ldots, n) \qquad (3)$$

where ϕ represents the distribution function of a normal standard rule.

The figure 1 shows that ϕ^{-1} returns the point into the abscissas axis, but the value that indicates the punctual probability is *p_hat*, i.e. the area below ϕ^{-1} in the normal rule function. Therefore, to find the correct value we need to integrate the next function:

$$p\_hat = \int_{-\infty}^{\phi^{-1}} \frac{1}{\sqrt{2\pi}} e^{\frac{-x^2}{2}} dx \qquad (4)$$

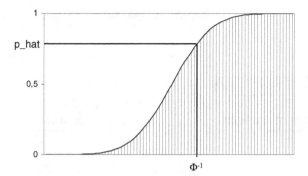

Fig. 1. N(0,1) Distribution function

3 First Version of *Higiεα*

The figure 2 depicts an example of an interface screen of *Higiεα*. Notice that a region in the mammogram has been selected in order to perform the whole analysis process on it. From this region of interest, a new image is generated that contains the results of the segmentation.

During the analysis process, the user has always the possibility to choose which algorithm is being used at each step, such as figure 3(a) shows. The process ends when a classification algorithm is selected, as is shown in figure 3(b), which enables to issue a risk factor associated to the analyzed region. At the moment, *Higiεα* uses a predictive statistical model based on the shape features of the microcalcifications.

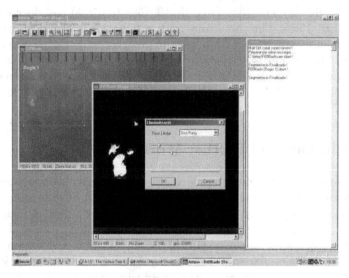

Fig. 2. Interface screen of *Higiεα*

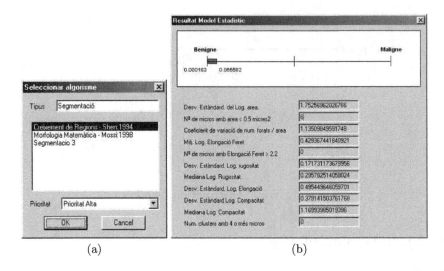

Fig. 3. Dialogs of *Higiεα*

As a final performance evaluation, the classification scheme provided by the model was compared with the diagnosis issued by three expert radiologists, which indicated the malignant character of the mammogram based on the microcalcifications appearance. Tables 2a and 2b tabulate the results obtained from the prospective data for both diagnoses, considering a confidence interval of 99%.

Over the 49 benignant mammograms diagnosed by the radiologists, 2 cases (4.08%) were diagnosed incorrectly, 25 cases (51.02%) correctly, and for 22 cases (44.90%) no clear diagnosis could be established. The proposed model misclassifies 3 cases (6.12%), classifies correctly 19 cases (38.78%) and does not decide in 27 cases (55.10%). The same conservative behavior is observed over the 21 malignant mammograms that complete the prospective set: while the diagnosis provided by the radiologists is incorrect in 3 cases (14.29%), correct in 12 cases (61.90%), and does not decide in 5 cases (20.81%), the proposed model classifies incorrectly 2 cases (9.52%), correctly 9 cases (42.86%) and does not decide in 10 cases (47.62%).

4   Conclusions and Further Work

A first prototype of a mammographic analysis system has been presented. The system allows several possibilities to the user at each analysis step: image segmentation using region-growing, mathematical morphology or wavelet algorithms; use of shape-based features of the segmented microcalcifications; and finally, classification using a predictive statistical model. The final application has been built up in such a modular way that easily permits to add new modules at any step: inclusion of new features for the microcalcifications, not only related to

Table 2. Comparative results between the diagnosis predicted by *Higiea* first prototype and the diagnosis issued by 3 expert radiologists, for benignant (a) and malignant (b) mammograms (cell contents: counts, % of row, % of column)

		Predicted by *Higiea*			
		bb	bm	mm	All
Diagnosis from radiologists	bb	11	13	1	25
		44.00	52.00	4.00	100.00
		57.89	48.15	33.33	51.02
	bm	7	13	2	22
		31.82	59.09	9.09	100.00
		36.84	48.15	66.67	44.90
	mm	1	1	0	2
		50.00	50.00	-	100.00
		5.26	3.70	-	4.08
	All	19	27	3	49
		38.78	55.10	6.12	100.00
		100.00	100.00	100.00	100.00

(a) Benignant Mammograms

		Predicted by *Higiea*			
		bb	bm	mm	All
Diagnosis from radiologists	bb	0	3	0	3
		-	100.00	-	100.00
		-	30.00	-	14.29
	bm	1	2	2	5
		20.00	40.00	40.00	100.00
		50.00	20.00	22.22	23.81
	mm	1	5	7	13
		7.69	38.46	53.85	100.00
		50.00	50.00	77.78	61.90
	All	2	10	9	21
		9.52	47.62	42.86	100.00
		100.00	100.00	100.00	100.00

(b) Malignant Mammograms

their individual shape, but also related to the cluster's shape; inclusion of new abnormalities, such as masses and spicules; test of new classification algorithms, such as Case Based Reasoning (CBR). Early results using this technique show a promising direction [6], and a second version of the prototype will include this technique as a new feature.

Acknowledgments

This work was supported by the Fondo de Investigación Sanitaria of Spain, grant no. 00/0037, and the FI/FIAP program of the Generalitat de Catalunya.

References

1. H. Sari-Sarraf, S. S. Gleason, K. T. Hudson, S. S. Gleason and K. F. Hubner: A novel approach to computer-aided diagnosis of mammographic images. *IEEE Workshop on Applications of Computer Vision.* December 1996. 174, 175
2. J. Martí, X. Cufí, J. Regincós, J. Español, J. Pont, and C. Barceló: Shape-based features selection for microcalcification evaluation. In *Proceedings of the Medical Imaging 1998: Image Processing.* SPIE vol. 3338, pages 1215–1224. February 1998. 175
3. L. Shen, R. M. Rangayyan, and L. Desautels: Detection and Classification of Mammographic Calcifications. In *Series in Machine Perception and Artificial Intelligence,* vol. 9. June 1994. 175
4. J. M. Mossi, and A. Albiol: Mathematical morphology applied to detection of clusters of microcalcifications. In *Proceedings of the 4th International Workshop on Digital Mammography,* pages 475–476. June 1998. 175, 176

5. S. Yu, L. Guan, and S. Brown: Automatic detection of clustered microcalcifications in digital mammograms based on wavelet features and neural network classification. In *Proceedings of the Medical Imaging 1998: Image Processing*. SPIE vol. 3338, pages 1540–1546. February 1998.   175

6. J. Martí, J. Español, E. Golobardes, J. Freixenet, R. García, and M. Salamó: Classification of microcalcifications in digital mammograms using Case-Based Reasoning. In *Proceedings of the 5th International Workshop on Digital Mammography*. To appear. June 2000.   179

Improvement of a Mammographic CAD System for Mass Detection

Arturo J. Méndez[1], Pablo G. Tahoces[2], Celia Varela[3], María J. Lado[1], Miguel Souto[3], and Juan J. Vidal[3]

[1] Department of Computer Science, University of Vigo,
Campus Lagoas-Marcosende, 36200 Vigo, Spain
{mrarthur,mrpepa}@uvigo.es

[2] Department of Electronics and Computer Science, University of Santiago de Compostela, Campus Sur, 15782 Santiago de Compostela, Spain
mrpablo@usc.es

[3] Department of Radiology, University of Santiago de Compostela,
San Francisco 1, 15782 Santiago de Compostela, Spain
{mrcuca,mrmiguel}@usc.es

Abstract. A previously developed computerized scheme to detect masses has been further revised and several improvements were intended. Mammograms were digitized at a higher resolution with a mammographic laser scanner providing 12 bits. Some steps of the scheme, based on bilateral subtraction technique, were modified. Several new features were designed and a BPN neural network was used to reduce the number of false positives. Results obtained with the training set were encouraging, yielding a sensitivity of 85% and 1.54 mean number of false positives per image before applying false positive reduction. After applying false positive reduction, a sensitivity of 78.3% at a mean number of 0.4 false positives per image was obtained. The area under the AFROC curve was $A_1 = 0.808$.

1   Introduction

The detection of masses in mammograms is a difficult task due to the similarity between many of these radiopacities and breast tissue, and also to the low contrast of many cancerous lesions [1, 2]. Although mammographic screening programs have proven to be an effective method for early detection of breast cancer [3], some cancers are still being missed or misinterpreted [4]. As a help, computer-aided diagnosis (CAD) schemes have been suggested in order to improve the sensitivity and specificity of the radiologists [5, 6, 7].

Therefore, a lot of effort has been devoted to the development of CAD schemes for detection of breast masses and clusters of microcalcifications in digitized mammograms. At present, the R2 ImageChecker Mammographic CAD System (R2 Technology Inc., Los Altos, CA) is a well known scheme used in many hospitals around the

J. Crespo, V. Maojo, and F. Martin (Eds.): ISMDA 2001, LNCS 2199, pp. 181-185, 2001.

world. There are also other schemes, as Second Look (CADx Medical Systems Inc., Quebec, Canada) or MAMMEX TR (SCANIS Inc., Foster City, CA), reflecting the emerging interest and needs for advance in early breast cancer diagnosis.

We have previously developed a method to detect masses[6], which uses bilateral subtraction technique of corresponding left-right matched image pairs. It is based on the symmetry between both images, with asymmetries indicating possible masses [8, 9]. This method has been evaluated and improved in successive studies. The main modifications refer to breast border detection and false positive reduction. Furthermore, mammograms were digitized with 12 bits precision, using a high-resolution laser scanner. Results form the training set are shown. The system was evaluated using free-response receiver operating characteristic (FROC) analysis [10].

2   Materials and Methods

2.1   Acquisition of Digital Mammograms and Database Characterization

Sixty pairs of conventional mammograms in lateral and craniocaudal views were digitized at a resolution of 2000x2500 pixels, and 12 bits precision employing a Lumiscan 85 laser scanner (Lumisys Inc., Sunnyvale, CA). Each pair of mammograms contained a single biopsy proven malignant mass in either the left or right mammogram. Images were directly stored via SCSI interface on a magnetic disk array Sun StorEDGE A5100, and a Sun Ultra 80 Workstation (Sun Microsystems, Inc., Mountain View, CA), was used for all the calculations. The computer programs were written in C language.

All lesions were ranked by two experienced radiologists by consensus in a four-level decision scale, *level 1*, corresponding to obvious masses (8), *level 2*, for relatively obvious masses (30), *level 3*, corresponding to subtle masses (7), and *level 4*, for very subtle masses (15).

Contrast value and effective size for each mass were manually measured, based on the masses outlined by the radiologists. A mean effective size of 19.33±10.56 mm was obtained and the mean contrast was 0.28±0.11.

2.2   Detection Scheme

The general scheme for detection of masses consists on five steps:

a) Detection of the breast border and nipple. To segment the breast region from the original image, a tracking algorithm to detect the breast border was applied [11]. The nipple was also detected in order to align both left and right breast images. The original algorithm to detect the border was modified. Several aspects are pointed out:

-    thresholds values used to eliminate artifacts were calculated for each mammogram from the histogram of gray-levels,
-    the condition that a point (x, y) belonging to the border must satisfy was made stricter,

$$f(x_1, y_1) < f(x_2, y_2) < ... < f(x_7, y_7) \leq f(x_8, y_8) \leq f(x_9, y_9) \leq f(x, y) . \qquad (1)$$

became,

$$f(x_1, y_1) < f(x_2, y_2) < ... < f(x_7, y_7) < f(x_8, y_8) < f(x_9, y_9) < f(x, y) . \qquad (2)$$

with this modified condition the algorithm did not get confused with artifacts,
- when the tracking algorithm did not detect the border yielding spurious values, this values were not taken into account and neglected, these values were a source of error when sorting the coordinates of the border .

b) Alignment of mammograms. Mammograms were aligned before subtraction, employing the breast border and nipple as reference points.

c) Normalization of mammograms. Images were corrected to avoid differences in brightness between left and right mammograms due to the recording procedure.

d) Subtraction of mammograms. Images were subtracted and, as a result, two new images were generated, one composed of the positive values, and the other of the negative values. A threshold to obtain a binary image with the information of suspect areas was automatically calculated. These areas were extracted by an adaptive region growing algorithm.

e) Reduction of false positives. Size and eccentricity tests were used. Furthermore, a backpropagation neural network classifier was developed. This classifier used as inputs features extracted from the suspect regions. Two types of features were extracted: on the one hand, features based on the gray level value of the image pixels and on the other hand features based on contrast measures.

3   Results

The 60 pairs of mammograms of our study were analyzed to detect possible masses employing the automated detection scheme described above. Figure 1 shows an example of the results of the detection procedure of a mammogram containing one mass in the right breast.

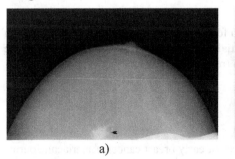 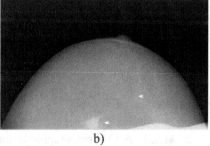

a)   b)

Fig. 1. a) An original mammogram containing a mass (indicated by the black arrow), and b) Results of the detection process (indicated by white arrows): the detected mass, and the presence of a false positive

The system achieved a sensitivity of 85% with a mean number of 1.54 false positives per image before applying false positive reduction. After applying false positive reduction, a sensitivity of 78.3% at a mean number of 0.4 false positives per image was obtained. The area under the AFROC curve was $A_1 = 0.808$.

4   Discussion

Because of the fact that the radiographic appearance of the right and left breasts of a given patient tends to be similar, radiologists hung films on the view box in a mirror image configuration and they scan the breasts searching for asymmetry. This is the reason to design CAD schemes based on bilateral subtraction. The bilateral-image subtraction method may help to reduce the number of false positives and may yield better performance after classification [12]. However, it may lack for high-sensitivity, it implies more intermediate steps (detection of the nipple, alignment), and it is limited in real clinical applications (e.g. mastectomy) [12]. Therefore we are also investigating other methods based on single-image segmentation, bearing in mind that bilateral subtraction may be useful in early cancer detection by using time comparison on the same breast.

In a previous study [6], we have developed the method to detect masses in digital mammograms. We have obtained a sensitivity of 71% at a false positive of 0.67 per image. In this work, our sensitivity has increased up to 78.3%, and the mean number of false detections have decreased to 0.4 per image. Our results suggest that the method could help radiologists in their daily work. Comparing with other studies, as the clinical results of the R2 ImageChecker that achieved a 75% sensitivity [13], it seems that the scheme obtained an acceptable sensitivity, however the scheme must be evaluated in a large database or in a clinical situation.

Although it would be desirable to improve the true-positive rate, the low average number of false positives per image indicates that our method would not confuse the radiologists by suggesting normal regions as masses.

Acknowledgments

The authors are grateful to Roberto Patiño for his technical assistance in the edition of this manuscript. This work has been partially supported by Secretaría de Estado de Universidades, Investigación y Desarrollo (ref. 1FD97-0147).

References

1.   Sickles, E. A.: Mammographic features of early breast cancer. Ameriacan Journal of Roentgenology 143 (1984) 461-464
2.   Tabar, L., Dean, P. B.: Teaching Atlas of Mammography. Georg Thieme Verlag/Thieme, Sttugart (1985)

3. Feig, S. A.: Decreased breast cancer mortality through mammographic screening: results of clinical trials. Radiology 167 (1988) 659-665
4. Bird, R. E., Wallace, T. W., Yankaskas, B. C.,: Analysis of cancers missed at screening mammography. Radiology 184 (1992) 613-617
5. Kegelmeyer, W. P., Pruneda, J. M., Bourland, P. D., Hillis, A., Riggs, M. W., Nipper, M. L.: Computer-aided mammographic screening for spiculated lesions. Radiology 191 (1994) 331-337
6. Méndez, A.J., Tahoces, P.G., Lado, M.J., Souto, M., Vidal, J.J.: Computer-aided diagnosis: Automatic detection of malignant masses in digitized mammograms. Medical Physics 25 (1998) 957-964
7. Lado, M.J., Tahoces, P.G., Méndez, A.J., Souto, M., Vidal, J.J.: A wavelet-based algorithm for detecting clustered microcalcifications in digital mammograms. Medical Physics 26 (1999) 1294-1305
8. Winsberg, F., Elkin, M., Macy, J., Bordaz, V, Weymouth, W.: Detection of radiographic abnormalities in mammograms by means of optical scanning and computer analysis. Radiology 89 (1967) 211-215
9. Yin, F. F., Giger, M. L., Doi, K., Metz, C. E., Vyborny, C. J., Schmidt R. A.: Computerized detection of masses in digital mammograms: analysis of bilateral-subtraction images. Medical Physics 18 (1991) 955-963
10. Chakraborty, D.P., Winter, L.H.L.: Free-response methodology: Alternate analysis and a new observer-performance experiment. Radiology 174 (1990) 873-881
11. Méndez, A.J., Tahoces, P.G., Lado, M.J., Souto, M., Correa, J., Vidal, J.J.: Automatic detection of breast border and nipple in digital mammograms. Computer Methods and Programs in Biomedicine 49 (1996) 253-262
12. Zheng, B., Chang, Y.-H., Gur, D.: Computerized detection of masses in digitized mammograms using single-image segmentation and a multilayer topographic feature analysis. Academic Radiology 2 (1995) 959-966
13. Doi, T., Hasegawa, A., Hunt. B., Marshall, J., Rao, F., Roehrig, J., Romsdahl, H., Schneider, A., Sharbaugh, R., Wang, B., Zhang, W.: Clinical Results with the R2 ImageChecker Mammographic CAD System. Computer-Aided Diagnosis in Medical Imaging, Elsevier Science (1999)

Classification of Gene Expression Data in an Ontology

Herman Midelfart[1], Astrid Lægreid[2], and Jan Komorowski[1]

[1] Department of Computer and Information Science
{herman,janko}@idi.ntnu.no
[2] Department of Physiology and Biomedical Engineering,
Norwegian University of Science And Technology, N-7491 Trondheim, Norway

Abstract. Prediction of gene function from expression profiles is an intriguing problem that has been attempted with both unsupervised clustering and supervised learning methods. By the incorporation of prior knowledge concerning gene function, supervised methods avoid some of the problems with clustering. However, even supervised methods ignore the fact that the functional classes associated with genes are typically organized in an ontology. Hence, we introduce a new supervised method for learning in such an ontology. It is tested on both an artificial data set and a data set containing measurements from human fibroblast cells. We also give an approach for measuring the classification performance in an ontology.

1 Introduction

DNA microarray technology makes large gene expression studies possible, but it generates vast amounts of data about complex biological phenomena. One of the goals for the analysis of this data is to classify unknown genes with respect to their biological function. The problem is rather intricate since a gene may have more than one function, functionally related genes may be anti-correlated in their expression profiles, and similarly expressed genes need not share the same function. This has been pointed out, for example, by Shatkay et al. [9]. We believe that this problem should be approached with *supervised* learning methods. Supervised learning offers a possibility to include prior (e.g. biological) knowledge in the learning process. Expression profiles of known genes can be associated with the corresponding gene function and used to induce a classifier.

However, there has been little work on supervised learning of gene expression data. Brown et al. [2] is one notable exception though. They used support vector machines to predict functional classes for the gene expression data analyzed in Eisen et al. [5]. Still, there are some problems left open by them. For instance, no attempt was made to induce a complete classifier. Instead, they predicted only five functional classes that were already known to cluster well. These classes covered only a minor part of the data set, and many genes that belonged to other classes, were not classified. Moreover, they did not take into account the fact that the classes associated with known genes form an ontology. More recently,

J. Crespo, V. Maojo, and F. Martin (Eds.): ISMDA 2001, LNCS 2199, pp. 186–194, 2001.

Hvidsten et al. [6] used standard Rough Sets methods to predict 16 biological processes from gene expression profiles. These processes were selected from an ontology by picking those having at least 10 genes, but the approach did not treat the issue of learning in an *ontology*, and evaluating a classifier that classifies in an ontology.

In this paper, we focus on the problem of classifying genes from expression profiles where the functional classes are organized in an ontology. We present a rule learning approach that uses the fact that the set of classes is not flat, as it is usually assumed in learning, but rather it is structured where a class may be an instance of another one. We also introduce numerical measures to assess the quality of such learning.

2 Methods

We used a rule learning approach similar to AQ [8] and CN2 [3] systems. One advantage of this approach over other methods, such as neural nets and support vector machines, is that it produces rules that characterize the decision class. In our problem, these rules can be interpreted to get an impression of the common behavior of the genes participating in the same process.

A simple example is given in Fig. 1. Each row in the table describes a gene annotated with one or more processes. We assume that the expression level of the gene has been measured at several time points, and the expression profile is represented by the direction of the slope between two adjacent time points[1]. From the table we wish to find rules. Fig. 1 includes some possible examples. A rule consists of a condition which is a conjunction of attribute-value pairs, and a conclusion. If a gene satisfies the conditional part, the conclusion gives the class, i.e., the process, to which the gene belongs. We say that a rule *covers* a gene if the gene satisfies the conditional part.

The classes assigned to the genes are taken from the ontology above the table. Notice that the genes are annotated with both leaf and non-leaf classes. If we ignore the ontology and use a standard algorithm directly on the table, it will try to discriminate between super- and subclasses such as "transport" and "cytoplasmic transport". This may lead to very specific rules and make the algorithm sensitive to noise. Hence, we risk overfitting the rules and may get a poor prediction result. Therefore, it is not possible to ignore the ontology as it would have been had the genes been only annotated with leaf classes. One possibility though would be to "flatten" the set of classes by selecting the most general ones containing any genes (e.g, "cell growth & maintenance" and "cell adhesion" in Fig. 1) and move the annotations from the subclasses to these classes. However, the detail of the annotations would be lost.

It follows that rule learning in an ontology should use all classes, and not discriminate between the super- and subclasses. At the same time it should retain as much as possible of the detail of the predictions without losing precision.

---

[1] If the absolute value of the slope was less than 0.03 (after log_2-transformation and normalization), *const* was assigned as value.

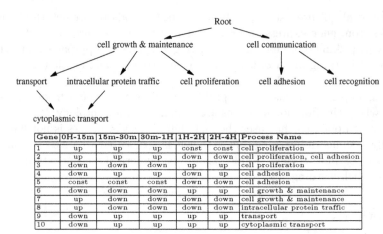

Gene	0H-15m	15m-30m	30m-1H	1H-2H	2H-4H	Process Name
1	up	up	up	const	const	cell proliferation
2	up	up	up	down	down	cell proliferation, cell adhesion
3	down	down	down	up	up	cell proliferation
4	down	up	up	down	up	cell adhesion
5	const	const	const	down	down	cell adhesion
6	down	down	down	up	up	cell growth & maintenance
7	up	down	down	down	down	cell growth & maintenance
8	up	down	down	down	down	intracellular protein traffic
9	down	up	up	up	up	transport
10	down	up	up	up	up	cytoplasmic transport

Goal: Find rules like
0H-15m(up) & 15m-30m(up) & 30m-1H(up) → cell proliferation
0H-15m(down) & 15m-30m(down) → cell proliferation
0H-15m(down) & 15m-30m(up) → cell adhesion
1H-2H(down) & 2H-4H(down) → cell adhesion

Fig. 1. Rule Learning

However, when the annotations are spread throughout the whole ontology, the data in a class may be too sparse to learn a good classifier. Each class may hold only a few examples of genes that may have quite different expression profiles. This may make it difficult to find distinguishing properties in the expression profiles and will often result in rules with poor performance.

In our method, we correct this by including not only genes annotated with the class, but also genes annotated with subclasses when rules are learned for each class. In this way, there will be more genes to learn from. However, the genes of a class are now covered by the rules of this class as well as the rules of its superclasses, and we resolve the conflict with a voting scheme where a class inherits votes from its superclasses. Hence, a prediction is not only based on a single class, but also on the superclasses. This reduces the risk of an incorrect prediction and increases the quality of the classification. A correct prediction will typically be supported by all the superclasses and will get a higher vote, while an incorrect prediction will not be supported by the superclasses, and its vote will be smoothed out by them.

The method is an ensemble approach [4]. It produces a classifier that really consists of multiple classifiers, since alternate classifiers could be constructed by using the rules from a subset of the classes. For example, if all the genes were annotated at the leaves, a full classifier could be constructed by selecting a set of classes where all other classes in the ontology were either a super- or a subclass of a class in this set. The granularity of the predictions made by the classifiers would vary depending on the classes being chosen. However, all genes would be covered by some rule in the classifier.

Algorithm 1 The learning part

Input: A set of annotations A, a DAG $\langle C, E \rangle$, and an accuracy threshold α.
Output: A set of rules RS.

$RS = \emptyset$
for all $c \in C \backslash \{Root\}$ **do**
  $\mathcal{P} = \{g \mid \langle g, d \rangle \in A \text{ and } c \succcurlyeq d\}$
  $\mathcal{N} = \{g \mid (\langle g, d \rangle \in A \text{ and } c \not\approx d) \text{ and } (\neg \exists (\langle g', d' \rangle \in \mathcal{P} : vec(g) = vec(g')))\}$
  $R = \{r_g \mid r_g \text{ is the most specific rule for } g \in \mathcal{P} \text{ with all attribute-value pairs}\}$
  while two rules in R can be merged into the rule r such that $\frac{|\mathcal{P}_r|}{|\mathcal{P}_r| + |\mathcal{N}_r|} \geq \alpha$ **do**
    select the two most similar rules $r_1, r_2 \in R$ and remove them from R
    merge r_1 and r_2 into r by deleting all dissimilar attribute-value pairs
    add r to R
  end while
  add R to RS
end for

Before presenting the algorithm in detail, we first introduce necessary notation. Let G be a set of genes, C be a set of classes, and A be a set of annotations. Each gene $g \in G$ has a vector $vec(g)$ containing its attribute values and is annotated with one or more classes. $\langle g, c \rangle \in A$, if gene $g \in G$ is annotated with class $c \in C$. The classes form a Directed Acyclic Graph (DAG) $\langle C, E \rangle$ where E is a set of edges such that $\langle a, b \rangle \in E$ is an edge from a to b if a is a superclass of b. We define a partial order on the DAG where p is *more general than* r, denoted $p \succcurlyeq r$, if $p = r$, or there is a $q \in C$ such that $p \succcurlyeq q$ and $\langle q, r \rangle \in E$. $p \approx q$ denotes that classes p and q are on the same branch, i.e., $p \succcurlyeq q$ or $q \succcurlyeq p$. p is strictly more general than q, denoted $p \succ q$, if $p \succcurlyeq q$ and $p \neq q$. If r is a rule and P is a set of genes, P_r denotes the genes in P covered by r.

The learning algorithm is given in Alg. 1. A set of rules is found for all the classes in the ontology except the root. For each class c, the genes are divided into a positive set $\mathcal{P}$ containing the genes that should be covered by the rules and a negative set $\mathcal{N}$ containing the genes that should not be covered. $\mathcal{P}$ contains all genes annotated with c or a subclass of c. $\mathcal{N}$ basically contains the genes from

---

Algorithm 2 The prediction part

Input: A gene g, a set of rules RS, a DAG $\langle C, E \rangle$, and a threshold t.
Output: A set P of class predictions for g.

  for all $c \in C$: $v_c = \begin{cases} 1 \text{ if there is a rule in } RS \text{ covering } g \text{ and predicting } c \\ 0 \text{ otherwise} \end{cases}$
  for all $c \in C$ **do**
    if $v_c = 1$ and there is no d such that $c \succ d$ and $v_d = 1$ **then**
      $Paths(c) = \{\{c_1, \ldots, c_n, c\} \mid root \succ c_1 \succ \ldots \succ c_n \succ c\}$
      $votes_c = \max_{P \in Paths(c)} \sum_{d \in P} v_d$
    end if
    else $votes_c = 0$
  end for
  $P = \{c \mid \frac{vote_c}{Norm} > t\}$ where $Norm = \sum_{c \in C} votes_c$

---

the classes that are not c or a sub- or superclass of c. However, a gene may have several annotations (e.g., gene 2 in Fig. 1) since its product participates in several processes, and none of theses should be excluded. Therefore, the algorithm does not try to find rules that discriminate between different annotations of the same gene; it rather makes a separate rule for each possible class of the gene. Hence, genes that otherwise would be in $\mathcal{N}$, are excluded if they also are annotated both with c or a subclass of c. Moreover, a gene may have an expression profile indiscernible from another gene annotated with c or a subclass of c. Such genes are not included in the negative set since the rules should not discriminate between them either. The rules are then found by searching the hypothesis space consisting of conjunctions of attribute-value pairs in a bottom-up fashion. A most specific rule are generated for each gene in the positive set. These rules are later merged into more general rules by dropping dissimilar attribute-value pairs.

Predicting the class(es) of a gene is done by voting. The voting scheme is shown in Alg. 2. Each class with a rule that covers the gene in question receives one initial vote. It obtains an additional vote for each class that occurs on the path to the root and has an initial vote. If there are several paths to the root (since the ontology is a DAG), the highest vote among the paths is chosen. If a class has a subclass with an initial vote, the subclass is preferred, and the class is given no votes. The votes are normalized, and the classes having a normalized vote higher than a given threshold are returned as the predicted classes.

3   Results

Our method was evaluated on a data set provided by Iyer et al. [7]. In their experiment, the response in human fibroblast cells to serum was measured at 12 time points during the first 24 hours after serum was added to starved cells. They found that only 517 of genes showed any significant changed, and these constituted the data set. Since this set did not contain any annotations for the genes, we annotated the genes by manually extracting relevant information from the literature and molecular biology databases. The annotation classes were taken from process ontology of the Gene Ontology Consortium [1], and process information was found for 323 of the genes in the data set. 203 of these were annotated with more than one class. Furthermore, only the subset of the classes containing annotated genes (and their superclasses) was used in our evaluation. Hence, a total of 234 classes was used where 157 were leaf classes, and 113 classes had only one gene. We used a similar representation to the one present in Fig. 1. However, not only features constructed from adjacent time points were used, but also features constructed from intervals stretching over 3 to 6 time points[2].

We also used an artificial data set. We constructed first a DAG and assigned model profiles to each leaf class. Gene profiles were then created for the model

---

[2] In this case, an additional requirement was set that the slope between adjacent time points in the interval could not be below -0.02 (above 0.02) for an increasing (decreasing) feature.

profiles and assigned at random to the leaf class or one of its superclasses. Noise was added to each profile by changing each attribute value with probability p. With $p = 0.10$, the probability of at least one change in a profile was $1 - (1 - p)^{11} = 0.69$ since it contained 11 values.

The performance of supervised learning methods is usually measured by accuracy. However, this measure assumes that there is only one prediction per gene. In our case, there may be several correct predictions for a gene and a gene may be annotated with several classes. Hence, we propose some new criteria. We report the ratio RA of annotations that are predicted, and the ratio RP of predictions that are correct, i.e., those that correspond to annotations: $RA = |MA|/|A|$ and $RP = |MP|/|P|$ where A is the set of annotations, P is the corresponding set of predictions, $MA = \{\langle g,a \rangle \in A \mid \langle g,p \rangle \in P \text{ and } a \approx p\}$, and $MP = \{\langle g,p \rangle \in P \mid \langle g,a \rangle \in A \text{ and } p \approx a\}$

However, these measures do not take the ontology into account. For instance, if a prediction is made to "cell communication" for a gene annotated with "cell adhesion", the prediction has lost some of the detail, but it is still correct. To capture this loss, we find the depth from the root by counting the edges from a class to the root and measure the depth of a prediction p relative to the depth of a annotation a as defined by $d(a,p)$: $d(a,p) = depth(p)/depth(a)$ if $p \succcurlyeq a$, 1 if $a \succ p$, and 0 otherwise. $DA = \sum_{\langle g,a \rangle \in A} \max_{\langle g,p \rangle \in P} d(a,p)/|MA|$ gives the average relative depth of the best matching prediction for each matched annotation, indicating how well the annotations are reproduced. $DP = \sum_{\langle g,p \rangle \in P} \max_{\langle g,a \rangle \in A} d(a,p)/|MP|$ gives the average relative depth for each prediction, indicating how the well all the predictions match in case there are more predictions for each annotation.

We tested the method using 10-fold cross validation on both data sets. The results are shown in Tab. 1. Most of the annotations were predicted in the fibroblast, and most of the predictions made by the classifier were correct. However, the predictions have lost a lot of the original detail. We believe that this is due to the nature of the fibroblast data.

Obviously, it is easier to learn the classes at the top. Fewer classes must be discerned, and more examples are available. However, the variation in the data may be insufficient to distinguish between all the classes. Iyer et al. found only 10 major clusters in the data indicating that only 10 classes could be distinguished. Even though our results suggest that present variation is sufficient to allow distinction between more than 10 classes, it is unlikely that all 157 leaf classes in our annotations may be discerned. This is partly due to the noise produced by the microarray technology, which makes it difficult to tell whether all of the measured variation is really significant. However, genes participating in different processes may simply be similarly expressed in the experiment of Iyer et al., and further experiments may be required to distinguish between the classes of those genes. Thus, the coarse classes at the top of the ontology may better capture the essential variations in the fibroblast data.

Our algorithm tries to predict the most detailed classes, but if the rules at a detailed class do not fire for a gene, the rules in a coarser class may. Therefore, the algorithm is capable of adjusting the granularity of the prediction to an

Table 1. Results

Data	PA	RP	DA	DP
Fibroblast data ($\alpha = 0.70, t = 0.3$)	0.714	0.691	0.293	0.339
Artificial data, $p = 0.01$ noise ($\alpha = 1.0, t = 0.0$)	0.937	1.0	0.992	0.992
Artificial data, $p = 0.05$ noise ($\alpha = 0.80, t = 0.0$)	0.821	0.967	0.948	0.948
Artificial data, $p = 0.07$ noise ($\alpha = 0.80, t = 0.0$)	0.822	0.992	0.932	0.932
Artificial data, $p = 0.10$ noise ($\alpha = 0.80, t = 0.0$)	0.744	0.976	0.915	0.915
Hvidsten et al. [6]	0.666	0.332	0.710	0.710

appropriate level of detail. If the data supports a level of detail in the original annotation, then the detail will be maintained in the predictions.

The results on the artificial data set confirm this conjecture. The DA/DP measure shows that the algorithm is capable of reproducing the detail of the original annotation as long as variations in the data is sufficient to support this level of detail. The RP level is nearly constant with increasing noise, and very few incorrect predictions are made. However, it is a bit sensitive to noise since the PA level falls a bit when the noise is increased. This is due to the rule generating part of the algorithm that searches the hypothesis space in a bottom-up fashion.

Tab. 1 also gives a comparison with Hvidsten et al. [6] who used the fibroblast data and learned rules for 16 classes. That work reported only sensitivity and specificity for each class, but a general impression of the performance is difficult to assess from these measures in the case of multiple classes. For any given class, the positive set, containing the genes annotated with the class, is much smaller than the negative set, containing genes annotated only with other classes. The errors from these classes add up since several predictions can be made for each gene. So even with seemingly high specificity, the number of false predictions to the class may be much higher that the number of true predictions, resulting in a low RP.

Tab. 1 gives estimates for the approach of Hvidsten et al. using our new criteria. From this it is evident that more of the annotation detail level was retained with that approach, but the ratio of predictions that were correct was rather low and unsatisfactory. In fact, about 2/3 of the predictions that were made, were incorrect. The main reason is that they used a slightly different representations where a feature consisted of at least 3 consecutive time points showing the same behavior. This forced the learning algorithm to make quite general rules for the detailed classes that they had picked, but resulted in many incorrect predictions. In our approach, we have chosen a less strict representation, but the rules in the detailed classes became too specific and do not fire in most cases. In this way, we have traded detail for prediction precision. However, this was necessary to get an acceptable RP.

4   Conclusions and Future Work

The task of predicting gene function from expression profiles creates new challenges for rule learning: The processes are typically organized in an ontology, and hence new learning algorithms are required. We have presented a method for learning in such a structure and shown than it gives accurate predictions – even when the data is scattered around the ontology. Supervised learning in our framework has been given a different dimension. Although, it is supervised, the classes to be predicted are not fixed, but defined dynamically by adjusting the detail in the predictions to an appropriate level relative to the data in question. Furthermore, approaches for learning in an ontology must be evaluated which requires new measures. We have proposed four measures, and we believe that they should give a good assessment of the performance of an algorithm.

There is still room for improvement. One possible source of the inaccuracy of the algorithm is the assumption that genes with similar expression profiles contribute to the same biological processes. This assumption does not always hold and may lead to incorrect predictions. The problem may be solved by including additional information about the gene. One possibility would be to identify specific transcription factor binding sites in the promoter region of the genes and to construct Boolean attributes where true (false) denotes the occurrence (lack) of such binding sites in a gene. Another possibility would be to use microarray data from several experimental conditions assuming that genes coexpressed under one condition are not necessarily coexpressed under another. Moreover, the data produced by the microarray is very noisy. Using replications of the experiment should reduce this noise and give better predictions.

Our method uses genes for the subclasses in the rule learning process and moves in this way genes upwards in the ontology. Another question that emerges in the ontology is whether it is possible to move genes downwards by finding rules that produce predictions that are more detailed than the original annotations (at least for the more general annotations). We are currently investigating this.

References

1. The Gene Ontology Consortium. Gene ontology: tool for the unification of biology. *Nature Genetics*, 25(1):25–29, 2000. 190
2. M. P. S. Brown, W. N. Grundy, D. Lin, N. Cristianini, C. W. Sugnet, T. S. Furey, M. Ares, Jr., and D. Haussler. Knowledge-based analysis of microarray gene expression data by using support vector machines. *PNAS*, 97(1):262–267, 2000. 186
3. Peter Clark and Tim Niblett. The CN2 induction algorithm. *Machine Learning*, 3(4):261–283, 1989. 187
4. Thomas G. Dietterich. Ensemble methods in machine learning. In Proc. of MCS-2000, LNCS 1857, pp. 1–15. 188
5. M. B. Eisen, P. T. Spellman, P. O. Brown, and D. Botstein. Cluster analysis and display of genome-wide expression patterns. *PNAS*, 95:14863–14868, 1998. 186
6. T. R. Hvidsten, J. Komorowski, A. K. Sandvik, and A. Lægreid. Predicting gene function from gene expressions and ontologies. In *Proc. of PSB-2001*, pp. 299–310. 187, 192

7. W. R. Iyer, M. B. Eisen, D. T. Ross, G. Schuler, T. Moore, J. C. F. Lee, J. M. Trent, L. M. Staudt, J. Hudson, M. S. Boguski, D. Lashkari, D. Shalon, D. Botstein, and P. O. Brown. The transcriptional program in the response of human fibroblasts to serum. *Science*, 283:83–87, 1999. 190

8. R. S. Michalski. A theory and methodology of inductive learning. In Michalski, Carbonell, and Mitchell (eds), *Machine Learning: An Artificial Intelligence Approach*, vol. 1, pp. 83–129. Morgan Kaufmann, 1983. 187

9. H. Shatkay, S. Edwards, W. J. Wilbur, and M. Boguski. Genes, themes and microarrays: Using information retrieval for large-scale gene analysis. In *Proc. of ISMB-2000*, pp. 317–328. 186

Feature Selection Algorithms Applied to Parkinson's Disease

M. Navío[1], J. J. Aguilera[2], M. J. del Jesus[2], R. González[3],
F. Herrera[4], and C. Iríbar[5]

[1] Ramón y Cajal Hospital, Madrid, Spain
mnavioa@hrc.insalud.es
[2] Dept. of Computer Science, University of Jaén
23071-Jaén, Spain
{jjaguile,mjjesus}@ujaen.es
[3] Dept. of Medicine, University of Granada
18071-Granada, Spain
[4] Dept. of Computer Science and A.I., University of Granada
18071-Granada, Spain
[5] Institute of Neuroscience, University of Granada
18071-Granada, Spain

Abstract. In Parkinson's Disease an analysis of Medical Data could highlight some symptoms, which can be used as a complementary tool in an early diagnosis. This paper analyses some Filter and Wrapper Feature Selection Algorithms and combinations of them that determine some relevant features in relation to this problem. The experimentation carried out with a data set of patients allows us to determine a set of different premorbid personality traits that can be considered in the early diagnosis of Parkinsonism.

1 Introduction

As a clinical-pathological entity, Parkinson's Disease (PD) is characterised by the presence of the symptoms of progressive Parkinsonism, which include a set of cardinal motor manifestations such as resting tremor, bradykinesia or akinesia, rigidity and alteration of postural reflexes. At present there exists general consensus at the Parkinson's Disease Foundation regarding the fact that the presence of at least two of these symptoms are considered to be a necessary requisite in order to diagnose Parkinsonism.

The possibility of an early diagnosis has been suggested [2] on the basis of the hypothesis of Langston et al. regarding to the existence of three phases in the natural history of the disease: a phase prior to the disease in which the risk factors making it potentially vulnerable are at work; a second phase (presymptomatic phase) ranging from the beginning of the disease up to the moment the typical signs of PD appear. The patient, although asymptomatic, has the illness. It is in these two phases that some authors have located the presence of premorbid

J. Crespo, V. Maojo, and F. Martin (Eds.): ISMDA 2001, LNCS 2199, pp. 195–200, 2001.

personality traits. The third or symptomatic phase is the one in which we find Parkinsonian motor signs.

Furthermore, some studies have compared groups of patients having an affected relative with patients having sporadic apparition of PD for the purpose of clarifying whether the same disease is involved and to find possible differences, if any. The so- called premorbid personality is present in all age groups. Its observation in this kind of study could support the hypothesis of one single nosological entity. Our intention is to determine whether these distinctive personality traits, studied in this case when the illness is evident, exist. If their existence is proven, they could serve as a tool to complement the diagnosis of the disease.

In order to do this, we will consider this problem as a classification problem where there is a patient (an example) with a set of symptoms (a set of features) and we must give a diagnosis about a disease (a class). So, with the set of distinctive personality traits we will apply some Feature Selection Algorithms to select a set of relevant personality features in the diagnosis of Parkinsonism.

The article is organised in this way: In Section 2, we define Feature Selection Algorithms. The application of Feature Selection Algorithms is described in Section 3. The results obtained in the experimentation carried out and their analysis are shown in Sections 4. Finally, the conclusions and future works are exposed in Section 5.

2   Feature Selection Algorithms

A Feature Selection Algorithm (FSA) starts with a set of examples and searches the most relevant features for the classification problem to solve, considering the complete set of features [8,11,12]. An FSA is composed of: a search algorithm that explores the space of feature subsets; an evaluation function that gives a measure of the feature subset adaptation for the classification task; and a performance function that validates the feature subset finally selected by the FSA. Many FSAs have been proposed, and they can be classified into two categories [11,12], filter and wrapper methods, which are briefly described in the following subsections.

2.1   Filter Approach

In this kind of FSAs, the evaluation function is calculated by class separability measures based on distance, information, dependency or consistency measures, and sieves the irrelevant and/or redundant features before the inductive learning process [12]. These FSAs are an efficient alternative to obtain a feature subset independent of the learning process used to obtain a model to classify. It can be a negative aspect due to the model ignores the heuristic and bias of the learning process in the feature selection.

2.2   Wrapper Approach

The FSAs included in this group use as evaluation function the estimation of accuracy obtained by the classification process with the model based on the selected features [11,12]. The computing of this value implies to learn the model for the candidate feature subset. This is the reason that wrapper feature selection process is slower than the filter. This approach is not as general as the filter model because it selects the data to fit the learning algorithm, it is restricted by the time complexity of the learning algorithm and it may cause a problem with some learning algorithms.

3   Application of Some Feature Selection Algorithms to the Parkinson Problem

There are different proposals for the FSAs depending on the objective of the feature selection process and the design of the algorithm components. In this medical problem the objective is to determine a small set of features which can help us as a complementary tool in the early diagnosis of Parkinsonism, if it is possible. Taking it into account, we have used two FSAs that searches for a feature subset with a previously fixed cardinality:

- A filter FSA based on a greedy search and on a function evaluation by means of the Mutual Information Measure, developed by Battiti [1].
- A wrapper FSA based on a Genetic Algorithm (GA) [10] as search algorithm and an accuracy estimation as evaluation function. The GA implemented is a Steady State GA developed by the authors [4] in which every chromosome represents a set of M features by using a set of M integer numbers.

Nevertheless, it is difficult to determine an appropriate value of the feature set cardinality for a specific problem. Therefore, it can be useful to apply some FSAs that select feature subsets with variable cardinality:

- A filter probabilistic algorithm based on the inconsistency measure, called Las Vegas Filter Algorithm (LVF) which uses the probabilistic technical Las Vegas as search algorithm, developed by Liu and Setiono [12].
- A wrapper FSA with a GA [10] as search process and accuracy estimation as evaluation function. This wrapper FSA uses binary code to represent in a chromosome the complete set of features symbolising with a 1 in the i-th position if the i-th feature is selected and with a 0 in other case.
- Two wrapper FSAs based on a forward and backward greedy search process with an evaluation function calculated by an accuracy estimation.

In this work, the accuracy in the diagnosis is calculated with the K-nearest neighbour's rule [6]. It is an efficient classification method with no learning time, which determines the class (diagnosis) based on the information provided by the k patients with a set of symptoms more similar to the patient to diagnose. For the k parameter, we use the values employed frequently in the specialised bibliography ($k = 1, 3, 5$).

We must note the set of FSAs applied to this problem select feature subsets using different evaluation measures (inconsistency, mutual information and accuracy measures) with different search algorithms (GAs, Las Vegas, Greedy forward and backward).

4 Experimentation

We have used a data set with the following characterictis: There are 96 examples, with 76 features for each example and 3 classes: family Parkinson, nonfamily Parkinson and cerebrovascular disease, each one consisting of 32 patients matched by sex, age and level of incapacity who came from the outpatient Neurology department of the Hospital Clínico San Cecilio of Granada (Spain). Once patients satisfied criteria for inclusion, they were assessed by means of a clinical, neuropsychological and personality study. The clinical study included epidemiological data as well as data from the Unified Parkinson's Disease Rating Scale (UPDRS). The neuropsychological and personality study included the following scale and Test: Mini-Mental State Folstein (MME) [9], Depression scale Zung-Conde, Personality Questionary H.J. Eysenck (EPQ-A) [7], Factorial Personality Questionary (16 PF) [5], ôBig FiveöQuestionary (BFQ) [3]. We must note that in this paper we do not focus the study in the nosological differentiation, if it could be possible, between family and non-family Parkinson patients.

To validate the selected features and to estimate their accuracy in the diagnosis, we have used the leaving one out technique [13] with the k-NN rule.

We have executed the Greedy and integer coded GA FSAs with cardinality 3, 4, 6 and 8. The results obtained by them are shown in Table 1, rows 1-8.

As we can see the wrapper FSA give us a feature set with a better prediction capacity than filter.

In addition, the experimentation does not remark the best cardinality feature subset for this problem. This is the reason we have applied FSAs that search for variable cardinality sets. Their results are shown in Table 1, rows 10-13. The use of this kind of FSAs does not highlight a unique proper size; it depends on the direction of the search, on the evaluation function and on the search algorithm employed by the FSAs.

The LVF FSA provides us a set of twenty features that have no inconsistencies. We can use this information in order to select a set of twenty features with the integer coded GA. So, we combine the information provided by a class separability measure (the inconsistency measure) with an accuracy one. The result is shown in Table 1, row 9.

The best result has been obtained with the binary coded GA, a wrapper FSA without limitation in the final number of features to select. This GA FSA makes a parallel search and it has not the limitation of the search direction as wrapper forward and backward FSAs have.

Nevertheless, sometimes is necessary to know a fix number of relevant symptoms and in this situation, we can use the integer coded GA FSA with previous information related to an adequate cardinality calculated by some class separability measure. The combination of filter and variable size with wrapper and fixed size FSAs allows us to obtain a small set of features with accurate behaviour.

An analysis of selected features in Table 1 and their descriptions (see the Appendix) points out the relevance of features 8, 10, 17-18, 20, 24, 34, 55, 62-63.

Table 1. Feature subsets and correct classification percentages for PD

Algorithm	Number of features	Selected Features	% Correct classification
Greedy	3	24,32,62	69.79
Greedy	4	10,24,32,62	72.92
Greedy	6	8,10,11,24,32,62	66.67
Greedy	8	6,8,10,11,24,29,32,62	69.79
Integer coded GA	3	18,20,62	84.87
Integer coded GA	4	17,20,24,43	81.25
Integer coded GA	6	17,24,34,63,67,71	75.00
Integer coded GA	8	10,18,20,22,28,30,60,62	84.38
Integer coded GA	20	8,17,18,25,27,28,29,30,31,32, 33,34,44,51,55,57,59,61,62,63	90.63
LVF	20	0,2,8,16,17,18,21,34,52,53,55, 56,57,58,61,66,67,69,71,75	68.75
Binary coded GA	30	3,8,10,13,16,21,22,25,26,27,29, 30, 31,32,34,35,37,38,39,44,47, 50,51,52,55,56,58,59,60,65	91.67
Wrapper forward	6	24,28,33,50,55,62	83.33
Wrapper backward	70	The complete set except 4,9,35,36,45 and 54 features	77.08

5   Concluding Remarks and Future Works

In this work we have applied a set of FSAs for the PD problem. These FSAs have selected a set of personality traits, which could be used as a complementary tool in an early diagnosis of PD. Considerations about the nosological differentiation between family and non-family PD have not been analysed.

As future work, we want to develop a hierarchical FSA, which could help us to confirm the hypothesis of both forms of the disease correspond to the same nosological entity. This FSA at a first level will select the relevant features considering not only an accuracy measure but also some class separability ones, with the objective to help in the early diagnose of PD. Finally it will work with the selected feature set to check if there are relevance differences between patients having sporadic PD and those presenting family aggreation.

For this problem, the design of a multiclassifier, which uses different feature sets in the diagnosis of PD can be considered. So, different feature sets could serve as a tool to complement diagnosis when the information is incomplete.

References

1. Battiti, R. Using Mutual Information for Selecting Features in Supervised Neural Net Learning. IEEE Transactions on Neuronal Networks **5:4** (1994) 537-550 197

2. Blesa, R. Diagnóstico precoz de la enfermedad de Parkinson. In:Obeso J., Martí-Massó J. (eds.):Enfermedad de Parkinson. McGraw-Hill (1993) 33-42 195
3. Caprara, G. V., Barbaranelli, C., Borgogni, L. Cuestionari ôBig-Fiveö TEA (1995) 198
4. Casillas, J, Del Jesus, M.J, Herrera, F. : Genetic Feature Selection in a Fuzzy Rule-Based Classification System Learning Process for High Dimensional Problems. Information Sciences **136** (2001) 135-137 197
5. Cattel, R. B. Cuestionario factorial de personalidad TEA(1992) 198
6. Dasarathy, B. V. Nearest Neighbour (NN) Norms: NN Pattern Classification Techniques. IEEE Computer Society Press (1990) 197
7. Eysenck, H. J., Eysenck, S. Cuestionario de Personalidad para Adultos TEA (1997) 198
8. Ferri, F. J., Pudil, P., Hatef, M., Kittler, J. Comparative Study of Techniques for Large-Scale Feature Selection. Pattern Recognition in Practice **IV** (1994) 403-413 196
9. Folstein, M., Folstein, S., McHugh, P. R. Mini-Mental State a practical method for grading the cognitive state of patients for the clinician. Journal of Psychiatry Research **12** (1975) 189-198 198
10. Goldberg, D. E. Genetic Algorithms in Search, Optimisation and Machine Learning. Addison-Wesley (1989) 197
11. Kohavi, R., John, G. H. Wrappers for Feature Subset Selection. Artificial Intelligence **97** (1997) 273-324 196, 197
12. Liu, H., Motoda, H. Feature Selection for Knowledge Discovery and Data Mining. Kluwer Academic Publisher (1998) 196, 197
13. Weiss, S., Kulikowski, C. Computer Systems that Learn. Morgan Kaufmann (1991) 198

Appendix

Table 2. Feature descriptions

N.	Description	N.	Description	N.	Description	N.	Description
0	Sex	19	Hardness	38	Blood pressure	57	C. of emotions-T
1	Age	20	Hardness-PC	39	Extraversion-16	58	Cont.of impulses
2	Evolution time	21	Sincerity	40	Anxiety	59	C. of impulses-T
3	Beginning age	22	Sincerity-PC	41	Hardness-16	60	Cultural opening
4	Tobacco	23	Affability	42	Independence	61	Cult. opening-T
5	Alcohol	24	Reasoning	43	Self-control	62	Exper. opening
6	Coffee or tea	25	Stability	44	Dynamism	63	Exp. opening-T
7	Water	26	Dominance	45	Dynamism-T	64	Energy
8	Toxic	27	Encouragement	46	Dominance-Five	65	Energy-T
9	Education	28	Normal attention	47	Dominance-T	66	Affability Five
10	Grey hair	29	Audacity	48	Co-operation	67	Affability-T
11	Antidepressant	30	Sensitivity	49	Co-operation-T	68	Firmness
12	Anxiolytic	31	Alertness	50	Cordiality	69	Firmness-T
13	Depression	32	Abstraction	51	Cordiality-T	70	Emotion Stability
14	M. M.E	33	Privacy	52	Meticulousness	71	Emot. Stability-T
15	Emotional	34	Apprehension	53	Meticulousness-T	72	Mental opening
16	Emotional-PC	35	Op. to the change	54	Perseverance	73	Ment. opening-T
17	Extraversion	36	Self-sufficiency	55	Perseverance-T	74	Distortion
18	Extrav.-PC	37	Perfectionism	56	Contr. of emotions	75	Distortion-T

A New Model for AIDS Survival Analysis

Jesus Orbe, Eva Ferreira, and Vicente Núñez-Antón

Departamento de Econometría y Estadística,
Universidad del País Vasco-Euskal Herriko Unibertsitatea,
Avda. Lehendakari Agirre, 83, E-48015 Bilbao, Spain
etporlij@bs.ehu.es
http://www.springer.de/comp/lncs/index.html

Abstract. In this work we present a new methodology proposed to study the survival time of Acquired Immune-Deficiency Syndrome diagnosed patients. This methodology is very flexible because it does not need the assumption of proportional hazards and the estimation is carried out without assuming any probability distribution for the variable of interest. The inference in the model has been put forward using bootstrap techniques. The main conclusion of the study is that the age of the patients and the period of diagnosis are relevant variables to explain the survival time for these patients.

1 Introduction

In this paper we study the survival time for AIDS (Acquired Immune-Deficiency Syndrome) diagnosed patients. Our dataset contains information about the survival time for patients who have lived in the Basque Autonomous Community and the Autonomous Community of Navarra in Spain.

A review of the literature on survival studies on AIDS (see, for example, some references in [1]) shows that practically all of the references focus on the study of the length of time for the "incubation" period, that is, the period starting with the seroconversion and lasting until the diagnosis of AIDS. This is the largest period in the evolution of the Human Immunodeficiency Virus (HIV) and it is at this time when the infected individual is classified as seropositive. For studies covering the same time period as the one in our sample, we have found that approximately 50% of the infected individuals develop the illness within ten years. During the "pre-antibody" stage, a period occurring right before the "incubation" period, infected people spend several months (less than two months for half of these individuals) before generating antibodies. In our study, instead of concentrating on these periods, we are interested in the last step of the illness, that is, the survival time starting with the diagnosis of the illness which begins when the infected individual develops some of the symptoms necessary to him/her an AIDS patient.

Survival data are very often censored and, usually, present asymmetric probability distributions. Because of these special characteristics, some specific methodologies for this kind of data have been developed. Among these, two major classes

J. Crespo, V. Maojo, and F. Martin (Eds.): ISMDA 2001, LNCS 2199, pp. 201–206, 2001.

of models are represented by the Cox model [2] and its various generalizations, mainly used in the medical and biostatistical fields, and the Accelerated Failure Time (AFT) models (see, for example, [3]), mainly used in reliability theory and industrial experiments. The models proposed by Cox is the most frequently used one because it offers the possibility to estimate the parameters of interest without assuming any probability distribution for the duration variable. However, the main drawback of this methodology lies on the need to have the restrictive assumption of proportional hazard functions. On the other hand, the usual estimation process for the AFT models implies the need to assume a given probability distribution for the duration variable.

The methodology used in this study is a flexible one because it does not require the knowledge of the probability distribution for the duration variable and, in addition, it does not need the assumption of proportional hazard functions. Moreover, this methodology allows us to estimate the direct effect of the covariates on the mean value of the duration, allowing for the possibility of specifying the effect of one of the covariables in a nonparametric way.

2   The Data

The dataset used here has been kindly provided by the "Centro Nacional de Epidemiología del Instituto de Salud Carlos III". This dataset contains information about a sample of 461 patients diagnosed with AIDS from 1984 until December 31, 1990. We followed these patients up until December 31, 1992. The survival time variable measures, in quarters, the lifetime from the diagnosis time up to the end of the study or up to death. Therefore, as it usually happens with this kind of data, we have some censored observations (right censoring). In order to explain this variable, we have information about personal characteristics of the patients and variables related to the illness. Thus, we can study the importance of those characteristics to explain the survival time of the patients.

We begin by indicating that the variables related to the characteristics of the individuals are the age and the gender of the patient. The variables related with the AIDS illness, in particular with the sort of disease at the diagnosis time are: the variable *Illa*, taking the value one if the patient has been diagnosed with AIDS through an opportunistic infection, and zero otherwise; the variable *Illb*, taking the value one if the AIDS diagnosis is produced by a Kaposi's sarcoma or some lymphoma, and zero otherwise; and the variable *Illc*, taking the value one if the patient has been diagnosed through an HIV encephalopathy or a HIV wasting syndrome, and zero otherwise. We also have information about the transmission via and, in order to code this effect, we have used five dummy variables: *Sexual, Drugs, Blood, Motherchild* and *Others*, taking value one if the transmission category is the indicated one, and zero otherwise (i.e., *Illc* and *Others* are the reference levels).

In addition, we have information about the time of diagnosis and, thus, we define another covariate that takes into account the diagnosis time (*Diagtime*). This covariate takes value one if the diagnosis takes place in the second quarter of 1984 (the first diagnosis), and value twenty seven for patients diagnosed in the last quarter of 1990. By using this variable, we can analyze the evolution of the survival time of the patients from the beginnings of the illness until 1990. In this evolution, we are particularly interested in studying the effect of the introduction of the Zidovudine (AZT) medicine on the survival time. The administration of AZT started in July 1987. In a previous work [4], we have tried to estimate this effect by using a dummy variable taking value one if the diagnosis had taken place after 1987, and zero otherwise. However, we think that it is more realistic to assume that the real effect of the administration of this medicine is more gradual than the sudden effect specified by a dummy variable. In addition, we have to point out that in [4] we assumed that the probability distribution of the duration followed a Weibull regression model. However, in this paper we use a new methodology that does not assume any probability distribution and, in addition, allows us to capture the gradual effect of the AZT treatment through a nonparametric specification of the *Diagtime* covariate.

3   The Model

We now briefly describe the model and the new methodology, based on the one proposed by Stute [5] for regression models with censored data. In summary, we will see that our methodology generalizes his.

Let us assume that we have a sample of observations (D_i, C_i, X_i) for $i = 1, \ldots, n$, where $D_1, \ldots, D_n$ are independent observations of the variable of interest, the duration variable, having some unknown distribution function F_D. $C_1, \ldots, C_n$ are independent observations of the censoring variable having some unknown distribution function F_C. In addition, we assume that D and C are independent variables and that $X_i = (X_{1,i}, \ldots, X_{k,i}, Z_i)$ is the $(k+1)$-dimensional vector of covariates for the i-th individual. Our goal is to be able to explain the relation between D and X using a regression model but, for our particular study, we need a semiparametric regression model. Thus, in the parametric component, assuming a linear relation, we introduce the first k covariates $(X_1, \ldots, X_k)$ and, in the nonparametric component, without assuming any functional form, we capture the effect of the covariate Z (in our example the *Diagtime* variable) on D. Due to the censoring, not all of the $D's$ are available; that is, rather than observing D_i, we observe O_i, the observed duration variable that is the minimum between the duration D_i and the censoring C_i. In addition, we know through an indicator variable I if each observation is censored or not. Thus, I_i takes value one if the i-th observation is not censored (i.e., $D_i \leq C_i$), and I_i takes value zero if the i-th observation is censored (i.e., $D_i > C_i$).

If we assume additive effects of the covariates on the logarithmic of the duration variable, we have the following model:

$$\log D_i = \beta_1 X_{1,i} + \ldots + \beta_k X_{k,i} + g(Z_i) + \mu_i \qquad \text{for} \qquad i = 1, \ldots, n \quad (1)$$

The estimation of the effect of the covariates can be carried out by minimizing the following expression:

$$\sum_{i=1}^{n} W_{in} [\log O_{(i)} - \beta_1 X_{[1,i]} - \ldots - \beta_k X_{[k,i]} - g(Z_{[i]})]^2 + h \int [g''(z)]^2 dz, \quad (2)$$

where $\log O_{(i)}$ is the i-th ordered value of the observed duration variable $\log O$, $(X_{[1,i]}, \ldots, X_{[k,i]}, Z_{[i]})$ is the concomitant vector of covariates associated with $\log O_{(i)}$, h is the smoothing parameter and W_{in} are the Kaplan-Meier weights, defined by:

$$W_{in} = \hat{F}_D(\log O_{(i)}) - \hat{F}_D(\log O_{(i-1)}),$$

and $\hat{F}_D$ is a Kaplan-Meier estimator [6] of the distribution function F_D.

As can be seen from (2), in order to estimate the model in (1), we have to consider several issues: (i) the goodness of the fit, (ii) the smoothness of the proposed function to model the effect of the covariate included in the nonparametric component, and (iii) the presence of censored observations. As for the goodness of the fit, this is controlled through the sum of the weighted squared residuals using the Kaplan-Meier weights. Thus, by using these weights, we take into account the existence of censored observations in the sample. As for the smoothness, we measure it in the usual way by using the integral of the square of second derivatives. The degree of smoothness is determined by h, the smoothing parameter. Large values of h produce smoother curves, while smaller values produce more wiggly curves. When h is close to zero, the penalty term becomes not relevant and the solution tends to an interpolating one. However, when h is large enough, the penalty term dominates and, thus, we obtain the weighted least squares solution.

It can be shown that the solution of the minimization problem for the function g is a natural cubic spline. Therefore, by using the value-second derivative representation of a natural cubic spline presented in Section 2.1 of [7], we can rewrite (2) and, thus, we can take derivatives in this new expression, with respect to β and $\mathbf{g}$ (where $\mathbf{g}$ is the vector of values $g_j = g(z_j)$ for $j = 1, \ldots, m$ and m is the number of distinct values for the covariate Z), obtaining the solution for β and g. For more details about the complete estimation process see [8]. We would like to add that [8] contains a simulation study, using different censoring levels and several sample sizes, to verify that the proposed estimation methodology to estimate the semiparametric censored regression model produces good estimates for the parametric component and for the nonparametric one, even in the case of a complicated function.

4   Empirical Results and Conclusions

In this section we fit model (1) by using the proposed methodology to our AIDS diagnosis patients dataset. In the parametric component, we introduce, specifying a linear effect, all the covariates except the diagnosis time (*Diagtime*), which is introduced in the nonparametric component. Thus, we estimate the model following the estimation procedure presented above. Table 1 and Figure 1 contain the results of the analysis for the parametric and nonparametric components, respectively. We have to point out that the confidence intervals and the variance of the estimators have been calculated by using bootstrap techniques. In addition, to obtain both the confidence intervals and variances, we have developed a new and flexible bootstrap resample generating procedure adequate for regression models with censored observations. This procedure is a flexible one, because is does not assume any relation between the censoring and the covariates (for more details about the proposed bootstrap procedure see [8]).

Table 1. Estimates of the β coefficients and 95% confidence bootstrap intervals

Variable	β	Variance	Lower Limit	Upper Limit
Constant	0.5266	0.1859	-0.3611	1.3357
Motherchild	0.3877	0.3110	-0.6330	1.5835
Blood	0.0702	0.0872	-0.4866	0.6971
Drugs	-0.0430	0.0472	-0.4722	0.3779
Sexual	-0.1201	0.0635	-0.6020	0.3610
IIIa	-0.0154	0.0745	-0.5672	0.5080
IIIb	-0.0508	0.1114	-0.6882	0.6272
Gender	0.0348	0.0203	-0.2501	0.3106
Age	-0.0177	0.00004	-0.0313	-0.0052

With regard to the estimation for the parametric component, we can conclude that the age of the patient has a negative significant effect on the survival time of the patient. The rest of the covariates: gender, transmission via and diagnosis illness turned out to be non statistically significant to explain the survival time. If we analyze the results for the nonparametric component (Figure 1), we can see that, when we move from the beginning of the illness, the survival of the patient increases, and this increment has a strong acceleration several quarters before the beginning of AZT administration (i.e. $z = 13$). Therefore, this acceleration can explain the positive effect of the treatment by increasing the survival time. In addition, this positive effect is previous to the introduction of AZT because patients whose diagnosis time was several quarters before starting the administration of AZT also receive the treatment. As for the estimation of g at the last diagnosis quarters, we want to mention that this final drop is caused by the data, because the distance from these quarters to the end of 1992 is not big enough to observe the duration in all of the cases and, therefore, the maximum reachable duration is smaller when we are approximating the last quarters in the sample.

Finally, in order to summarize our proposals, we have to mention that we have used a flexible model without assuming any probability distribution for the duration variable, which must indeed be done when using the AFT models, and

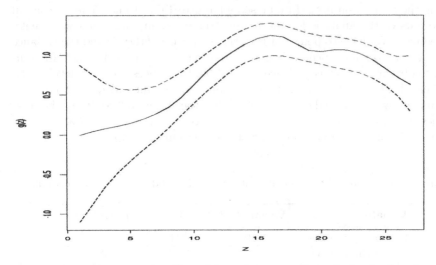

Fig. 1. The estimation and 95% confidence bootstrap intervals for the function g introduced in the nonparametric component of the semiparametric model

without assuming proportional hazard functions, as required when using Cox's models. In addition, to be able to estimate the effect of the administration of AZT on the survival, we have introduced this effect in a flexible form using a nonparametric term, so that it is possible to capture its gradual effect on the duration variable.

References

1. Brookmeyer, R., Gail, M.H.: AIDS Epidemiology a Quantitative Approach, Oxford University Press, Oxford (1993)
2. Cox, D.R.: Regression models and life-tables. Journal of the Royal Statistical Society-Series B Vol. **34** (1972) 187–220
3. Lawless, J.F.: Statistical Models and Methods for Lifetime Data. John Wiley and Sons, New York (1982)
4. Orbe, J., Fernández, A., Nuñez-Antón, V.: Análisis de la supervivencia en enfermos de SIDA residentes en la Comunidad Autónoma del País Vasco y Navarra. Osasunkaria Vol. **12** (1996) 1–8
5. Stute, W.: Consistent estimation under random censorship when covariables are present. Journal of Multivariate Analysis Vol. **45** (1993) 89–103
6. Kaplan, E.L., Meier, P.: Nonparametric estimation from incomplete observations. Journal of the American Statistical Association Vol. **53** (1958) 457–481
7. Green, P.J., Silverman, B.W.: Nonparametric Regression and Generalized Linear Models, Chapman and Hall, London (1994)
8. Orbe, J., Ferreira, E., Nuñez-Antón, V.: Survival Analysis using a Censored Semiparametric Regression Model. Documentos de Trabajo (Biltoki) D.T. 2000.07, Universidad del País Vasco-Euskal Herriko Unibertsitatea (2000)

A Frequent Patterns Tree Approach for Rule Generation with Categorical Septic Shock Patient Data

Jürgen Paetz[1,2] and Rüdiger Brause[1]

[1] J. W. Goethe-Universität Frankfurt am Main, Fachbereich Biologie und Informatik,
Institut für Informatik, AG Adaptive Systemarchitektur
Robert-Mayer-Straße 11-15, D-60054 Frankfurt am Main, Germany
[2] Klinikum der J.W. Goethe-Universität, Klinik für Allgemein- und Gefäßchirurgie
Theodor-Stern-Kai 7, D-60590 Frankfurt am Main, Germany
{brause,paetz}@cs.uni-frankfurt.de
http://www.medan.de

Abstract. In abdominal intensive care medicine letality of septic shock patients is very high. In this contribution we present results of a data driven rule generation with *categorical septic shock patient data*, collected from 1996 to 1999. Our descriptive approach includes preprocessing of data for rule generation and application of an efficient algorithm for frequent patterns generation. Performance of generated rules is rated by frequency and confidence measures. The best rules are presented. They provide new quantitative insight for physicians with regard to septic shock patient outcome.

1 Introduction

A septic shock during a stay in an intensive care unit affects outcome in a negative manner [1], [2]. This phenomenon is related to mechanisms of the immune system [3]. Our approach to reduce letality of septic shock patients is the automated, intelligent search of information in already documented patient records without looking at additional costly measurements of immune system reactions and markers. We analysed the data of 362 patients by 30 boolean variables, including almost all the usually documented categorical data like relevant diagnoses, medicaments and therapies. For technical reasons operations were not included in this analysis. Data was collected in a german hospital from 1996 to 1999. 14.9% of all the patients are deceased. Our analysis of categorical data carries on the analyses already done for metric septic shock patient data with another data base in [4] and [5]. To find interesting rules within the high number of all the rules coming from subsets of 30 variables we used a tree search algorithm based on [6] which is described in Sect. 2. Subsequently, in Sect. 3 achieved results are presented.

J. Crespo, V. Maojo, and F. Martin (Eds.): ISMDA 2001, LNCS 2199, pp. 207–213, 2001.
© Springer-Verlag Berlin Heidelberg 2001

2   Frequent and Confident Patterns by FP-Trees

If you have medical – or economical, geological, biological, etc. – categorical variables (in database language called *attributes*) with different possible values like
{high, middle, low}, {yes, no} or {A, B, C, ...}, i.e. n different variables $v_1, \ldots, v_n$,
each variable v_i takes one of the m_i different values $a_{i,1}, \ldots, a_{i,m_i}$, it could be
interesting to find out which combinations of attribute values could be observed
with respect to one class c like the class of deceased patients. Therefore, all the
patients P_j are listed with their attribute values and their outcome, e.g. $P_1 :=$
(high,yes,...,C,no;deceased), $P_2 :=$ (low,yes,...,D,no;survived), etc. Now we are
looking for rules of the form "**if** $v_{l_1} = a_{l_1,k_1}$ **and** ... **and** $v_{l_s} = a_{l_s,k_s}$ **then**
class c" that contain a small number s of variables. Rule R is better than a
rule S if it is valid for more samples (patients), and R is also better than S if it
produces less misclassifications. For this purpose the *frequency* and *confidence*
of a rule are defined in Sect. 2.1.

There exist a lot of different approaches to solve the combinatorical problem
of finding appropriate rules efficiently, e.g. [7], [8]. Ref. [7] combines the elemen-
tary attributes to more complex combinations, evaluating the frequencies of the
emerged patterns (*association rules*). [8] starts using the complex patterns P_j,
melting them to less complex rules (*generalization rules*). Both algorithms are
based on *frequent patterns*, i.e. frequent occurences of equal attribute values in
different samples. So, here we base our algorithm on a frequent patterns approach to generate rules, improving it by additional confidence calculations, see
Sect. 2.2.

2.1   Frequency and Confidence of Rules

Now, we define the common rule performance measures *frequency* and *confidence*.

Definition 1: (Frequency and Confidence)
Let N be the number of all the samples and let R be a generated rule of class c
with $\leq n$ attribute values b_k for variables v_k. Let $\sharp$ denote the number of elements
of a set.
a) The **frequency** freq$(R) \in [0, 1]$ of R is the number of samples $P_j = (d_1, \ldots, d_n; \tilde{c})$ that induces rule R divided by N, i.e.

$$\text{freq}(R) := \frac{\sharp\{P_j \mid \forall k \ (b_k \text{ is attribute value of } R \text{ and } b_k = d_k)\}}{N} . \tag{1}$$

b) The **confidence with respect to c** conf$(R, c) \in [0, 1]$ of R is defined as
the number of all the samples of class c inducing R divided by the number of
samples P_j of any class that induces rule R,[1] i.e.

$$\text{conf}(R, c) := \frac{\sharp\{P_j = (d_1, \ldots, d_n; c) \mid \forall k \ (b_k \text{ is attrib. value of } R \text{ and } b_k = d_k)\}}{\sharp\{P_j \mid \forall k \ (b_k \text{ is attribute value of } R \text{ and } b_k = d_k)\}} . \tag{2}$$

---

[1] Multiplied by 100 the measures could be interpreted as a percentage.

The aim of our rule generation process is now to find all the sufficient *frequent* and *confident* rules R, those with $\text{freq}(R) \geq \text{min}_{\text{freq}}$ and $\text{conf}(R, c) \geq \text{min}_{\text{conf}}$ using predefined thresholds min_{freq} and min_{conf}. These thresholds must be high enough to provide interesting, significant rules and low enough to generate a sufficient number of rules. So an expert of the application area – in medical applications a physician – has to be involved in order to design proper thresholds for useful results.

To extract all the frequent patterns fast without scanning the database several times we use the FP-tree structure.

2.2   The FP-Tree Approach

For convenience of the reader we repeat shortly the ideas behind the basic algorithm with an example. We refer to [6] for more formal, extensive definitions, proofs and explanations. Basic knowledge of data structures for algorithms [9] is required. For our purpose we changed the algorithm slightly and added the last step 7.

1. Let us assume, our database D consists of three patient records, each with 3 variables: $P_1 = (\text{yes}, \text{high}, \text{low}; \text{deceased})$, $P_2 = (\text{yes}, \text{middle}, \text{low}; \text{deceased})$ and $P_3 = (\text{no}, \text{high}, \text{middle}; \text{survived})$. For technical reasons, encode the attribute values so that no attribute value of one variable is equal to one of another variable. For our example, we encode the attribute values with letters: $P_1 = (A, G, L; \text{deceased})$, $P_2 = (A, H, L; \text{deceased})$ and $P_3 = (B, G, M; \text{survived})$. We choose $\text{min}_{\text{freq}} := 2/3$ and $\text{min}_{\text{conf}} := 0.6$ for class "deceased".
2. For generating a FP-tree for class "deceased" in step 3, we have to count the frequency of all attribute values related to this class and order the attributes in a descending list. For our small database of three patients we get: (A:2), (L:2), (G:1), (H:1), (B:0), (M:0). Then we re-order the attributes in the samples with respect to this list: $P_1 = (A, L, G; \text{deceased})$, $P_2 = (A, L, H; \text{deceased})$ and $P_3 = (G, B, M; \text{survived})$.

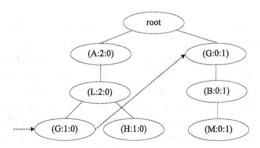

Fig. 1. FP-tree for database D with node information. Here, only G's link list is shown (dotted arrows)

3. We build up a prefix-tree with an additional link list pointer for every attribute and attached basic information (attribute value, frequency count "deceased", frequency count "survived") to every node, see Fig. 1. This prefix-tree is called a **FP-tree**. So, the data base is very efficiently stored, avoiding redundancy (*database compression*). You can efficiently reconstruct all the samples and their frequencies for the class "deceased".

4. For every attribute construct a **conditional database**, i.e. walk through the link lists of the items and build up (from attribute node to root) lists of all prefix paths with maximal possible frequency for the classes "deceased" and "survived" in the path. For our example, this means for item A the path (<root>), for item L the path (<(A:2:0), root>), for G the paths: (<(L:1:0), (A:1:0), root>, <root>), for H: (<(L:1:0), (A:1:0), root>), for B: (<(G:0:1), root>) and for M: (<(B:0:1), (G:0:1), root>). After step 4 we have a set of conditional databases.

5. We chose $\min_{\text{freq}} = 2/3$ for class "deceased" in step 1, so without the trivial path <root> we only have to consider the path L: (<(A:2:0), root>), because all the other paths do not fulfill the frequency threshold condition (*frequency pruning*).

6. For all conditional databases – generated in step 4 – that contain more than one single path, build a (sub-)FP-tree using items and frequencies from the paths. Then, repeat steps 4 and 5 separately for every (sub-)FP-tree (recursion). For conditional databases with only a single path go on with step 7. In our simple example we need no recursion for the single conditional database L: (<(A:2:0), root>).

7. Calculate the confidence for combinations – that represent the rules – in each single path, i.e. for the resulting rules. For this purpose in our example we set $R_1 := (A, L)$, $R_2 := (A)$ and $R_3 := (L)$. Then, we have $\text{conf}(R_1,\text{deceased}) = 1$, $\text{conf}(R_2,\text{deceased}) = 1$, $\text{conf}(R_3,\text{deceased}) = 1$. Select confident rules with respect to $\min_{\text{conf}}$. Here, all three rules are confident. However, we generate longer rules only if the confidence is better, but this depends on the application. So only $R_2 = (A)$ and $R_3 = (L)$ - meaning "yes" resp. "low" – are given out, i.e. we have generated two rules R_2 "**if** $\text{var}_1 = $ yes **then** class deceased" and R_3 "**if** $\text{var}_3 = $ low **then** class deceased", both with confidence 1 for class "deceased" and frequency 2/3.

Of course, the whole procedure could be applied for class "survived". The algorithm performs efficiently if and only if there are a lot of common long subpatterns in most of the samples of the database, so that there is no explosion of recursive calls of the steps 4 and 5. Due to the fact that we have only binary variables and patients with a very individual behaviour the algorithm is not very performant, but until now it is one of the few algorithms that can find *all* frequent and confident rules in acceptable time. Other algorithms could be more inefficient due to a *combinatorical explosion* in the search space.

3 Results

Before we will present the results of our application of the FP-tree approach, we give a short description of the database with respect to preprocessing steps.

3.1 Data Preprocessing

Our database consists of 362 septic shock patients. Because it is often difficult to get a verification of an infection in time, this criteria was not presumed in the septic shock definition. The data of each patient was given as admission data (e.g. chronic diagnoses) and daily measurements (e.g. acute diagnoses, medicaments and therapies). We extracted binary values from *time series* in the following manner: If someone developed an organ failure during a stay at the hospital we set this binary variable to "true" for this patient. So the dynamical behaviour of the time series is lost; the analysis of dynamical behaviour of 30 synced variables is not yet possible. – Another problem are *missing values*: A maximum of 30, a minimum of 12 and a mean of 25 variables was available for every patient. For this reason some technical adaptations were necessary in the FP-tree algorithm. In fact, preprocessing of multivariate time series with missing values – the usual case in medical databases – is very time consuming but although very important [5], [10].

3.2 Generated Rules

Now, let us give examples of frequent and confident rules. We chose $\min_{\text{freq}} = 0.020$ and $\min_{\text{conf}} = 0.750$ for class "deceased". Because the database of survived patients is easier to describe with rules we set $\min_{\text{freq}} = 0.165$ and $\min_{\text{conf}} = 0.980$ for class "survived". We generated 1284 rules for class "deceased" and 9976 rules for class "survived" that are frequent and confident with respect to the thresholds. Two of the best rules for survival and death are listed below.

1) "**if** peritoneal lavage = no **and** thrombocyte concentrate = no **and** haemodialysis = no **then** class survived **with** confidence 0.980 **and** frequency 0.420"

2) "**if** haemofiltration = no **and** reoperation = no **and** acute renal failure = no **and** liver cirrhosis = no **then** class survived **with** confidence 0.990 **and** frequency 0.290"

3) "**if** minimal use of three different antibiotics = yes **and** artificial respiration = yes **and** tube feeding = no **then** class deceased **with** confidence 0.818 **and** frequency 0.030"

4) "**if** organ failure = yes **and** antiarrythmics = yes **and** haemodialysis = yes **and** peritoneal lavage = yes **then** class deceased **with** confidence 0.800 **and** frequency 0.028"

Although the rules are frequent and confident enough to indicate survival and death of patients and the rules have mostly conditions for only a few of the 30 variables, the number of rules is surely too high. A physician can not consider all the rules for practical use. So future work have to be done to find a smaller rule basis that describes the patient data sufficiently.

4   Conclusion

Our aim was the extraction of information from categorical septic shock patient data. For this purpose we applied an efficient improved frequent patterns algorithm to generate frequent and confident rules. We obtained a lot of performant rules for the classes of deceased and survived patients. Such rules give good hints for physicians. The remaining problem is the high number of interesting rules – due to the individual behaviour of the patients – that have to be reduced technically with the support of experts to obtain a human understandable rule basis. Also it is desirable to combine an approach for categorical data with an approach for metric rule generation to build up a warning system. Finally, we plan to analyse multicenter data to get more representative results.

Acknowledgement

Our work was done within the DFG-project MEDAN (Medical Data Analysis with Neural Networks). The authors like to thank Mr. Slomka who implemented the FP-tree algorithm and all the participants of the MEDAN working group especially Prof. Hanisch.

References

1. Wade, S., Büssow, M., Hanisch, E.: Epidemiologie von SIRS, Sepsis und septischem Schock bei chirurgischen Intensivpatienten. Der Chirurg **69** (1998) 648–655   207
2. Schoenberg, M. H., Weiss, M., Radermacher, P.: Outcome of Patients with Sepsis and Septic Shock after ICU Treatment. Arch Surch **383** (1998) 44–48   207
3. Fein, A. M. et al. (eds.): Sepsis and Multiorgan Failure, Williams & Wilkins Baltimore (1997)   207
4. Hamker, F., Paetz, J., Thöne, S., Brause, R., Hanisch, E.: Erkennung kritischer Zustände von Patienten mit der Diagnose "Septischer Schock" mit einem RBF-Netz. Interner Bericht 04/00, FB Informatik, J. W. Goethe-Univ. Frankfurt am Main, Germany (2000)   207
5. Paetz, J., Hamker, F., Thöne, S.: About the Analysis of Septic Shock Patient Data. 1st Int. Symp. on Medical Data Analysis (ISMDA). Frankfurt am Main, Germany. LNCS Vol. 1933. Springer-Verlag (2000) 130–137   207, 211
6. Han, J., Pei, J., Yin, Y.: Mining Frequent Patterns Without Candidate Generation. ACM SIGMOD Int. Conf. on Management of Data. Dallas, USA (2000) 1–12   207, 209
7. Agrawal, R., Skrikant, R.: Fast Algorithms for Mining Association Rules. 20th Int. Conf. on Very Large Databases (VLDB). Santiago de Chile, Chile (1994) 487–499   208
8. Brause, R., Langsdorf, T., Hepp, M.: Neural Data Mining for Credit Card Fraud Detection. 11th IEEE Int. Conf. on Tools with Artificial Intelligence (ICTAI). Chicago, USA (1999) 103–106   208
9. Sedgewick, R.: Algorithms in C. Addison Wesley (1992)   209
10. Tsumoto, S.: Clinical Knowledge Discovery in Hospital Information Systems: Two Case Studies. 4th European Conf. on Principles of Data Mining and Knowledge Discovery (PKDD). Lyon, France. LNAI Vol. 1704. Springer-Verlag (2000) 652–656   211

Analysis of Medical Diagnostic Images via the Implementation and Access to a Safe DICOM PACS with a Web Interface: Analysis of Contrast-enhanced CT Imaging of Oral and Oropharyngeal Carcinomas.

Javier Pereira[1], Alejandro Lamelo[1], Jose Manuel Vázquez-Naya[1], Mario Fernández[1], Julián Dorado[2], Antonino Santos[2], Jorge Teijeiro[1], and Alejandro Pazos[2]

[1] Medical and Diagnostic Radiologic Image Laboratory (IMEDIR Lab.), A Corunha University. Spain.
javierp@udc.es; {alamelo, jose}@mail2.udc.es; {mmff, jtv}@udc.es
http://www.imedir.udc.es

[2] Artificial Neural Networks and Adaptative Systems (RNASA//GIB Lab.). Department of Information and Communications Technology, A Corunha University. Spain.
{julian, nino, ciapazos}@udc.es

Abstract. The implementation of an Information System of medical images with safe Internet access and with an interface which allows visualization, analysis, processing and advanced visualization, will enable the radiologist to access those clinical cases he wishes to consult, both within the hospital Intranet and also from an extranet.

Freeware software has been used for its implementation and the analysis, processing and advanced visualization module is easily integrated in the existing equipment of the organization. This system also allows for the production of multi-centre epidemiological studies.

An analysis of radiological data from patients with head and neck cancer were carried out in order to validate the system. This system has automatic link devices with the medical modality equipment for a safe and restricted acquisition, storing, and access. This allows its integration within the existing RIS at the medical centres.

1 Introduction

As in any other research field, in the medical environment the present developments of software applications tend to be designed for their use within the Net, making the most of the Internet infrastructure.

The development of an information acquisition, storing and management system which can be accessed from remote spots and which possesses an ergonomic and user-friendly interface is necessary when we try to carry out a medical study. In the present case, our study uses diagnostic images (also known as modalities), such as Computerized Tomography (CT), Digital Substraction Angiography (DSA), Nuclear Medicine (NM), Magnetic Resonance Imaging (MRI) or ultrasounds (US)[1][2][3] [4].

A research was carried out in order to validate the system, in which information and communication technologies were applied to the digital access and treatment of

J. Crespo, V. Maojo, and F. Martin (Eds.): ISMDA 2001, LNCS 2199, pp. 213–218, 2001.

CT images, in order to obtain certain parameters. The results were later compared to the anatomic-pathology findings and to the survival of a series of patients suffering from epidermis carcinoma of the oral pharynx cavity.

The present paper introduces an Information System of Medical Diagnostic Images which can be accessed from the Web, and which integrates a set of digital analysis and processing tools which allow to carry out multi-centre studies, regardless of the number of participants and their geographical location.

The system developed centralizes all the modalities of a medium-sized hospital. Restricted access is permitted according to the access privileges, in order to produce reports or just to check results.

2 Material and Methods

2.1 System's Architecture

One of the main goals established when planning the design of the system was that of achieving a final product as open and compatible as possible. That is the reason why a PC in NT Windows environment was used as hardware platform.

With regard to the software used for the implementation, Apache v.1.3.12[5] was used as web server, a freeware server widely used on the Internet[6]. MySql was used as Data Base manager, being a freeware data base engine which is also widely used on the Internet at present[7]. PHP4 was installed for the implementation of dynamic web pages, which is also a freeware tool[8].

2.2 Image Acquisition Mechanism

Once the communication network is analysed, the equipment may be divided into three different types: DICOM compatible and non-compatible[9].
a) An application with the services Query/Retrieve and Storage was designed for the acquisition of images with the DICOM equipment, acting as SCU (Service Class User), and being able to acquire and introduce the images into the PACS. The equipments are consulted every 24 hours.
b) With non-compatible DICOM madalities, they are acquired through a programmed FTP, being transformed form their proprietary format to the DICOM standard via a software which has been developed for that purpose.

2.3 Development of the Output Interface

It was defined which information would be shown via the web pages, the look of the screens and the basic functions of the pages accessed through the Internet.

2.4 Security Devices

User profiles and safe data transmission. At this stage it was decided which information is of public access and which restricted. In order to maintain the privacy of data in the Internet transmissions, it is necessary to use a safe protocol.

2.5 Visualization and Analysis Tools

The image analysis functions allowed by traditional web pages are very limited. A JAVA technology was developed in order to access the image source and to apply various digital processing techniques. It also provides the user with a series of tools, which try to assist with the acquisition of a more accurate report. There are several possibilities: outlining, softening, pseudo-colour, application of standard protocols for visualizing grey windows, equalization, modification of brightness and contrast, manual outlining of edges and visualization of the histogram of the 3D image.

2.6 Description and Analysis of the Clinical Series

Both for the development of the system and for the evaluation of the method, a retrospective sample of patients from the ENT department of Juan Canalejo Hospital is used. 38 patients with oral and oropharyngeal carcinoma were included in the sample, with a follow-up from 22 to 89 months.

The contrast used in Computerized Tomography (CT) was Iohexol (Omnipaque) for every case, according to the existing protocol for head and neck tumours.

All surgical pieces and preparations were reviewed by 2 observers from Pathology department.

The images used are the contrast tomographical studies carried out on the patients before surgical treatment.

Preparation of the samples were carried out with the tools supplied by the system:

a) three slices with a good visualization of the whole tumoral mass were chosen. The artefacts usually come form the patients' metallic tooth fillings

b) the density of the muscle obtained from sampling the posterior muscles of the neck, and these will be used as a reference for tumour parameters. Equalizing of the tumoral image will increase the contrast of the tumour structures to reach the maximum definition of the tumoral border. Finally, the 3D histogram is calculated in order to visualize the 256 grey levels and to facilitate the manual segmentation of the tumour in CT scan. Once the tumour profile is obtained for each of the three slices selected for each patient, the following data is calculated: number of segmented pixels, range, average, mode, standard histogram deviation, percentage value at 50(p50), 75(p75), 90(p90) and 100 (p100). Finally, the following parameters are defined for each patient: patient tumour average (XP), patient tumour medium (LP), p75 patient (LXXVP), p90 patient (XCP), p100 patient (CM), patient tumour average dif. – patient muscle average (XD), dif.p75 patient tumour - patient muscle average (LXXVD), dif.p90 patient tumour - patient muscle average (XCD), dif. p100 patient tumour - patient muscle average (CD), % pixel threshold below muscle density (VIABLE)

3 Results

3.1 System's Functioning

The huge size of these data makes their Internet transmission slow. With the purpose of reducing the waiting time, a fast visualization icon (preview) is generated for each image in JPG format (around 50 kb). These icons allow the medical doctor to have a first rapid glimpse of the study, so that a specific image can be selected to be analysed or reported. Then the original DICOM image (full size) is visualized. The DICOM files are validated after being acquired by the sending equipment, their preview is generated and they are stored in the database as BLOB data (Binary Large Object), thus respecting the standard.

The access interface to the system is via web pages. This environment is familiar to the doctors, which facilitates their acceptance, avoiding usage-learning time.

3.2 Implementation of Security Devices

In order to guarantee the confidentiality of data avoiding their access by non-authorized personnel, user profiles have been defined: there are users who have access to certain information, others who may access the whole information but cannot modify it, while others are able to check studies, to analyse them and to register modifications.

The SSL protocol (Secure Sockets Layer) was used for a safe Internet transmission, which guarantees the privacy and integrity of the transmitted data, and the identity of the Web server [10].

3.3 Analysis of Medical Data

Among the tools used for segmentation, those designed for facilitating the manual segmentation tasks have proved to be completely satisfactory. Image equalization and 3D histogram segmentation were the chosen procedures for segmentating most tumours. Other procedures, such as pseudo-colour, have been discarded due to lack of information about the correlation between each tissue type and their radiological density.

With regard to the correlation between anatomic-radiology and survival, those poorly differentiated tumours had lower proportions of tumour mass below the muscle density threshold (83,4%) with regard to those which were moderately or well differentiated (94,1%). This difference proved to be statistically significant. The poor histological differentiation has been independently related to a lower global survival rate (13,5% v. 44,3 months), cause-specific survival (13,5 v. 46,9 months), and shorter disease-free period (5,2 v. 36,6 months). The *viable* parameter has been significantly different in the tumours of deceased patients (90,6%) with regard to survivors (97,2%), and also among those patients who died from the illness compared to the rest (90,5% v. 96,4%). Those patients with more than 90% of threshold tumour had a greater survival rate (48,8 months) than those with less than 90% (19,6 months) ($p<0,05$). For cause-specific survival, it was found that those tumours with more than

95% had a greater survival rate, with an average life of 54 months, compared to the 25,6 months of those with less than 95% (p<0,05).

The tumour average did not show any relationship with pathological parameters or prognosis. However, the difference of the tumoral average density with the muscle reference (XD), which stands for the tumour contrast in relation to the tissue with a relatively homogeneous uptake level in time, has shown certain qualities. The measurement clearly represents other data, given that the medium muscle variable has shown a high variability among the patients (107,8, ranging from 128,7 to 236,5 (ED:25,15)). This big variability among patients justifies the need to obtain individualized figures for each patient. XD has been statistically related to microvascular infiltration of tumours. Those tumours with microvascular infiltration had an average XD of 42,9, while those tumours without it did not influence the statistical survival of our patients. However, infiltration is associated with a poorer prognosis in most publications in head and neck cancer.

The maximum contrast concentration (CM) was higher in the group of patients who have developed a local relapse with regard to those who have not (246,5 v. 239,9).

4 Discussion

The information demand, both from external and internal sources, occurs once the PACS is implanted. The answer to these demands is easily solved by means of using Web technology.

The system was developed with medium-low cost tools: PC hardware and freeware software. The performance is acceptable for a medium-sized hospital (around 100 beds) such as the one used for the clinical research. If the hospital was bigger, commercial tools would have to be used, which guarantee reasonable response times regardless of the work load, the concurrent access of a great number of users and a fault-tolerant hardware.

With regard to scalability, the system's storage requirements will increase indefinitely. It is necessary to devise a mechanism which will enable old studies (for instance, more than four year old) to be restored in low-cost storage systems (DLT.DDS4, etc.).

With regard to the results of the clinical study, the findings serve to state that the distribution of hydrosoluble contrast media such as Iohexol, in neck and head carcinomas is different among tumours. And this heterogeneity may have a pathological basis.

5 Conclusions

Image diagnosis researchers will have the chance to access clinical studies from any computer linked to the Internet. This opens the field of medical studies, which require the use of clinical series with a huge number of cases. It is possible to create clinical series among several centres by means of Information Systems such as the one introduced in the present paper, series which can be analysed by different doctors in a simple manner.

According to the requirements of the Spanish legislation, certain security levels for information access have been implemented, together with a communication protocol, which guarantees the safe transmission of data[11][12].

This system is user-friendly and has a low cost, while DICOM modalities are automatically acquired. Freeware tools are used, with a widespread Internet use and a great number of servers.

Acknowledgments

This work was supported in part by the Spanish Department of Science and Technology (MCYT). Reference TIC2000-0120 -P4-03.

References

1. Fernandez-Bayo J, Barbero O, Rubies C, Sentis M, Donoso L. Distributing medical images with internet technologies: a DICOM web server and a DICOM java viewer. Radiographics. 2000 Mar-Apr;20(2):581-90
2. McColl R, Lane T. The DICOM-WWW gateway: Implementation, configuration, security and privacy. [Last access 04/01/2001]. Available URL *http://www.rad.swmed.edu/PhysWeb/dicom.htm*
3. Grevera GJ, Feingold E, Horii SC. A WWW to DICOM interface. [Last access 04/01/2001]. Available URL *http://oasis.rad.upenn.edu/~grevera/papers/spie /mi96/www.paper.html*
4. Lou SL, Hoogstrate, Huang HK. Automated PACS image adquisition and recovery scheme for image integrity based on the DICOM standard. Comput Med Imag Graph 1997;21:209
5. Apache secured by SSL [Last access 05/01/2001]. Available URL: *http://www.apache-ssl.org/*
6. The Netcraft Web Server Survey [Last access 05/02/2001]. Available URL: *http://www.netcraft.com/survey/*
7. MySQL Official Homepage [Last access 05/01/2001]. Available URL: *http://mysql.com/*
8. Sæther Bakken S, Aulbach A, Schmid E, Winstead J, Torben Wilson T, Lerdorf R et. al. PHP Manual [Last access 05/02/2001]. Available URL: *http://www.php.net/manual/*
9. DICOM Standard Status. Base Standard - 2000. [Last access 04/01/2001] Available URL: http://www.dclunie.com/dicom-status/status.html
10. OpenSSL Official Homepage [Last access 05/02/2001]. Available URL: *http://www.openssl.org/*
11. Ley Orgánica 15/1999, de 13 de diciembre, de Protección de Datos de Carácter Personal (Boletín Oficial del Estado, número 298, de 14 de diciembre de 1999)
12. Real Decreto 994/1999, de 11 de junio, por el que se aprueba el Reglamento de medidas de seguridad de los ficheros automatizados que contengan datos de carácter personal (Boletín Oficial del Estado, número 151, de 25 de junio de 1999)

Classification of HEp-2 Cells
Using Fluorescent Image Analysis and Data Mining

Petra Perner

Institute of Computer Vision and Applied Computer Sciences
Arno-Nitzsche-Str. 45, D-04277 Leipzig, Germany
ibaiperner@aol.com
http://www.ibai-research.de

Abstract. The cells that are considered in this application for an automated image analysis are Hep-2 cells which are used for the identification of antinuclear autoantibodies (ANA). Hep-2 cells allow for recognition of over 30 different nuclear and cytoplasmic patterns, which are given by upwards of 100 different autoantibodies. The identification of the patterns has recently been done manually by a human inspecting the slides with a microscope. In this paper we present results on image analysis, feature extraction, and classification. Starting from a knowledge acquisition process with a human operator, we developed an image analysis and feature extraction algorithm. A data set containing 162 features for each entry was set up and given to a data mining algorithm to find out the relevant features among this large feature set and to construct the classification knowledge. The classifier was evaluated by cross validation. The results show the feasibility of an automated inspection system.

1   Introduction

In this paper, we present results on the analysis and classification of cells using image analysis and data mining techniques. The kinds of cells that are considered in this application are Hep-2 cells, which are used for the identification of antinuclear autoantibodies (ANA). ANA testing for the assessment of systemic and organ specific autoimmune disease has increased progressively since immunofluorescence techniques were first used to demonstrate antinuclear antibodies in 1957. Hep-2 cells allow for recognition of over 30 different nuclear and cytoplasmic patterns, which are given by upwards of 100 different autoantibodies.

The identification of the patterns has up to now been done manually by a human inspecting the slides with the help of a microscope. The lacking automation of this technique has resulted in the development of alternative techniques based on chemical reactions, which have not the discrimination power of the ANA testing. An automatic system would pave the way for a wider use of ANA testing.

We present our results on image analysis, feature extraction, and classification based on images that were taken by an digital image acquisition unit under real

J. Crespo, V. Maojo, and F. Martin (Eds.): ISMDA 2001, LNCS 2199, pp. 219-224, 2001.

clinical conditions (see Sect. 2). Starting from a knowledge-acquisition process with a human operator (see Sect. 3), we developed an image analysis and a feature extraction algorithm, described in Sect. 4 and Sect. 5. A data set containing 162 features for each entry was set up and given to our data mining tool to find out the relevant features among this large feature set and to construct the structure of the classifier, see Sect. 6. The classifier was evaluated by cross validation. The results show the feasibility of an automatic inspection system (see Sect. 7).

2   Image Acquisition

The images were taken by a digital image-acquisition unit consisting of a microscope AXIOSKOP 2 from Carl Zeiss Jena, coupled with a color CCD camera Polariod DPC [1]. The digitized image were of 8-bit photometric resolution for each color chanel with a per pixel spatial resolution of 0.25 μm. Each image was stored as a color image on the hard disk of the PC. Form there it was accessed for further calculation.

3   Knowledge Acquisition

For our experiment we used fluorescence images from six different classes (see Fig. 1).

In a knowledge-acquisition process [2] with a human operator, using an interview technique and a repertory grid method, we acquired the knowledge of this operator, while classifying the different cell types. Some of this knowledge is shown in table 1. The symbolic terms show that a mixture of different image information is necessary for classification. The operator uses the color intensity as well as some texture information. In addition, the appearance of the cell parts within the cells are of importance, like "dark nuclei", which also requires spatial information.

We started out to develop the image analysis procedure and constructed a feature set, which seems to be powerful enough to describe this symbolic knowledge. It is left to the data mining experiment to find out the relevant features for classification and to show us gaps in our description of the domain.

Table 1. Some knowledge about the class description given by a human operator

Class	ClassName	Description
Homogeneous nuclei fluorescence	Class_1	Smooth and uniform fluorescence of the nuclei. Nuclei appear sometimes dark. The chromosome fluorescence is weak up to very intense
Fine speckled nuclei fluorescence	Class_2	Dense fine speckled fluorescence
...	...	...
Nuclei fluorescence	Class_6	Nuclei are weakly homogenous or fine grained and can be hardly discerned from the background

4   Image Analysis

The color image has been transformed into a gray level image. Automatic thresholding has been performed by the algorithm of Otsu [3]. The algorithm can localize the cells with their cytoplasmatic structure very well, but not the nuclear envelope itself. We then applied morphological filters like dilation and erosion to the image in order to get a binary mask for cutting out the cells from the image. Since there are only cells of one type in an image, overlapping cells have not been considered for further analysis.

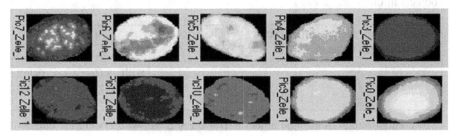

Fig. 1. Examples of Cell Images for 10 different Classes

The gray levels ranging from 0 to 255 are quantized into 18 intervals t. Each subimage $f(x,y)$ containing only a cell gets classified according to the gray level into t classes, with $t=\{0,1,2,..,18\}$. For each class a binary image is calculated containing the value "1" for pixels with a gray level value falling into the gray level interval of class t and value "0" for all other pixels. The quantization of the grey level into 18 intervals was done based on a logarithmic characteristic curve. We call the image $f(x,y,t)$ in the following class image. Object labeling is done in the class images with the contour following method [4]. Then features from these objects are calculated for classification.

5   Feature Extraction

For the objects in each class image features are calculated for classification. The first one is a simple Boolean feature which expresses the occurrence or none occurrence of objects in the class image. Then the number of objects in the class image is calculated. From the objects the area, a shape factor, and the length of the contour are calculated. However, not a single feature of each object is taken for classification, but a mean value for each feature is calculated over all the objects in the class image. This is done in order to reduce the dimension of the feature vector. We also calculate the frequency of the object size in each class image. The list of features and their calculation is shown in table 2.

Table 2. List of Features and their Calculation

Description	Name	Type	Formula
Object occurred in class image t	Gray_t	boolean	yes or no
Number of objects in class image t	Count_t	numerical	n(t)
Mean area of objects in class image t	Area_t	numerical	$\overline{A}(t) = \dfrac{1}{n(t)} \sum_{i=1}^{n(t)} A_i(t)$
Relative mean area of objects in class image t to area of cell	Rarea_t	numerical	$RA(t) = \dfrac{\overline{A}(t)}{A_{cell}}$
Mean shape factor for objects in class image t	Form_t	numerical	$\overline{F}(t) = \dfrac{1}{n(t)} \sum_{i=1}^{n(t)} 10 \cdot \dfrac{A_i(t)}{u_i(t)}$ with $u_i(t)$ contour being the length of the i-th object in class image t.
The contour length of a single object is $u = l + \sqrt{2} \cdot m$ with l being the number of contour pixels having odd chain coding numbers and m being the number of contour pixels having even chain coding numbers.			
Mean contour lenght of objects in class image t	Length_t	numerical	$\overline{u}(t) = \dfrac{1}{n(t)} \sum_{i=1}^{n(t)} u_i(t)$

6   Learning of Classifier Knowledge

For each of the six classes, we had 19 data sets; each data set contained 162 features, obtained from each of the eigthteen class images. The whole data set has 105 samples. Based on that data set we acquired the knowledge for classification. We used a binary [5] and n-ary decision tree induction algorithm [6] realized in our data mining tool *DECISIONMASTER* [7]. The n-ary decision tree can split up a numerical feature into more than two intervals which leads sometimes to a better performance than the one of a binary decision tree. The learning algorithm selects from the data set the most promising features and constructs the structure of the classifier during the learning phase. The resulting decision tree is shown in Fig. 2. The true error rate was estimated by cross validation [8], which works properly on small sample sets. The error rate for both classifier is shown in table 3. The unpruned binary decision tree shows the best result.

Table 3. Error Rate for the Classifier estimated with Cross Validation

Method	Unpruned Tree	Pruned Tree
Binary Tree Induction	13.33 %	15.24 %
N-Ary Tree Induction	20.00 %	20.00 %

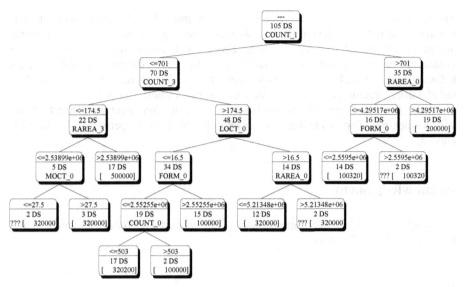

Fig. 2. Resulting Decision Tree

7   Results and Discussion

The learning algorithm only recognizes 10 features as relevant features. The most discriminating feature is the feature *count_1*, which means that there occur or do not occur objects in the class image one. This goes conform to what we can see in the class images for all cell types. There are classes having lighter objects within the cell and there are other classes having darker objects within the cell. The next important feature is the number of objects in class three and the relative area of objects in class_0, which can also be confirmed by looking at the class images.

The error rate of 13.33 % is a very good result. For the type of application presented in this paper there has not existed any automated feature extraction and classification system up to now.

Recently, we are collecting more samples for all classes as soon as the class occurred in practice. Beyond that we want to improve the accuracy of the system by defining new features and incorporating these features in our data mining experiment.

8   Conclusions

In this paper, we have shown the feasibility of an automatic system for Hep-2 cell analysis and classification. The classification problem is a multi-class problem. In our application 6 classes have to be distinguished. We developed an image analysis and a feature extraction algorithm, which classifies the subimage containing only the cells into 18 class images and calculates from each class image features for classification.

The resulting data set has 162 features for each entry. Based on this data set, it is possible to obtain the relevant features with data mining techniques. Only 10 features are necessary in order to classify nine classes with an accuracy of 86,67%. We evaluated our result with cross validation. We have shown that data mining techniques are powerful techniques for determining the relevant features as well as the classifier structure. Furthermore, they can work on small data sets.

Further work will be done to improve the classification accuracy. Therefore, we will develop new features that can better describe the basic properties of the different classes.

Acknowledgement

The work presented in this paper is part of the project *LernBildZell* funded by the German Ministry of Economy.

References

1. U. Sack, Digital Image Acquisition Unit for Fluorescent Images, IBaI Report 2000
2. P. Perner, A knowledge-based image inspection system for automatic recognition, classification, and process diagnosis, Machine Vision and Applications (1994) 7:135-147.
3. Otsu, N., A threshold selection method from gray-level histograms, IEEE Trans., vol. SMC-9, Jan. 1979, p. 38-52.
4. H. Niemann, Pattern Analysis and Understanding, Springer Verlag 1990.
5. J.R. Quinlain,"Induction of Decision Trees," Machine Learning 1(1986): p. 81-106.
6. P. Perner and S. Trautzsch, Multinterval Discretization for Decision Tree Learning, In: Advances in Pattern Recognition, A. Amin, D. Dori, P. Pudil, and H. Freeman (Eds.), LNCS 1451, Springer Verlag 1998, S. 475-482
7. Data Mining Tool Decision Master http://www.ibai-solutions.de.
8. S.M. Weiss and C.A. Kulikowski, Computer Systems that Learn: Classification and Prediction Methods from Statistics, Neural Networks, Machine Learning, and Expert Systems. Morgan Kaufmann, San Mateo, 1990.

Multitask Pattern Recognition Algorithm for the Medical Decision Support System

Edward Puchala and Marek Kurzynski

Wroclaw University of Technology, Division of Systems and Computer Networks,
Wybrzeze Wyspianskiego 27, 50-370 Wroclaw, Poland
puchala@zssk.pwr.wroc.pl

Abstract. The paper presents algorithms of the multitask recognition for the decomposed dependent approach. First one, with full probabilistic information and second one, algorithms with learning sequence. We have focused our attention on the multitask recognition technique and its application to the computer aided diagnostic and therapeutic decision in non-Hodgkin lymphoma disease. Adequate computer system was projected. This system has been practically implemented in Department of Hematology if Wroclaw Medical Academy in Poland.

1 Introduction

The classical pattern recognition problem is concerned with the assignment of a given pattern to one and only one class from a given set of classes. Multitask classification problem refers to a situation in which an object undergoes several classification tasks. Each task denotes recognition from a different point of view and with respect to different set of classes. For example, such a situation is typical for compound medical decision problems where the first classification denotes the answer to the question about the kind of disease, the next task states recognition of the stadium of disease, the third one determines the kind of therapy, etc.

In the present paper we have focused our attention on the concept of multitask classification and application this technique to the decision making in medicine.

2 Multitask Recognition: Full Probabilistic Information

Let us consider N-task recognition problem. We shall assume that the vector of features $x_k \in X_k$ and the class number $j_k \in M_k$ for the k-th recognition task of the pattern being recognized are observed values of random variables $\mathbf{x_k}$ and $\mathbf{j_k}$, respectively [5]. When *a priori* probabilities of the whole random vector $\mathbf{j} = (\mathbf{j_1}, \mathbf{j_2}, ..., \mathbf{j_N})$ denote as $P(\mathbf{j}=j) = p(j) = p(j_1, j_2, ..j_N)$ and class-conditional probability density functions of $\mathbf{x} = (\mathbf{x_1}, \mathbf{x_2}, ..., \mathbf{x_N})$ denote as $f(x_1, x_2, ..x_N / j_1, j_2, ..j_N)$ are known then we can derive the optimal Bayes recognition algorithm minimizing the risk function [3], [4]:

J. Crespo, V. Maojo, and F. Martin (Eds.): ISMDA 2001, LNCS 2199, pp. 225-230, 2001.
© Springer-Verlag Berlin Heidelberg 2001

$$R = E\ L(i, j) \tag{1}$$

i.e. expected value of the loss incurred if a pattern from the classes $j=(j_1,j_2,....,j_N)$ is assigned to the classes $i=(i_1,i_2,...,i_N)$.

In the case of multitask classification, we can define the action of recognizer which leads to so-called decomposed dependent approach. [1].

In this instance, an object is classified in a successive manner for particular recognition tasks and now the decision algorithm Ψ_k for the k-th classification uses not only features x_k but also additionally the results of former classifications, that is:

$$\Psi k : Xk \times M1 \times M2 \times Mk\text{-}1 \Longrightarrow Mk. \tag{2}$$

This concept denotes the decomposition of the whole problem, but now the successive classification tasks are mutually dependent and fully describe real situations occurring in the computer-aided medical diagnosis tasks (Fig. 1.).
Minimization of the risk function R with loss function:

$$L\ [(\ i_1,\ i_2,..i_N\ ),(\ j_1,\ j_2,..j_N)] = n \tag{3}$$

leads to the following optimal algorithm for k-th task (using the dynamic programming method):

$$\Psi_k^*(x_k, i_1, i_2,..i_{k-1}) = i_k \tag{4}$$

if

$$p(i_k/x_k,\ i_1,\ i_2,...,i_{k\text{-}1}) + \sum_{n=k+1}^{N} P_{C_n}\ (i_1,\ i_2,...,i_k) =$$

$$= \max_{i_k} p(\ i_k^{'}/x_k,i_1,i_2,...i_{k\text{-}1}) + \sum_{n=k+1}^{n} P_{C_N}\ (i_1,i_2,...,i_k^{'}\ ) \tag{5}$$

where:

$p(i_k/x_k,i_1,i_2,..,i_{k\text{-}1})$ - denotes *aposteriori* probability

$P_{C_n}\ (i_1,\ i_2,...,i_k)$- denotes average probability of correct classification in n-th recognition task for decisions $i_1,i_2,..i_k$.

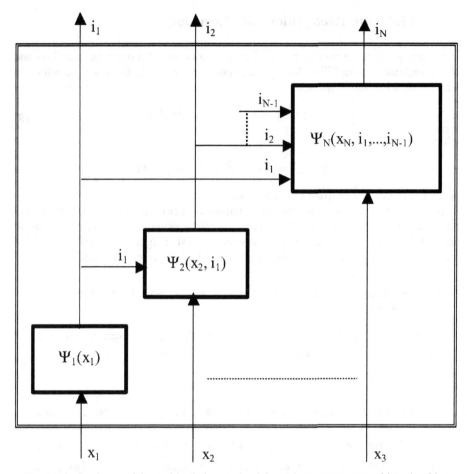

Fig. 1. Block scheme of the multitask decomposed dependent pattern recognition algorithm

Let us assume that decisions for first (n-1) tasks are correct. In this case, we can determine *aposteriori* probability, like below:

$$p(i_k/x_k,i_1,i_2,..,i_{k-1}) = \frac{f(x_k/i_1,i_2,...,i_{k-1},i_k)p(i_1,...,i_k)}{f(x_k/i_1,...i_{k-1})p(i_1,...i_{k-1})} \tag{6}$$

Therefore, beginning at the end, recognition algorithms for all tasks are calculated after a following order:

$$\Psi_N^* \Rightarrow P_{C_N} \Rightarrow \Psi_{N-1}^* \Rightarrow P_{C_{N-1}} \Rightarrow ... \Rightarrow \Psi_2^* \Rightarrow P_{C_2} \Rightarrow \Psi_1^* \tag{7}$$

3   Multitask Recognition with Learning

In the real world there is often a lack of exact knowledge of *a priori* probabilities and class-conditional probability density functions. For instance, there are situations in which only a learning sequence:

$$S_L = (x^1, j^1), (x^2, j^2),...,(x^L, j^L) \qquad (8)$$

where:

$$x^k = (x_1{}^k,...,x_N{}^k) \in X, j^k = (j_1{}^k,...,j_N{}^k) \in M \qquad (9)$$

as a set of correctly classified samples, is known.

In this case we can use the algorithms known for conventional pattern recognition, but now algorithm must be formulated in the version corresponding to above concepts. As an example let us consider nearest neighbour (NN) recognition algorithm for decomposed dependent approach, which is presented below.

```
Decomposed dependent multitask NN algorithm (for the
k-th task):

Notation: i₁,i₂,...,iₖ₋₁ - results of recognition for
the first (k-1) tasks



1.Measure features xₖ of the pattern to be recognized,

2.Find the nearest neighbour (in the space Xₖ ) to xₖ
from among learning patterns for which jⁿ consists at
the first (k-1) positions the sequence (i₁,i₂,...,iₖ₋₁)
(let say xₖᵐ),

3.Assign the recognized pattern into the class jₖᵐ.
```

The superiority the decomposed dependent NN algorithm over the classical pattern recognition one demonstrates the effectiveness of this concept in such multitask classification problems for which the decomposition is necessary from the functional or computational point of view (e.g. in medical diagnosis)

4   Decision Problem in Non-Hodkin Lymphoma

Above we have discussed the concepts of multitask classification. Now the application of this technique in medical diagnosis problem will be presented.

The non-Hodgkin lymphoma is a common dilemma in hematology practice. It provides a physician with many difficult decision problems. For this medical problem we can utilise the decompose dependent approach of multitask classification (this is caused by the structure of the decision process), which leads to the following scheme.

In the first task of recognition, using the algorithm $\Psi_1(x_1)$, we arrive at a decision $i_1 \in M_1 = \{1,2,3,4,5\}$ about the lymphoma type. $i_1=1$ means that the degree of lymphoma malignancy is small; $i_1=2$ - the degree of malignancy is moderate; $i_1=3$ - there is a highly malignant immunoblastic lymphoma; $i_1=4$- the lymphoma is lymphoblastic of high degree of malignancy; and $i_1=5$ denotes a Burkitt-type lymphoma. The features x are results of cytological examinations of cells as well as results of examinations of lymphoma structure (e.g. diffuse, nodulous).

After the type of lymphoma has been determined, it is essential for diagnosis and therapy to recognize its stage. To that end we use the algorithm $\Psi_2(i_1,x_2)=i_2$. The values of decision i_2 denote the first, the second, the third and the fourth stage of lymphoma development, respectively. The vector of features x_2 has components that determine the degree to which particular nodes, tissues, and organs are affected. Apart from that, each stage of lymphoma may assume two forms. Which of such forms occurs is determined by the algorithm $\Psi_3=i_3$, where $M_3=\{1,2\}$. If $i_3=1$, then lymphoma assumes the form A (there are no additional symptoms). For $i_3=2$, lymphoma takes on form B (there are other symptoms, as well).

Decisions i_1, i_2, and i_3 are arguments for the algorithm $\Psi_4=i_4$ which determines therapy, that is one of the known schemes of treatment (e.g. CHOP, BCVP, COMBA, MEVA, COP-BLAM-I). A therapy (scheme of treatment) cannot be used in its original form in every case. Because of the side effects of cytostatic treatment it is necessary to modify such a scheme. Decision about modification is taken by the last algorithm $\Psi_5=i_5$, $M_5=\{1,2,3,4,5\}$. If $i_5=1$, the scheme remains unchanged, if $i_5=2$, 75 percent of the cytostatic dose recommended in the scheme is administered; if $i_5=3$ - 50 percent; if $i_5=4$ - 25 percent and if $i_5=5$, the chemotherapy is stopped. The features of the vector x_5 determine whether the side effects occur or not. As algorithms Ψ_1 - Ψ_5 MC rules in the decomposed dependent form with Parzen estimator [2] were used.

References

1. Kurzynski, M., Puchala, E., :Algorithms of the multiperspective recognition. Proc. of the 11th Int. Conf. on Pattern Recognition, Hague (1992)
2. Puchala, E., Kurzynski, M.,: A branch-and-bound algorithm for optimization of multiperspective classifier. Proceedings of the 12th IAPR, Jerusalem, Israel, (1994) 235-239
3. Parzen, E.,: On estimation of a probability density function and mode. Ann. Math. Statist., (1962) Vol.33, 1065-1076

4. Duda, R., Hart, P.,: Pattern classification and scene analysis. John Wiley & Sons, New York (1973)
5. Fukunaga, K., : Introduction to Statistical Pattern Recognition, Academic Press, New York (1972).

The Analysis of Hospital Episodes

David Riaño[1] and Susana Prado[2]

[1] Universitat Rovira i Virgili,
Carretera de Salou s/n, 43006 Tarragona, Spain
drianyo@etse.urv.es
[2] Informàtica El Corte Inglés,
Bolivia 234, 08020 Barcelona, Spain
susana_prado@ieci.es

Abstract. A file of episodes stores data about the patients that are admitted to a hospital. This structure can be analyzed to obtain clinical, supervision and normative knowledge about the hospital functioning. HISYS1 is a system that integrates graphical and artificial intelligence techniques to automatically generate hospital decision support systems that organize and use the above knowledge to predict the evolution of the new patients. The system has been proved with the patients of the Hospital Joan XXIII in Tarragona (Spain) for six diagnoses.

1   Introduction

Hospitals are complex systems where patients, physicians, hospital managers, and public health-care administrations interact[1]. The well functioning of a hospital depends not only on the health aspects as instruments, activity protocols (treatments and tests), etc., but also on the structural organization as the hospital budget, resource optimization (number of beds and available operating theaters), etc.

Whereas patients and physicians are concerned about the best medical care, managers and public administrations go after the cost reduction, mainly. These two points of view give rise to faced up decisions as whether an expensive drug must be prescribed or whether a medical test must be done or not. Therefore, many hospital decisions are a trade off between excellence and cost.

The application of computer-based intelligent data analysis to the personal, clinical, and logistic data that the Hospital Administration Departments store about the admitted patients can be used to discover knowledge that could be useful to physicians (*clinical knowledge*), managers (*supervision knowledge*), and public administration (*normative knowledge*).

In the next sections we describe the sort of data that we want to study, the sort of knowledge that we can discover, the tool used to analyze the data, the tests performed on the Hospital Joan XXIII in Tarragona (Spain), and some conclusions and future work.

---

[1] Private companies that supply outsourcing services and product dealers are not considered here.

J. Crespo, V. Maojo, and F. Martin (Eds.): ISMDA 2001, LNCS 2199, pp. 231–237, 2001.

2   The File of Episodes

An episode is described as the structure that contains all the new data introduced between the moment that a patient arrives to a hospital department and the moment that the patient leaves it. According to the attention received, hospitals have three access types: external consulting, emergencies and hospitalization.

In external consulting (EC) the family doctor sends a patient to the hospital with a particular request for an expert call. When the request arrives to the hospital it is given a date and an hour for the first call (*examination call*) and a patient episode is opened. After the first EC call, some other complementary calls and tests can follow in order to confirm or to determine the patient diagnosis and to have a medical treatment. Each EC call is related to an episode line in which some basic data are stored (episode number, date, sort of call -first or second-, test performed, etc.).

In emergencies (ER) the process is simpler because it only involves one patient call with the related tests and medication. Emergency inputs conclude with the patient admission or discharge. ER episodes are single lines containing information about the episode number, arriving date and time, moment of the first contact with a practitioner, input time in boxes, input reason and origin, input and output diagnoses, sort of output (hospitalization, home, exitus, transfer, etc.), and output time.

Finally, hospitalizations (H) include programmed admissions (surgical operations) and ER transfers of seriously ill patients. When a patient is admitted in a hospital he is given an episode number and he is inscribed into one of the hospital departments. Complex treatments that involve several hospital departments are represented as a temporal sequence of H episodes. Each episode contains information about the episode number, the department, the physician, the primary diagnosis and procedure, the secondary diagnoses and procedures, the date and the time of the patient input and output, the discharge reason, the related costs, etc. All this information is stored in a *file of episodes* which can be used to learn and predict the evolution of the patients in the hospital: average stay and cost in a department, sort of patients arriving to and leaving from a department, analysis and comparison of hospital protocols, etc.

In this work we extend the file of episodes with data about hospitalized patients: *personal data* (age, sex, address, telephone number, bank account, etc.), *clinical data* (case history, test results, daily evolution parameters, etc.), *actuation data* (procedures applied, medicines provided, costs, etc.) and *logistic data* (bed number, hosting department, involved physicians, etc.). These episodes describe the clinical activities of the hospital in a period of time, and it can be a source of knowledge about the hospitalization protocols, costs and effectiveness.

3   The Knowledge Learned

The file of episodes represents all the patient evolutions and, therefore, the internal behavior of the hospital in a period of time. An intelligent analysis of these files can find some knowledge about the hospital and staff activities. Table 1 displays the kind of new knowledge grouped in *clinical knowledge* (useful to physicians and nurses), *supervision knowledge* (useful to the hospital managers and administration) and *normative knowledge* (useful to the public administrations and politicians).

Table 1. Knowledge elicitation from a file of episodes

Clinical Knowledge to
analyze the patient behaviors for specific pathologies.
use the acquired experience to predict patient evolutions and risk situations.
aid in the education and training of inexperienced physicians.
study and compare population groups in time.
Supervision Knowledge to
analyze the hospital behavior.
compare the techniques used by different physicians and their efficiency.
compare the real costs by procedure with the established theoretical costs.
detect economic deviations and their possible causes.
organize more efficiently the logistic and human resources.
Normative Knowledge to
compare the techniques used by different hospitals and their efficiency.
determine the hospital specialization.
control the activity and functioning of different hospitals.
finance hospitals according to their real situation.

In order to achieve all these goals several data mining techniques have been developed and integrated within an intelligent analysis tool called HISYS1.

4   The Analysis Tool

HISYS1 [5] is a tool that combines the static and the dynamic data about the patients that are admitted to a hospital. The patient transitions are represented as a path in a flowchart where nodes represent admissions, hospital services and discharge reasons, and arrows represent single transitions within the hospital departments. Each node stores accumulated information about the number of patients visiting the node, the number of days, cost of all the stays, and the sets of secondary diagnoses, procedures and physicians involved. Each arrow stores the detailed information of the patients that have passed through it: admission number, sex, age, ZIP code, cost, physician in charge, number of days, and the sets of secondary diagnoses and procedures.

HISYS1 uses the data stored in the arcs of the flowchart to obtain knowledge about the hospital functioning. For each non terminal node of the graph with more than one outgoing arc a rule set is generated that distinguishes between the patients that leave the node following different arcs.

There are two main representations of symbolic knowledge: decision trees [2] and production rules [4]. CN2 [1] is an inductive learning program that makes IF-THEN rules to classify elements. This program has been integrated with HISYS1 to construct rules that predict the behavior of the patients at the nodes of the graph [3].

The rules obtained by HISYS1 are integrated in a knowledge-based system. See figure 1. There we can distinguish in vertical lanes the primary diagnoses that we want the system to predict. For each lane, there is a set of rules describing each one of the hospital departments involved in the treatment of the diagnosis. This organization of the rules describes a decision support system (DSS) that HISYS1 generates automatically for the primary diagnoses that the user indicates. When a DSS is active, HISYS1 is able to predict the behavior of new patients by means of a "question & answer" interface. It is possible to generate several DSS and store them separately.

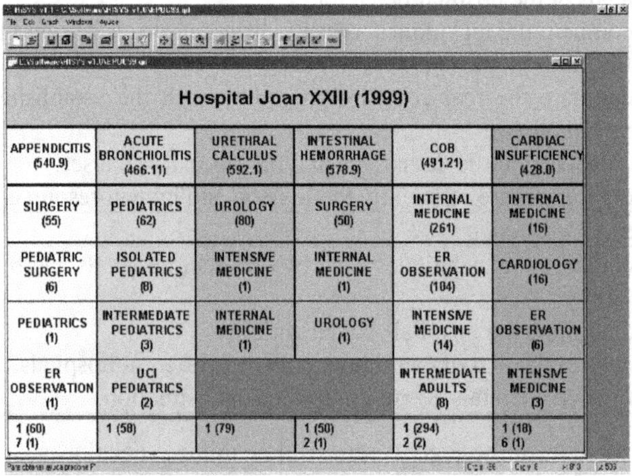

Fig. 1. Knowledge-based prediction tool

5   Tests and Results

Some of the uses of HISYS1 to achieve the goals in table 1 have been tested by the staff of the Hospital Joan XXIII in Tarragona (Spain). HISYS1 was applied to a set of six diagnoses: appendicitis (Cod. 540.9), acute bronchiolitis (Cod. 466.11), urethral lithiasis (Cod. 578.9), digestive hemorrhage (Cod. 592.1), chronic obstructive bronchitis or COB (Cod. 491.21), and cardiac insufficiency (Cod. 428.0). For each diagnosis, we have studied the patients in 1998 and 1999. Figure 2 shows the flowcharts of the six diagnoses for the patients in 1999.

There were 23,158 episodes in 1998 and 18,787 episodes in 1999, from which we selected those related to the above six diagnoses. Table 2 shows the number of episodes and patients, for each particular diagnosis. The episodes were taken from the hospital databases in 1998 and 1999 and they contained quantitative and qualitative data: admission number, sex, age, ZIP code, primary and secondary diagnoses, primary and secondary procedures, physicians, costs, and number of days. There were not missing or noise data and only a simple pretreatment of the data was required: due to the hospital functioning, secondary diagnoses and procedures are introduced in the last episode, when the patients are discharged. Since this is an important information, we extended them to all the episodes of the patient admission for HISYS1 to be able to generate knowledge about the secondary diagnoses and procedures.

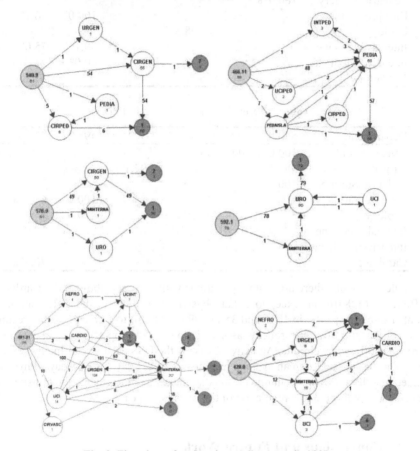

Fig. 2. Flowcharts for six primary diagnoses in 1999

Moreover, two DSS were made. The first one was trained with patients in 1998 and tested with patients in 1999, and the second one the opposite. The predictive accuracy, defined as the proportion of rule hits, was studied separately for the hospital services as tables 3 and 4 show. Empty dark spaces represent departments that do not attend the respective primary diagnosis.

Table 2. Accuracy of the prediction in 1998

Department	540.9	466.11	570.9	592.1	491.21	428.0
Pediatric Unit	100.0%	91.7%				
Surgery	98.0%			96.0%		
Pediatric Surgery	100.0%					
ER observation					100.0%	66.7%
Urology			98.8%			
Internal Medicine					89.1%	75.0%
Intensive Medicine					50.0%	
Cardiology						87.5%

Table 3. Accuracy of the prediction in 1999

Department	540.9	466.11	570.9	592.1	491.21	428.0
Pediatric Unit	100.0%	100.0%				
Surgery	98.8%			92.1%		
Pediatric Surgery	100.0%					
ER observation					100.0%	67.9%
Urology			99.0%			
Internal Medicine					89.5%	78.9%
Intensive Medicine					35.5%	
Cardiology						70.6%

Tables show that there are many predictions with accuracy above 90%. Cardiac insufficiency (428.0)is an exception, that physicians attribute to the difference in the number of patients (102 in 1998 and 35 in 1999) and also to a change in the treatment protocol that the flowchart reflects as a variation in the proportion of patients in the cardiac insufficiency circuits. An extreme case is the DSS accuracy of Intensive Medicine. This has passed from an average patient stay of 8.3 days to 3.35 days. Physicians argued that there was an economic reason that makes them to change the transfer criterion. That explains the low prediction of the rules in this case.

6   Conclusions and Future Work

HISYS1 have been proved to be an efficient tool to generate clinical, supervision, and normative knowledge within a hospital framework that can be used to analyze the data of the patients that are admitted to a hospital. The tool is currently being working in the Pediatric Unity of the Hospital Joan XXIII in Tarragona (Spain) where there are several physicians testing and proposing modifications and extensions to the system. The authors are also working to increase the cost analysis functions of HISYS1 and also to incorporate alternative efficiency measures that could help physicians, hospital managers and public health-care organizations to detect anomalies in the hospital daily clinical practice. The work has been partially supported by the *Agència d'Avaluació de Tecnologia Mèdica (AATM)*.

References

1. Clark, P., Niblett, T.: The CN2 Induction Algorithm. Int. J. Mach. Lear. 3 (1989) 261–283
2. Quinlan, J.R.: Induction Decision Trees. Int. J. Machine Learning 1 (1986) 81–106
3. Riaño D., Prado, S.: Improving HISYS1 with a Decision Support System. In: Artificial Intelligence in Medicine. LNAI 2101, Springer-Verlag, (2001) 140-143
4. Riaño, D. On the Process of Making Descriptive Rules. In: Padget, J. (eds.): Collaboration Between Human and Artificial Societies. LNAI 1624. Springer-Verlag, (1999) 182–197
5. Riaño, D., Prado, S.: A Data Mining Alternative to Model Hospital Operations: Filtering, Adaptation and Behavior Prediction. In: Brause, R.W., Hanisch, E. (eds.): Medical Data Analysis. LNCS 1933. Springer-Verlag (2000) 293–299

Electroshock Effects Identification Using Classification Based on Rules

Jorge Rodas[1], Karina Gibert[2], and J. Emilio Rojo[3]

[1] Department of Computer Science, Technical University of Catalonia, Jordi Girona
Salgado 1-3, Modul C6, D-201, 08034 Barcelona, Spain
jr@lsi.upc.es
[2] Department of Statistics and Operational Research, Technical University of
Catalonia, Pau Gargallo 5, 08028 Barcelona, Spain
karina@eio.upc.es
[3] Psychiatry Service, Hospital of Bellvitge, (Bellvitge) Barcelona, Spain
jrojo@csub.scs.es

Abstract. This article focuses on results obtained from a hierarchical
classification applied to a repeated short time series data in a medical
ill-structured domain. The analyzed information is relative to patients
−with major depressive disorders or schizophrenia− under ECT treatment; as a consequence, this information contains data corresponding to
measures taken at different time, throughout a 24-hour period after an
electroshock application to the patient. . . .

Keywords: Classification, Short Series, Curve Analysis, ill-structured
domains.

1 Introduction

A great quantity of medical information is obtained from domains without structure and when we need to make a decision about what is good knowledge and
what is not is a very difficult problem. These kind of domains are named by [2] as
ill-structured domains. Some of their features are : *heterogeneous data, additional
knowledge of the domain,* and *partial and non-homogeneous knowledge.*

In the data of our case study it is possible to find features of ill-structured
domains (mentioned above) and others, such as time series. Then, finding the
way to handle them, extract useful information from them, and find profiles in
this kind of data is our goal.

The structure of the paper is as follows: Firstly, a very brief summary of
Electro-Convulsive Therapy is introduced in section 2 where its effects are also
described. Section 3 describes the data used in the analysis. In section 4 we
present the problem description and main goals. In section 5 we show the classification results of baseline data and give some observations about resultant
classes. In section 6 we present the results obtained from applying the classification based on rules to a modified dataset. In addition, we present the classification results and give some observations about resultant classes. Finally, in

J. Crespo, V. Maojo, and F. Martin (Eds.): ISMDA 2001, LNCS 2199, pp. 238–244, 2001.

section 7 we draw conclusions about analysis results and point to various directions for future work.

2 Application Domain

An interesting psychiatric study field corresponds to therapies for depressive disorders or schizophrenia. The "Electro-Convulsive Therapy" (ECT) is a safe, effective, fast, valuable and widely used treatment for serious depressive illnesses and other psychiatric disorders [4]. ECT is based on electroshocks. An electroshock is an electrical current through the brain in order to induce seizures (convulsions) and improve the psychiatric condition. ECT is a moderately complex procedure where an adequate seizure is necessary for therapeutical response; yet the brain biological events related to its efficacy are still unknown.

The neuropsychological effects of ECT are cognitive changes involving orientation, attention and calculation, memory loss, and recall (see [1]).

Many works have studied the physiological response of ECT through heart rate, blood pressure, electrocardiogram effects, cardiac enzymes, electroencephalogram effects or hormonal response. However, at the moment, a formalized technique applied to this therapy does not exist and there are a few works done about the neuropsychological effects of ECT on psychophysiological parameters such as reaction times (RT). We are trying to study the effects of ECT application to both visual and audible reaction times and if there exists a formal profile from reaction times, we want to know what kind of variables have a direct influence on cognitive patient's state to formalize a general analysis methodology for this kind of domains.

3 Data Description

In this study, 13 patients with major depressive disorders or schizophrenia and under ECT treatment are monitorized. The present standard practice optimizes the therapeutic ratio, in selecting electrical stimulus parameters such as: energy level, stimulus duration, pulse width and pulse frequency. In addition, multiple responses from patient are monitorized by ElectroEncephaloGram (EEG), ElectroCardioGram (ECG), and ElectroMioGram (EMG). We also try to make a rigorous evaluation of patient's neuropsychological effects.

The evaluation of psychophysiological variables was done with Vienna Reaction Unit at 2, 4, 6, 12, and 24 hours after every ES application.

The Vienna Reaction Unit is a visual and audible stimulus unit. Four tests were carried out: Simple Visual (S5), Simple Audible (S6), Complex Visual (S7), and Complex Visual-Audible (S8). The following measures were registered: wrong decisions, wrong reactions, no reactions, incorrect reactions, right reactions, decision times, reaction times, and motor times. Besides that, there is additional information about each patient such as: age, weight, education, blood and urine analysis, VIENNA protocol baseline results, electroencephalograms, electrocardiograms, and electromiograms. For more details about vienna unit, tests, measures, datasets and others see [5] and [3].

4   Problem Description and Goals

There are different levels of drawbacks due to the particular data structure. Firstly, we have a representation problem.

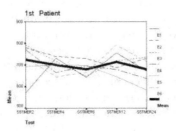

Fig. 1. Curves of Test S5 from 1st patient

Figure 1 shows lines joining the simple visual test (S5) reaction times measured at 2, 4, 6, 12 and 24 hours after an ES applied to the 1st patient. This patient receives an ECT of 6 electroshocks and each bend represent his/her reaction-time evolution.

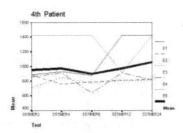

Fig. 2. Curves of Test S5 from 4th patient

Figure 2 shows the 4th patient ECT evolution for the simple visual test (S5) reaction times. The patient receives an ECT of 5 electroshocks.

As we could observe in these figures, to obtain a unique prototype curve from mean reaction times (thick line) as a representation of patient's evolution is a non optimal process; however, this mean could give us an idea of a generalized patient's evolution trend.

Due to the fact that there is not an standard about the quantity of ES application to a patient, the patients' information reduction is not possible.

Then, we must have all the curves of all the patients and take into account this factor for the analysis.

The objective of this work is finding useful information to discover features of possible patient's profiles under ECT treatment using data mining techniques, even this non optimal process.

In this fashion, and interesting challenge consist in finding a methodology to obtain a efficient process for handle this kind of data.

5   Classification of Baseline Reaction Times

A hierarchical method was used to classify the patients considering their baseline reaction times, because these times represent the patients' initial condition test set (the method was exactly a reciprocal neighbors hierarchical method with Ward's criterion of aggregation and euclidean distances between patients). Next, we search for relevant features from each group that allow us to obtain understandable logic rules.

The classification technique suggested the existence of three different groups of patients according to their baseline reaction times. Figure 3 shows the hierarchical organization of patients following the clustering process, where the vertical cut indicates which patients are included in each group, in figure 4 the general tendency of basal curves of each group is shown. This clearly indicates different initial conditions of the patients. By studying the distribution of the other variables locally to each class, it is remarkable the behaviour of Age, which is shown in figure 5. Where young patients are in A class (1), with baseline reaction times lower than B class (2), mature patients. C class (3) has only the 4th patient.

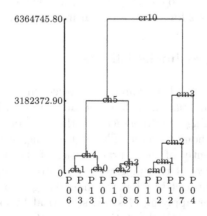

Fig. 3. A general tree from Baseline Classification

The expert considers omit 4th patient after he analyzed his/her singular behaviour. Therefore, taking this observation into consideration, we conclude

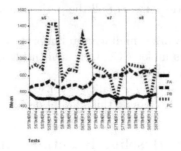

Fig. 4. 3 classes curves for tests S5 to S8

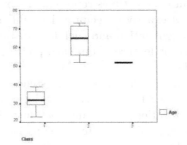

Fig. 5. Multiple Boxplot of Age

that there are 2 groups of patients described by young patients and mature patients. Then we obtained 2 simple rules, that make a clear description of A and B groups: 1. *If AGE ≤ 40 → young* and, 2. *If AGE > 50 → mature.*

From this result, we decided to include this information for posterior analysis, performing separate processes for young and mature patients.

6   Analysis of Electroshocks Effects

The analysis of the effect of the ECT should be analyzed through the comparison on the reaction times of each patient before and after a given ECT. So, a new database was built containing the differences on the reaction times of a given before and after each ES hour to hour. This data is measuring the effect of the ES by itself independently of the characteristics of the patient. This new data is only taking into account the improvement or worsening of the reaction time due to one ES with respect to what was happening before that ES. This data is bad conditioned for applying classical statistical hypothesis tests. An interesting proposal to overcome its limitations is *Classification Based on Rules* technique [2] so, it was used for classifying the "effects" of each ECT on reaction times. Basically, local clustering processes were performed for young patient's ECT and also for mature patient's ones. Finally both hierarchies are integrated together and a single partition of the ES was found (see Fig. 6).

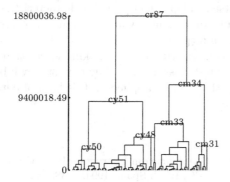

Fig. 6. A general tree from Classification

The analysis suggests four classes, whose general tendency on reaction times is represented in figure 7.

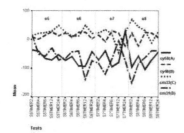

Fig. 7. 4 classes curves for tests S5 to S8

In figure 7 we can see that Classes B and C the effect of every electroshock is increasing the reactions times. That is why the differences between posterior and previous are positive, and this means that the reaction times are greater after the electroshock than before; as a result the patients in these classes have a deterioration trend. On the other hand, in Classes A and D, we found that reaction times decrease and differences between after and before are negative; then the patients in these classes have a positive trend.

7   Conclusion and Future Work

Some interesting conclusions can be established: 1. Two rules were derived and the groups of young and mature patients are delimited by them. 2. A Classification Based on Rules method was applied, using as Knowledge-Base the 2 rules obtained. We used the differences between RT because they measure the effect of the electroshock by itself independently of the characteristics of the patient. Four classes into 2 groups of patients (young and mature) were detected, the patients with deterioration or positive trend.

As a future work, it is interesting to see the kind of relation between others patients variables and the last classification. The next step will be the search for a standard methodology that can be applied on this kind of data.

References

1. Abrams, R. and Swartz, C.: Thymatron Instruction Man. US. 1985. 239
2. Gibert, K.: phD. thesis. UPC, BCN, Spain. 1994. 238, 242
3. Rodas J., Gibert K., Rojo J.: TR (LSI-01-6-R). UPC, Spain. 2001. 240
4. Rojo J., Gibert K., Rodas J., Oms A., Pifarrè J. and Vallejo J. : The Time Course of Psichophysiological Effects During ECT. In press. 2001. 239
5. Schuhfried. G. : Wiener Testsystem. Vienna Reaction Unit. Austria. 1992. 240

Advanced Visualization of 3D data of Intravascular Ultrasound images

D.Rotger[1], C.Cañero[1], P.Radeva[1], J.Mauri[2], E.Fernandez[2], A.Tovar[2], V.Valle[2]

[1] University Autonoma of Barcelona, Computer Vision Center, Bellaterra
[2] Hospital Universitari Germans Trias i Pujol, Badalona

Abstract. Intravascular ultrasound images (IVUS) have allowed deepening in the knowledge of the true extension of the coronary vessel illness. Today, vessel diagnosis is limited to observation and measurements in the IVUS planes. For a bigger accuracy, 3D visualization is necessary to allow estimating the extension, localization and severity of the pathology. We develop tools for interactive 3D visualization to extend the views to any sailing angle through the cube of IVUS data. As a result, physicians are allowed to inspect and get 3D measurements about the vessel pathology from IVUS images.

1 Introduction

IVUS provide a unique 2D *in vivo* vision of the internal vessel walls, determining the extension, distribution and treatment of the atherosclerotic, fibrotic plaques and thrombus, and their possible repercussion on the internal arterial lumen. The main difference between the ultrasound and the angiography images (figure 1), as the most used image modalities for vessel diagnosis, deals with the fact that the most of the visible plaque lesions with IVUS are not evident with angiogram. Studies on intravascular ecography have shown that the reference vessel segment has the 35-40% of its sectional area occluded because of the plaque, although it appears as normal in the angiography Moreover, IVUS offer information about the composition of the internal lesion; in particular, about calcium deposits as the most important isolated predictors to evaluate if a particular lesion will respond to a catheter treatment. The possibility of visualizing directly the plaque by IVUS also benefits the receptors of a heart transplant; the IVUS have demonstrated that the 25% of the hearts to be transplanted are already ill.

IVUS are of particular interest in case of vessel therapy by stents. Intracoronary stent is a spiral metallic mesh that is implanted inside a vessel to save the stenosis effect (figure 1(b)) caused by a calcification or a grown of the intimal vessel layer. This mesh widens the vessel walls, recovering the necessary lumen for a good irrigation. The studies about stents carried out with IVUS show that the appearance in the angiography of a good stent deployment can hide two possible problems: the incomplete apposition (a portion of the stent is not making pressure on the vessel wall) and the incomplete expansion (a portion of the

J. Crespo, V. Maojo, and F. Martin (Eds.): ISMDA 2001, LNCS 2199, pp. 245–250, 2001.

stent remains closed although the expansion of the rest of the stent areas). Both problems are very significant since they can be worse than the problem they are trying to solve.

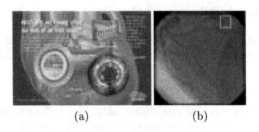

(a)   (b)

Fig. 1. (a) IVUS image (reprint). (b) Angiography of a vessel with stenosis.

One of the problems of dealing with IVUS is the fact that the images represent a 2D plane perpendicular to the catheter without any depth information. This IVUS property hides the real disease's extension and represents a very unnatural way of conceptualization. The foremost limitation of IVUS on the pre- and post-treatment studies is the lesion images correlation in the serial studies. This limitation is due to the lack of the third dimension that gives much more global information about the internal and external vessel structure [1]. The third dimension allows a better knowledge of the vessel, the lumen and the plaque, visualizing simultaneously multiple sections of the vessel and obtaining a longitudinal perspective [5, 6]. The vessel can be later studied under multiple formats and different cut axes to interpret, in the space, a certain discovery, hardly esteemed from the two-dimensional images. To see the real extension of the lesion, we propose a navigation method based on cutting planes. These cuts allow passing in a continuous way from the traverse views to the longitudinal ones. The 3D reconstruction allows, for example, a more precise calculus of the size of the stent or the balloon to be implanted or make easier the election of better interventional instruments and their sizes. Three-dimensional images are synthesized by the sequential apposition of the two-dimensional ones. This kind of reconstruction presupposes the coronary section that we are treating as a straight line with the catheter transducer in the middle, determining the center of the lumen.

Taking measures of the volumetric vessel information is also a very important point. To this purpose IVUS data are completed by vessel and stent models to extract volumetric measurements about the vessel structures. According to the medical experts collaborating in this work, measuring the volume of the lumen before and after an intervention is good to evaluate the positive and/or negative effects that the intervention has provoked [2]. It helps to decide about further stent or angioplasty balloon interventions.

The article is organized as follows: section 2 discusses the 3D visualization for "navigating" inside the vessel; section 3 explains the process of extracting volumetric measurements by vessel model and IVUS data; the article finishes with conclusions and future work.

2 3D Visualization of Coronary Vessels

2.1 Cutting Planes Generation

Let us assume the IVUS data as a sequence of parallel planes, it can be seen as a cube. Hence, we can generate cutting planes under any spatial angle for better identification of calcium plaque and intimal layer grown. The possibility of cutting the data cube under any navigation angle allows passing in a continuous way from the traverse views to the longitudinal ones (figure 2). In a longitudinal cut of the section to study, the physician has a more accurate idea of the real extension of the lesion as well as a possibility to measure the stent size by pointing an initial and ending point.

To generate the cutting planes, we use the two orthogonal vectors that are the generators of a plane containing the cut image. Initially, these two vectors have the X- and Y-axis direction of the central image of the cube. The intersection point of both vectors coincides with the catheter's center of this image. Applying rigid transformations (3D rotations and translations) to these two vectors, the physician is able to generate any plane contained in the data cube. [2]

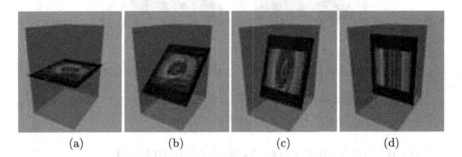

(a)   (b)   (c)   (d)

Fig. 2. Cutting planes generation: continuous pass from the traverse views to the longitudinal ones.

If we define the center of the catheter, the translation vector and the central plane vectors as follows:

$$c = (c_x, c_y, c_z), \quad t = (t_x, t_y, t_z), \quad v_x = \begin{pmatrix} 1 \\ 0 \\ 0 \end{pmatrix}, v_y = \begin{pmatrix} 0 \\ 1 \\ 0 \end{pmatrix}$$

we are able to calculate all the generating vectors by the formulas:

$$v_1 = \mathbf{Rz} * \mathbf{Ry} * \mathbf{Rx} * vx + t$$
$$v_2 = \mathbf{Rz} * \mathbf{Ry} * \mathbf{Rx} * vy + t \tag{1}$$

where $\mathbf{Rx}, \mathbf{Ry}, \mathbf{Rz}$ are the third order rotation matrix.

Taking into account the different horizontal and vertical calibration factors, we multiply each vector component by its calibration factor to assure the continuous way of passing from the short-axes images to the long-axes ones:

$$v\prime = \frac{v}{\|v\|}, \qquad v = (v_x' * c_H, v_y' * c_H, v_z' * c_V)$$

where c_H and c_V are the calibration factors.

When constructing the IVUS data cube, we should take into account the vessel dynamics at the time the catheter is doing its pullback i.e. the beating of the patient's heart. Ignoring the rotation of IVUS data in the image planes around the catheter leads to artifacts that can be appreciated in figure 3(a). This problem is avoided by estimating the rotation manually or automatically [4] and including it in the matrix Rz of formula (1). The correction of image rotation allows to obtain a continuous view of vessels in cutting planes under any spatial angle (figure 3(b)).

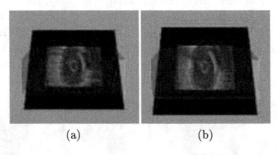

(a)   (b)

Fig. 3. (a) Cut plane without rotation correction. (b) Cut plane with rotation correction

3   Extracting Volumetric Vessel Measurements

A model of the vessel wall and of the stent is very useful in order to determine its morphology in space, to extract volumetric measurements and to take decision about stent implantation. These models have been implemented by B-Splines because of their nice properties (easy to adapt to the vessel wall and stent, local control, model compactness, etc.)[7]. The models can be easily generated by determining the B-Spline control points that define a B-Spline curve to adjust manually or automatically [3] to vessel and stent boundary in each of the IVUS images (figure 4).

3.1   Spatial Models

Once obtained B-Spline curves that represent vessel and stent boundaries, they are interpolated in space using B-Spline surfaces to construct a spatial model of the vessel and stent taking into acount the pullback speed (the distance between planes) and 2D control points (figure 5(a)). [1, 7]

3.2   Measures Between the Vessel Wall and the Stent

As discussed above, extracting volumetric information is very important in order to evaluate intervention effects. Until now, area and distance calculus in IVUS planes have been the only possible ones carried out with IVUS images. Having a B-Spline representation of vessel and stent, it is easy to estimate the distance between them using a filling algorithm (Y-X, for example) in the images with drawn vessel and stent models. Then, we can calculate the area of each model in pixels and infer the intersectional area (s):

$$s = c_H^2 * (a_v - a_s)$$

where c_H is the horizontal calibration, a_v and a_s are the vessel and the stent areas.

We extrapolate the area calculus to the space, using trapezoids, to get the volumetric measurement as follows:

$$V = |s_i - s_{i+1}| * c_V$$

where c_V is the vertical calibration defined by the pullback speed (the distance in millimeters between 2 images) and the s_i and s_{i+1} are the intersectional areas of two consecutive planes.

4   Results and Conclusions

The implemented tools for 3D interactive visualization of vessel morphology is of great clinical interest [2] making easier the conceptualization process of vessel diagnosis and therapy. Until now, clinical comparisons of different pullbacks of a patient limit to compare distances and areas of a selected IVUS image

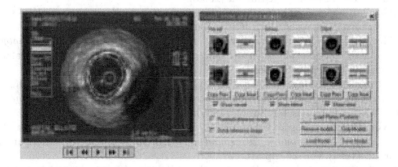

Fig. 4. Vessel wall and stent curve models.

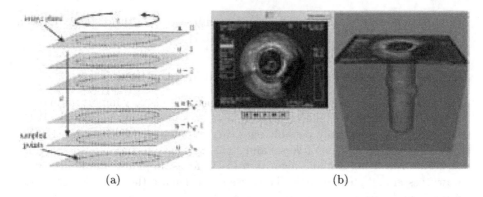

(a)   (b)

Fig. 5. (a) Two-dimensional B-Spline model space generalization. (b) Spatial model of the vessel wall (the intimal layer) and the stent.

trying to figure out the severity of vessel pathology in space. As a result of this work, the medical doctors have a tool to see the real extension of the coronary disease not in an image or a sequence but in space as well as to measure more accurately its effect. Currently, the project is under clinical validation, extracting information from a statistic number of patients and comparing previous results with the new ones to estimate the importance of volumetric vessel measurements. A natural extension of this work includes creating a virtual reality environment for realistic navigation and interaction with the vessel as well as simulating vessel interventions, implementing the automatic correction of the vessel rotation and automatic segmentation of the vessel layers.

References

1. Oriol Pujol: *Model-based Three Dimensional Interpolation of IVUS Images*. Computer Vision Center. (1999)
2. Mauri, FN, Valle, Esplugas, Cequier, Rotger et al.: *Ecografía Intracoronaria: Navegación Informática por el Cubo de Datos de las Imágenes*. Congreso de la Sociedad Española de Cardiología. Granada (2000).
3. D. Gil, P. Radeva, J. Saludes: *Segmentation of artery wall in coronary IVUS images: A probabilistic approach*. 15th ICPR. Barcelona, 4:352-355, (2000).
4. J. Mauri, E-F. Nofreras, D. Gil et al: *Moviment del vas en l'analisi d'imatges de ecografia intracoronaria: un model matematic*. Congrés de la Societat Catalana de Cardiologia. Barcelona (2000).
5. Von Birgelen C., Slager C., Di Mario C., de Feyter PJ., Serruys W.: *Volumetric Intracoronary Ultrasound "A New Maximum Progression-Regression of Atherosclerosis"*. Atherosclerosis 118 Suppl. (1995).
6. C. Von Birgelen, Mario C.D., Li W. Et al: *Morphometric Analysis in Three-Dimensional Intracoronary Ultrasound during Stent Deployment*. American Heart Journal. (1996) Vol.132, pp.516-527 .
7. Brian A. Barsky, Richard H.Bartels, John C.Beatty: *An Introduction to Splines for use in Computer Graphics and Geometry Modeling*. Morgan Kaufmann Publishers INC, (1987).

Investigations on Stability and Overoptimism of Classification Trees by Using Cross-Validation

Willi Sauerbrei

Institut für Medizinische Biometrie und Medizinische Informatik,
Universitätsklinikum Freiburg,
Stefan-Meier-Strasse 26, D- 79104 Freiburg

Abstract. Development of classification rules is often based on tree methodology. Using data from a diagnostic study where Doppler flow signals were measured to separate between malignant and benign breast tumors I will discuss issues of searching for the cutpoint of continuous variables with a minimal p-value and the necessity to correct this p-value because of multiple testing. Ignoring the correction will strongly favor continuous variables in tree development and may lead to useless trees. I will further investigate the influence of the complexity of a tree by estimating the overoptimism as the difference from the apparent error rates based on the original data to estimated error rates based on 5-fold crossvalidation. Furthermore I consider the use of predefined cutpoint on the development of trees and the resulting error rates.

1   Introduction

The method of classification and regression trees (CART) is one approach for modeling the relationship between a response or dependent variable and factors or explanatory variables possibly measured on different scales. CART is often used synonymous for different types of tree-based approaches, the book of Breiman et al. (1984) gives a detailed description of various aspects of the method. Several programs for different types of outcome variables (e.g. continuous, binary, survival time with censored data) are available and the list of applications is large. Nevertheless, for many issues there are no accepted standard approaches and substantially different trees can result with the approaches. Beside of users of tree methods, increasing in the last years because of data mining, the community of scientists being very skeptical is large because of several reasons, e.g. instability of trees developed, analysis of (small) subgroups, overoptimism concerning the separation of groups, uncertainty about the usefulness of stop criteria discussed, small final nodes giving results in contrast to medical knowledge, usefulness of pruning or amalgamation of complex trees etc.

I will investigate some of the aspects by using a diagnostic study in breast cancer. Several Doppler flow signals were measured in patients with the aim to differentiate between benign and malignant tumors (Sauerbrei et al 1998). For a binary

J. Crespo, V. Maojo, and F. Martin (Eds.): ISMDA 2001, LNCS 2199, pp. 251-257, 2001.
© Springer-Verlag Berlin Heidelberg 2001

outcome the general idea of the tree approach is to split the population into two parts with the aim to have a low percentage of patients with the outcome of interest in one subpopulation and a high percentage in the other. By using a cutpoint a continuous exploratory variable is split into two parts with values smaller and higher than the cutpoint, and for the resulting categorized explanatory variable a p-value is calculated by using the chi-square test of independence in a 2x2 table. To avoid very small groups with extreme values only, the possible cutpoints have to be restricted to a sensible range of the distribution function of the variable. All values within the range are investigated and the cutpoint that minimizes the p-value of the chi-square test is chosen for that variable. Therefore multiple testing is used for continuous variables, whereas only one test is possible for binary explanatory variables. All explanatory variables are investigated in this way and the minimal p-value over all variables with the corresponding cutpoint is used as the splitting criterion. Each of the two resulting subpopulations are investigated in the same way and splitted furthermore until some predefined stop criteria are reached. Stop criteria may be based on estimated misclassification rates estimated by crossvalidation, a predefined minimal allowable sample size for further splitting, significance level for the test, further criteria or combinations of some of them. Because of the structure of the analysis tree approaches are also called recursive partitioning methods.

If factors are measured on different scales development of the tree will favor continuous variables as several cutpoints are investigated resulting in too small p-values because of multiple testing. This problem is well known for a long time, e.g. Breiman et al. (1984, p 42) state 'variable selection is biased in favor of those variables having more values and thus offering more splits', but often ignored by the development of the tree. Analysing prognostic factors in patients with a brain tumor by a tree approach the severity of this issue is demonstrated in Lausen et al. (1994). In a study with 12 factors only age is measured on a continuous scale. In their original tree age is used as a split criteria in 7 (sub-)populations. Correcting for multiple testing results in a tree with a smaller number of nodes and age is used only two-times as a splitting criteria. Furthermore, using all cutpoints as possible split criteria for continuous variables increases the instability of trees substantially (Sauerbrei (1997)).

I will investigate the influence of different stop-criteria, correcting for multiple testing and using restrictions for allowable splits on misclassification rates in the breast cancer example. I will use 5-fold crossvalidation to investigate stability of the trees selected and to estimate the influence of the complexity of a developed tree on the overoptimism concerning error rates from classification rules.

2   Patients and Methods

Between July 1992 and February 1994, 458 consecutive women with breast disease, submitted for surgical biopsy with clinical symptoms, palpable, mammographic or sonographic findings, were examined at the Gynecology Department of the University of Freiburg. There was no preselection of patients as all of them received a Doppler examination. However, all patients were symptomatic. The final histologic or cytologic diagnosis was invasive carcinoma in 123 women and 10 in situ carcinoma, which were combined to a group of 133 patients with malignant tumor, and benign disease in 325 women. Beside of age the number of arteries and number of contralateral arteries were counted, flow velocities (3 continuous variables) and resistance index (2 continuous variables) were measured. For more details see Sauerbrei et al. (1998).

Concerning categorization of continuous variables and searching for the cutpoint with the minimal p-value Miller & Sigmund (1982) derive the asymptotic distribution of maximally selected chi square statistics in fourfold tables. They show that a nominal p-value of 0.05 from the chi-square distribution results in a p-value of 0.49 according to the asymptotic distribution of the maximally selected chi square statistic. Lausen & Schumacher (1992) derive the same asymptotic distribution for a wide range of two sample statistics. Using these results a corrected p-value can be obtained by

$$P_{cor} = \varphi(z)[z - 1/z]\log_e\left[(1-\varepsilon)^2/\varepsilon^2\right] + 4\varphi(z)/z$$

where φ denotes the probability density function and z is the $(1 - P_{min}/2)$-quantile of the standard normal distribution. P_{min} denotes the minimum P value of the tests. The selection interval is characterized by the proportion ε of smallest and of largest values of the continuous factor that are not considered as potential cutpoints. Altman et al. (1994) also propose a simple approximation.

$$P_{cor} \approx -1.63 \, P_{min}(1+2.35 \log_e P_{min}) \text{ for } \varepsilon = 10\% \text{ and}$$

$$P_{cor} = -3.13 \, P_{min}(1+1.65 \log_e P_{min}) \text{ for } \varepsilon = 5\%$$

More details are discussed in Lausen et al. (1994) and Altman et al (1994). I will develop trees with and without p-value correction and use $\varepsilon = 10\%$.

As stop-criteria I use a maximal allowable tree level of 7 in combination with a nominal selection level and a subgroup considered for further splitting must have a minimum number of patients. If any of the three criteria is violated splitting is stopped and the corresponding subgroup is considered as a final node of the tree. As nominal selection levels I use 5% and 16%, the latter corresponds to asymptotic results of the Akaike Information Criterion in selecting regression models and the similarity to selection by cross-validation. Corresponding to the $\sqrt{n}$ criterion, which is sometimes discussed as stop criterion in the tree development, I use 21 as a minimum number of patients. To investigate this issue I use furthermore 5 as a small value.

Restricting the allowable splits for continuous variables to some predefined, medically plausible values is the only way to avoid selecting cutpoints which were never used before in the literature. Pre-defining allowable cutpoints will also introduce stability concerning trees selected. Based on the distribution I define four cutpoints for each of the continuous variable.

I attribute the final node as 'benign' or 'malignant' by considering the percentage of malignant patients in this final node, and a cutpoint for this percentage. This gives a classification rule for which sensitivity is estimated as the percentage of correct classification of malignant tumors and specificity as the corresponding number of benign tumors. As often in these problems the loss of misclassification is considered more serious if a patient with a malignant tumor is misclassified. Therefore I will aim to reach a high sensitivity by using only 10% as the cutpoint for the attribution 'benign' respectively 'malignant' for the final node. As a further 'natural' cutpoint for this percentage I use the prevalence of malignant tumors in the study, which is 29%. For both cutpoints I also calculate the accuracy as the percentage of correct classifications in all patients. I estimate sensitivity, specificity and accuracy based on the original data and by using 5-fold crossvalidation. To asses the stability of trees selected and the amount of overoptimism concerning sensitivity and specificity of the resulting classification schemes, I use 5-fold crossvalidation (CV) in the following way. The data are randomly divided into 5 parts of equal size. Four parts are used as a 'training set' for building a tree, and to attribute 'benign' or 'malignant' to each final node, the remaining part is used to estimate sensitivity and specificity of the corresponding classification scheme. This process is repeated for all 5 parts, resulting in different classification schemes in each part and in the classification of each tumor as benign or malignant based on a rule, which is developed independently of the subject classified. Based on the true status, the cross-validated estimates of sensitivity and specificity are calculated and compared with the estimates from the usual classification schemes based on the original data.

3   Results

For all combinations of significant level, stop criteria and p-value correction the first and second split level is very stable. The number of arteries with a cutpoint of 3 is the split criterion in all combinations and in all cross validation runs. At the second split level the number of arteries is also the dominating factor (cutpoints 2 and 6). At the further levels trees developed by using the p-value correction are more stable than trees were correction for multiple testing is not done. For the 5 situations considered in table 1 the number of final nodes varies between 8 and 19. These differences are also reflected in the cross-validation runs. For the first situation the tree is very similar to the one presented in Figure 2 of Sauerbrei et al. (1998).

Using 0.10 as the cutpoint for the classification rule aims to classify correctly patients with a malignant tumor and to reach a very high sensitivity. For all combinations of stop criteria and p-value correction the estimated sensitivity is 97.0% or larger if the assessment is based on the original data. The corresponding specificities are between 89.5% and 95.9%. The number of final nodes is only 8 if p-value correction and strong stop-criteria are used, but increase to 19 for weak stop criteria and p-value correction ignored. Using only 5 as the minimum number of patients gives the best accuracy with apparent error rates of less than 5%. However, the cross-validation approach indicates the severe overoptimism with these complex trees.

Table 1 Based on the original data and by using 5-fold cross-validation estimates of sensitivity (sens), specificity (spec) and accuracy (accur) for different combinations of stop criteria (sig-significance level, minpat-minimum number of patients), with and without p-value correction (pcorr).

pcorr	sig	min pat	no. nodes	Original data			CV-difference			CV
				Sens	spec	accur	sens	spec	accur	accur
Cutpoint for the classification 0.10											
yes	5	21	8	97,7	89,5	91,9	2,2	1,2	-0,2	92,1
yes	5	5	10	97,7	91,4	96,2	2,2	0,9	1,3	91,9
yes	16	5	12	97,0	95,4	95,9	4,5	4,3	3,5	92,4
no	5	21	10	97,0	93,5	94,5	-0,7	4,6	3,1	91,4
no	16	5	19	98,5	94,2	95,4	3,0	3,5	3,3	92,1
Cutpoint for the classification 0.29											
yes	5	21	8	95,5	92,0	93,0	0,0	1,2	0,9	92,1
yes	5	5	10	97,7	91,4	93,2	6,7	1,2	1,1	92,1
yes	16	5	12	97,0	95,4	95,9	5,3	3,4	3,9	92,0
no	5	21	10	94,7	96,0	95,6	0,7	4,6	3,5	92,1
no	16	5	19	98,5	94,2	95,4	6,8	2,6	3,7	91,7

For the most complex situation the CV-difference (estimate based on original data – estimate based on 5-fold cross-validation) for sensitivity, specificity and accuracy is at least 3.0%. For a significance level of .16 the estimated error rate increases from 4.6% (accuracy based on original data) to 7.9% (accuracy based on cross-validation). This estimate is identical to the estimate from the cross-validation approach by using the most restrictive tree based on a significance level of 5%, a minimum number of 21 patients and by using the p-value correction. In contrast to the advantages of using 0.16 as significance level if accuracy is measured from the original data, the investigation shows that the apparent advantage is caused mainly by the overoptimism and that the results based on cross-validation are nearly identical for all five combinations considered.

Increasing the cutpoint to 0.29 results for some combination in an increase of the estimated specificity, but at the cost of a decrease in the corresponding sensitivity. Estimates of accuracy based on cross-validation are nearly unchanged.

The approach based on pre-defined cutpoints for continuous variables results in changes of the trees developed after the first level. These analyses identify age as the most important factor after the number of arteries. In general the error rates increase (data not shown). As already seen in the analyses without pre-defined cutpoints overoptimism is a less severe problem if stronger stop criteria are used.

4   Discussion

Often several variables are measured with the aim to develop classification rules in medicine. Regression models are generally considered as the method of choice, however approaches based on trees or neural nets are used as important competitors, in data mining issues they are even more popular. Although the approaches are conceptionally very different, they all share the common problem of overoptimism concerning the predictive ability, mainly if too complex 'final' models are developed. For a detailed discussion of this issue in regression models see Sauerbrei (1999). Concerning trees this issue may be more serious because the overall population is separated in smaller subpopulations. In essence, a final tree consists of a number of high-dimensional interactions and instability in tree development is a serious issue. As searching for high-dimensional interactions is a very difficult task in regression models, trees may be considered as a useful complement, provided that some aspects are taken into account in their development. Several approaches to improve classification based on trees have been proposed recently, e.g. bagging trees (Breiman 1996).

For continuous variables I consider to use corrected p-values in tree development as the most important issue. Because of the dominating effect of the number of arteries the difference between trees developed with and without p-value correction was less severe in this study than in other examples (Lausen et al. 1994, Sauerbrei 1997). Another issue is the complexity of trees developed. In contrast to other approaches I do not prefer to develop very complex trees which are simplified by pruning and amalgamating. Using strong stop criteria I prefer to develop only relatively simple trees. A further collapsing of nodes should also try to consider medical knowledge (Sauerbrei et al. 1997). For more discussion of issues in tree construction, pruning and recombination of nodes see LeBlanc (2001).

Using cross-validation I showed that overoptimism was no problem in situations with strong stop-criteria where trees were mainly based on the number of arteries and age. This result is in agreement with the analysis using the logistic model which included number of arteries, age and number of contralateral arteries. With cross-validation and bootstrap resampling it could be shown that stability and overoptimism is no serious problem for developed diagnostic rules from logistic regression models in these data (Sauerbrei et al. 1998). The ROC curves based on two logistic regression models and the tree approach show that the error rates of the different approaches are nearly identical (Figure 3 in Sauerbrei et al. 1998). The data were also analysed with a feed-forward neural network (Schumacher et al. 1996). With an increasing number of hidden units the authors were able to develop a perfect classification of benign and malignant tumors. However, they state that this result is caused by substantial overfitting, an issue which is considered as an important general drawback of neural networks.

Because of the importance in the growing field of data mining further investigations on the sensible use of tree methods are necessary. As for the development of regression models I consider the use of resampling approaches as a necessary step to assess the usefulness of any tree developed.

References

1. Altman DG, Lausen B, Sauerbrei W, Schumacher M: Danger of using "optimal" cutpoints in the evaluation of prognostic factors. Journal of the National Cancer Institute, 1994; 86: 829-835.
2. Breiman L: Bagging Predictor. Machine Learning 1996, 24:123-140.
3. Breiman L, Friedman JH, Olshen RA, Stone CJ: Classification and Regression Trees. Wadsworth: Monterey, 1984.

4. Lausen B, Sauerbrei W, Schumacher M: Classification and regression trees used for the exploration of prognostic factors measured on different scales. In: Dirschedl, P, Ostermann, R (Hrsg): Computational Statistics. Physica-Verlag, Heidelberg, 1994; 483-496.

5. Lausen, B, Schumacher M.: Maximally selected rank statistics. Biometrics, 1992; 48: 73-85.

6. LeBlanc M: Tree-Based Methods for Prognostic Stratification. In: Crowley, J (Ed): Handbook of Statistics in Clinical Oncology. Marcel Dekker, New York, 2001; 457-472

7. Miller R, Siegmund D: Maximally Selected Chi Square Statistics. Biometrics. 1982; 38: 1011-1016.

8. Sauerbrei W: On the development and validation of classification schemes in survival data. In: Klar, R, Opitz, O (Hrsg): Classification and Knowledge Organization Springer-Verlag, 1997; 509-518.

9. Sauerbrei, W: 'The use of resampling methods to simplify regression models in medical statistics', Applied Statistics, 1999; 48:313-329.

10. Sauerbrei, W, Hübner, K, Schmoor, C, Schumacher, M for the German Breast Cancer Study Group (1997): 'Validation of existing and development of new prognostic classification schemes in node negative breast cancer', Breast Cancer Research and Treatment, 42: 149-163; Corrigendum Breast Cancer Research and Treatment 1998; 48: 191-192.

11. Sauerbrei, W, Madjar, H, Prömpeler, HJ: Differentiation of benign and malignant breast tumors by logistic regression and a classification tree using doppler flow signals. Methods of Information in Medicine, 1998; 37: 226-234.

12. Schumacher M, Roßner R, Vach W: Neural networks and logistic regression: Part I. Computational Statistics & Data Analysis 1996; 21:661-682.

A Case-Based Approach for the Classification of Medical Time Series

Alexander Schlaefer[1], Kay Schröter[1], and Lutz Fritsche[2]

[1] Humboldt University Berlin, Department of Computer Science,
Artificial Intelligence Group, Unter den Linden 6, D-10099 Berlin, Germany
{schlaefe,kschroet}@informatik.hu-berlin.de
[2] University Hospital Charité, Department of Nephrology
Charité Campus Mitte, Schumannstr. 20/21, D-10117 Berlin, Germany
Lutz.Fritsche@charite.de

Abstract. An early and reliable detection of rejections is most important for the successful treatment of renal transplantation patients. A good indicator for the renal function of transplanted patients is the course over time of the parameter creatinine. Existing systems for the analysis of time series usually require frequent and equidistant measurements or a well defined medical theory. These requirements are not fulfilled in our application domain. In this paper we present a case-based approach to classify a creatinine course as critical or non-critical. The distance measure used to find similar cases is based on linear regression. Our results show that while having a good specificity, our sensitivity is significantly higher than that of physicians.

1 Introduction

Decision making is a vital task in medicine. Reasonable decisions on diagnostics and therapy require a complex domain knowledge. The values of many medical parameters, provided by different examinations, and the connections between these parameters have to be taken into account. Apart from general domain knowledge, decision making also depends strongly on individual experience. Decision support systems were developed to support especially less experienced physicians. Beside giving suggestions on possible diagnosises, such systems can give hints on useful examinations and can make treatment suggestions. New and improved examination methods lead to an increasing amount of available data. Even for the experienced physicians it becomes impossible to pay equal attention to all the information. Decision support systems can help to focus on relevant or critical information.[12]

Most of these systems rely on a complete and sound medical theory, so called expert knowledge. The medical experts have to define rules, patterns, states of functions etc. in order to make those systems work. In many cases this may be a promising approach, as long as the domain is well understood. Other domains are still developing and not as well founded yet. Furthermore it is not always easy to incorporate the expert knowledge into an electronic system.

J. Crespo, V. Maojo, and F. Martin (Eds.): ISMDA 2001, LNCS 2199, pp. 258–263, 2001.

Much of the data in the medical domain is time related, and often the course over time of some parameter is more interesting than its value at a certain point in time. This is especially true for the long term monitoring of patients who suffer from chronical diseases. When assessing the state of health of such patients, physicians have to compare a number of different parameter courses which may vary around the patients individual levels.

While there exist a various number of algorithms for the analysis of time series, most of them are designed for equidistant series with frequent measurements. These assumptions do not hold for many medical time series, since the frequency of examinations depends on the patients health and may vary. Especially when considering chronical patients, the interval between two medical examinations can be quite long.

There is some other work investigating the analysis of medical time series. TrenDx [3] was developed to detect conspicuous trends in a course. It requires patterns that describe typical, normal and critical courses of a parameter (trend templates). ICONS [7,8] is a case-based system that predicts the renal function of intensive care patients. The intensive care unit environment allows to make equidistant measurements. Only the values from a short period of time are considered. ICONS uses temporal abstractions as described in [10,11]. T-IDDM [1] analyses the blood sugar level of chronical diabetes patients. It is based on a well defined domain model and needs regular measurements. VIE-VENT [5] observes and controls the artificial respiration of newborns. This system works with high frequent measurements.

2 Domain and Data

Our project is located at the department of nephrology in the university hospital Charité. A major task of the nephrologists is the treatment of patients who underwent a kidney transplantation and live with a kidney graft. Although the physicians thoroughly check whether recipient and donor have compatible tissue types, there is virtually never a hundred percent match. Hence there is always the risk, that the immune system of the recipient attacks the graft and destroys it. The patients have to take drugs that suppress the immune system to prevent such rejections. Still the patients need to be monitored carefully, since an acute rejection may occur even months or years after a successful transplantation. Acute rejections can be treated by high doses of drugs. For a successful treatment it is of most importance to recognize an acute rejection as early as possible.

The circumstances that initiate an acute rejection and the symptoms that reliably indicate a rejection are not completely understood yet. A promising parameter, that is also used by the physicians, is the level of creatinine in the blood. Creatinine is a waste product of the metabolism that is excreted by the kidneys only. Hence it is a good indicator for the renal function, that decreases in the case of a rejection. The creatinine level should be almost constant between 0.6 an 1.2 mg/dl. For patients who live with a kidney graft the normal individual level can even be higher than the limit for healthy humans. Therefore not only the level at one point in time but rather the course of creatinine measurements over time is used to recognize a possible rejection.

A complete and correct set of all relevant medical data of a patient is necessary for a substantial decision. We use the electronic patient record TBase2 [4,9] to collect the data, obtained during the regular health checks of the patients. Among others TBase2 contains information on transplantations, rejections and laboratory results. All this information is associated with time stamps. For transplantations this is the date of the surgery, for rejections the beginning of the treatment and for laboratory results the date when the blood test was taken. As much data as possible is obtained electronically from the diagnostic unit. This increases the quality of the data and avoids time consuming and fault-prone manual input. Nevertheless the available data may be rare due to the long time intervals between two examinations.

3   Case-Based Reasoning

Case-based reasoning (CBR)[6] is a technology that has been successfully applied in different domains so far. Applications also include decision support systems in medicine like ICONS [7,8]. The idea behind case-based reasoning is to solve problems analogous to the way humans do: for a new problem the system retrieves similar cases from the case base and uses the solutions associated with these cases to construct a solution for the new problem. These steps correspond to the human processes of remembering and adaption. Case-based systems make experiences usable.

A case consists of a problem description and a solution. When looking at the course of creatinine the problem is the underlying time series. In a first stage the solution is just the classification of such a course into one of the two classes 'critical' and 'non-critical'. Ideally a creatinine course that is classified as 'critical' also indicates a beginning rejection.

A vital task during the development of a case-based system is to find an appropriate definition of similarity. We designed a CBR algorithm that uses a distance measure to compare two creatinine courses (see next section). A distance measure can be seen as an inverse similarity measure.

The design of our algorithm can be described as follows. In a first step the case base and the distance measure are initialized. When a new course is presented to the system, all cases of the case base are compared with that course and then ranked in order of ascending distance. The class of the k closest cases is used to determine the class of the new course. For our experiments we simply assigned the class of the majority of the k cases.

4   Distance Measure

In statistics and classical time series analysis exists a various number of algorithms to compare two time series. Most approaches expect the time series to consist of equidistant measurements and to be of equal length. Examples include 'correlation' and 'Euclidean distance', two common algorithms for comparing time series.

Both assumptions are not met by the creatinine courses we obtained from TBase2. In fact, the interval between two measurements depends on the patient and may range from a couple of days up to three month. The frequency of the measurements also varies, e.g. for inpatients.

In order to compare two creatinine courses we developed a distance measure based on linear regression. Essentially our algorithm compares the measured values of the two time series at time t, if both courses have a value at t. Otherwise the measured value of one of the courses is compared to the expected value of the other course.

We use the absolute value of the difference of the two values to determine their distance. The sum over all local distances is our raw distance measure. We divide this value by the number of considered pairs to obtain a normalized distance. Since the time series are chronologically ordered, this algorithm can be implemented in linear time ($O(n+m)$).

5 Evaluation and Testing

To evaluate our case based algorithm we used a test set with courses from TBase2. It consist of 102 creatinine courses of which 51 courses actually end with a rejection. The other 51 courses were randomly chosen from courses of all patients that never had a rejection. For our experiments we interpreted the existence of a rejection as a classification criterion. Courses that end with a rejection are considered to be critical courses, the other courses are considered to be non-critical.

We defined a valid course to have a maximum length of 360 days and to start not earlier than 90 days after transplantation. The second condition is necessary, since there is a significant difference in the course of creatinine shortly after the transplantation and later on. We also required at least four measurements per course. For the 51 courses that end with a rejection the last measurement has to be within two days before the rejection.

Instead of dividing the courses from our test set into a case base and a distinct test set, we used a leave-one-out approach to test our algorithm. We tested the algorithm on each course of the test set, but we excluded the tested course from our case base. Indeed, we also excluded one randomly chosen case from the other class, such that both classes were represented by an equal number of cases in the case base.

For our tests we used different values of k and differently sized case bases. In order to obtain valid means we rerun every test thirty times with independently chosen case bases of the same size. The results of our case based approach were compared with the results of medical experts. We showed the courses to eight experienced physicians who had to assess whether the course is likely to end with a rejection (critical course) or not (non-critical course).

6 Results

The results of our experiments are highly encouraging. The figures 1 and 2 show sensitivity and specificity for different case bases and for $k = 1$ and $k = 3$, respectively. Sensitivity is a measure to estimate the classification of critical courses. Specificity estimates the classification of non-critical courses. While the specificity is good but smaller than the average specificity of the eight physicians, the sensitivity achieved by our case based algorithm is generally much higher compared to the physicians average.

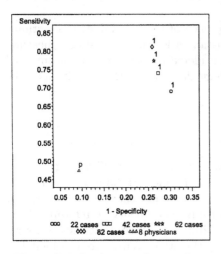

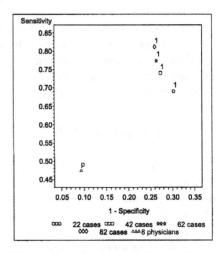

Fig. 1. Results for case bases of size 22, 42, 62, 82 and $k = 1$ compared with the results of physicians. The values are the means of 30 tests of the algorithm for each size of the case base and of 8 physicians, respectively

Fig. 2. Results for case bases of size 22, 42, 62, 82 and $k = 3$ compared with the results of physicians. The values are the means of 30 tests of the algorithm for each size of the case base and of 8 physicians, respectively

Both figures show that with increasing size of the case base the classification results improve. The gain in sensitivity for $k = 1$ (figure 1) is not matched by the gain in specificity for larger case bases. Figure 2 suggests that it is necessary to increase the size of k when the case base grows.

7 Conclusions and Further Work

The recognition of critical creatinine courses is essentially a screening problem. While it is not harmful if physicians do a detailed diagnosis even though there is no problem with the patients graft, it can be most dangerous for the patient if a beginning rejection is overlooked.

The algorithm we presented is able to classify critical courses with a sensitivity of up to 81% compared to the physicians average of about 47%. At the same time the specificity is higher than 70%, which means that the algorithm is well suited to support the physicians decision and to warn of critical situations. This is especially true since the physicians decisions are partly based on experience and intuition.

For our future work we plan to investigate other distance measures for the comparison of time series. Since the course of creatinine alone is to unreliable when classifying the courses with regard to a suspected rejection, we will also include other parameters into our distance measure. So far the retrieval step of our case based algorithm uses linear search. Although runtime is not an issue in our setting, there is related work that addresses this problem [2,7,8].

References

1. R. Bellazzi, C. Larizza, A. Riva: *Interpreting Longitudinal Data through Temporal Abstractions: An Application to Diabetic Patients Monitoring*. In Liu, Cohen, Berthold (Eds.) LNCS 1280, Springer , 1997. 259
2. L. Gierl, M. Bull, R. Schmidt: *CBR in Medicine*. In B. Bartsch-Spoerl, S. Wess, H.-D. Burkhard, M. Lenz (Eds.): Case-Based Reasoning Technology - from Foundation to Application, Springer, 1998. 263
3. I. J. Haimowitz, P. Phuc Le, I. S. Kohane: *Clinical monitoring using regression-based trend templates*. Artificial Intelligence in Medicine 7, 473-496, 1995. 259
4. G. Lindemann, L. Fritsche, K. Schröter, A. Schlaefer, K. Budde, H.-H. Neumayer: *A Web-Based Patient Record for Hospitals -The Design of TBase2*. In Bruch, Köckerling, Bouchard, Schug-Paß (Eds.): New Aspects of High Technology in Medicine, 2000. 260
5. S. Miksch, W. Horn, C. Popow, F. Paky: *Intensive Care Monitoring and Therapy Planning for Newborns*. In AAAI 1994 Spring Symposium: Artificial Intelligence in Medicine Europe: Interpreting Clinical Data, AAAI Press, 1994. 259
6. M. M. Richter: *Introduction*. In B. Bartsch-Spoerl, S. Wess, H.-D. Burkhard, M. Lenz (Eds.): Case-Based Reasoning Technology - from Foundation to Application, Springer, 1998. 260
7. R. Schmidt, B. Pollwein, L. Gierl: *Experiences with Case-Based Reasoning Methods and Prototypes for Medical Knowledge-Based Systems*. In W. Horn et al. (Eds.): AIMDM 99, LNAI 1620, Springer, 1999. 259, 260, 263
8. R. Schmidt, B. Heindl, B. Pollwein, L. Gierl: *Multiparametric time course prognoses by means of case-based reasoning and abstractions of data and time*. Medical Informatics, Vol. 22, No. 3, 237-250, 1997. 259, 260, 263
9. K. Schröter, G. Lindemann, L. Fritsche: *TBase2 - A Web-Based Electronic Patient Record*. Fundamenta Informaticae 43, pages 343-353, IOS Press, Amsterdam, 2000. 260
10. Y. Shahar: *Timing Is Everything: Temporal Reasoning and Temporal Data Maintenance in Medicine*. In LNAI 1620, Springer, 1999. 259
11. Y. Shahar, M. A. Musen: *Knowledge-Based Temporal Abstraction in Clinical Domains*. Technical Report SMI-95-561, Stanford University 1995. 259
12. E. H. Shortliffe: *Clinical Decision-Support Systems*. In E. H. Shortliffe, L. E. Perreault (Eds.): Medical Informatics - Computer Applications in Health Care, Addison-Wesley, 1990. 258

Binary Vector or Real Value Coding for Secondary Structure Prediction?
A Case Study of Polyproline Type II Prediction

Markku Siermala[1], Martti Juhola[1], and Mauno Vihinen[2]

[1] Department of Computer and Information Sciences,
33014 University of Tampere, Finland
[2] Institute of Medical Technology,
33014 University of Tampere, Finland

Abstract. Amino acid sequences are usually described using categorical variables which are difficult to change to a numerical form. We compare two numerical coding methods in polyproline type II secondary structure predictions, the frequently used binary vector coding method and our new real value coding method based on the PAM250 substitution table which consists of amino acid mutation information. The real value coding method has good properties such as space saving and illustrative form. Our first results are almost comparable to the results of traditional binary vector coding method.

1   Introduction

Our study deals with the protein sequence coding. The main question is how categorical variables could be changed to a numerical form. This is important, because in the field of secondary structure prediction there are few methods to code amino acid sequences and all of these methods have some shortcomings. The most popular coding method is the orthogonal binary vector coding, where a 20-dimensional binary vector with one 1 and 19 zeros represents one amino acids. The number of different amino acids is 20. A sequence of length k is represented by a binary vector whose length is k times 20 [1]. The fractal coding method uses properties of amino acids (hydrophobic and charges). It converts a sequence to a path through a quadratic area in a binary feature matrix of sequences [2]. Dummy coding [3], where a categorial variable is replaced with a set of binary variables, is often applied in statistics. We excluded it, because it resembles the binary coding technique.

We describe the real value coding technique and compare neural network results of this coding technique to our earlier results with the binary vector coding [1]. Starting from the well-known *PAM250* substitution table [4], we change the amino acid relations to the target distances with a genetic algorithm [5]. We then use the distances with the genetic algorithm to evaluate real value points which present amino acids in an Euclidean space. Amino acid sequences are encoded to present the polyproline type II (PPII) class and non-polyproline (non-PPII) class [1].

J. Crespo, V. Maojo, and F. Martin (Eds.): ISMDA 2001, LNCS 2199, pp. 264–269, 2001.

PPII secondary structures are quite rare (incidence 1.3 %) and they are, therefore, difficult to separate from other structures in the level of the sequence. There are also other problems, which make it difficult to predict those structures:

·   The sequence space is almost empty. In the uniform learning set there are about 9000 learning cases and the size of the sequence space is 20^{13} giving the load factor of $9000/20^{13}$.

·   PPII and non-PPII cases are badly mixed with each other in the 13-dimensional sequence space.

·   13-dimensional sequences are the longest we can use, because longer sequences would require more PPII cases for the learning.

The final aim of our research was to predict PPII structures with neural networks by taking advantage of amino acid sequences. The material was extracted from the Protein Data Bank [6].

2   Real Value Coding Method

We used genetic algorithm twice to produce real value coding for the neural networks. Firstly, relations were changed to the distances. Secondly, distances were transformed to the real value coordinates.

2.1   From Relations to Distances

The values of the *PAM250* substitution table [4] indicate how amino acids mutate to the each other. The substitution table probably includes information also of protein structures, such as PPII, and this information possibly increases prediction accuracy.

Relations in *PAM250* have many conflicts and, therefore, the coding task is difficult. Further, the relations of amino acids to themselves are problematic, because self-relations do not include the same values for every amino acid. This leads to conditions that must be taken into account in the fitness function of the genetic algorithm.

Let M be an upper triangle matrix (the actual data) for the *PAM250* matrix. We randomly initialised a new distance table *D250* that is also an upper triangle matrix. The fitness function of the genetic algorithm consists of two conditions.

The genetic algorithm must increase negative correlation between the *PAM250* table and the new distance table *D250*, because relations must be changed to the distances.

The genetic algorihtm should assign zero distances to the diagonal values of *D250*, because the self-distance for every amino acid must be zero.

The fitness function is

$$f = (\text{cor}(PAM250, D250) + 1) + \text{diagsum}(D250) \qquad (1)$$

where correlation between A and B ($\text{cor}(A,B)$) is calculated between vectors, which include upper triangle values of the matrices without diagonal values. The function diagsum(A) is the squared sum of the diagonal values of matrix A. If $D250$ fulfils both conditions, then f approaches zero. Populations, which the genetic algorithm evaluated, consisted of matrix presentations of the distances. We ran the genetic algorithm repeatedly in the Matlab environment until negative correlation stopped to increase. The best member of each prosess was inserted to the initial population of the next prosess. Minimum and maximum values in the genetic operations were 0 and 100. Values in Figure 1 and Tables 1 and 2 are also within this interval.

The optimization task was easy, because we got high correlation –0.9979 between values of $PAM250$ and values of $D250$. Distances are presented in Table 1.

Table 1. D250 distance matrix for amino acids after genetic algorithm processing

	A	C	D	E	F	G	H	I	K	L	M	N	P	Q	R	S	T	V	W	Y
A	1	32	62	48	62	31	62	47	48	47	47	63	47	48	47	18	30	32	77	62
C		0	77	92	62	77	78	47	77	46	47	78	78	77	77	47	47	47	62	61
D			0	3	77	47	49	77	47	93	77	16	47	31	62	32	48	78	92	77
E				0	77	62	33	78	17	78	63	32	47	1	32	31	47	63	78	62
F					0	77	47	32	78	31	33	77	92	78	77	62	62	48	16	0
G						0	62	93	62	93	78	32	62	62	62	32	62	78	62	78
H							0	77	48	78	63	17	62	32	32	47	62	77	62	3
I								0	77	2	17	77	77	77	78	62	47	0	78	47
K									0	63	46	31	47	17	3	32	47	61	78	63
L										0	2	77	78	63	62	63	47	17	62	47
M											0	62	62	32	48	48	47	17	49	47
N												0	63	32	32	17	32	79	92	62
P													0	47	62	47	47	63	93	77
Q														0	17	32	48	62	63	47
R															0	46	48	78	77	63
S																0	17	63	77	63
T																	0	33	59	63
V																		0	77	47
W																			0	0
Y																				0

2.2   From Distances to Coordinates

Next we generated floating point representations from Table 1. We used 3- and 5-dimensional presentations for amino acid sequences and 2-dimensional presentations to visualize their relations. Thus, 20 floating point values were randomly initialized and the genetic algorithm tried to find floating point positions in 2-, 3- and 5-dimensional Euclidean spaces. The genetic algorithm maximized positive correlation between floating point presentations and $D250$ distances. A member of population was one presentation of the amino acids in the Euclidean space and the population was a set of these members. Again, we used the genetic algorithm repeatedly.

We obtained quite good representations of the floating point values. The correlation with 2-dimensional points was 0.89, with 3-dimensional points 0.94 and with 5-dimensional points 0.95. We can see that conflicting distances work better in a space where the dimension is higher. Some floating point presentations are shown in Table 2. See also Figure 1 with 2-dimensional presentations of the amino acids.

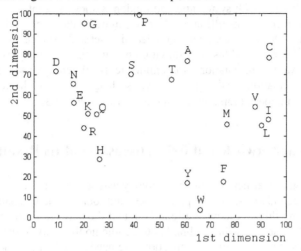

Fig. 1. 2-dimensional presentation of amino acids

3   Material for Neural Network

Learning material was taken from the Protein Data Bank having approximately 8600 macromolecules. We discarded such molecules which were not proteins, proteins which had a low resolution, and identical cases. Further we excluded proteins that had a relative in the same protein family and had a lower resolution than that of the relative. In this operation we used the sequence alignment and sequence identity measurements [7]. Finally, there were 1848 proteins for our real value coding and neural network tests.

Table 2. 5-dimensional presentations of amino acids

Dim.	A	C	D	E	F	G	H	I	K	L
1st	31.6	26.7	11.7	16.4	79.1	8.25	36.6	97.5	14.8	87.1
2nd	4.47	12.9	37.4	33.8	81.3	48.9	86	14.7	16	21.8
3rd	84.5	99.3	17.9	8.14	69	92.6	25.4	69.3	26.1	62.6
4th	53.1	22.6	97.2	66.7	21.8	94.8	52.3	19.4	35.3	1.01
5th	55.4	91	38	33.5	73.1	33.3	33.7	74.2	17	63.3
Dim.	M	N	P	Q	R	S	T	V	W	Y
1st	71.2	35.8	18.5	22.5	22.3	36.3	67.2	84.1	45.5	58.2
2nd	24	46.7	2.75	36.1	31.6	19.6	11.1	3.93	99.1	89.8
3rd	45.3	37.9	10.5	9.51	29.3	59.4	51.8	60	74.5	51.5
4th	9.96	83.2	75.8	41.8	24.6	78.1	75.8	30.7	22.8	27.4
5th	58.1	7.56	89.5	34.7	3.06	32.7	51.6	80	85.5	65.2

Five learning and test sets were selected as in [2]. We split the data into the learning (90% of the data) and test (10 %) sets. For the learning, PPII cases were separated from non-PPII cases. A length of the sequence was 13.

We had to discard, with systematic and random sampling, a lot of non-PPII cases, because the number of non-PPII and PPII cases must be the same in the learning set. Approximately 9000 cases remained in the learning set and 1200 cases in the test set.

Finally, the learning and test sets (having now uniform distribution) were recoded by using real value presentations for amino acids. When we used 3-dimensional amino acid presentations and sequences whose length was 13, the length of input vectors and the number of input nodes in the network were 13·3.

4   Neural Network and Brief Discussion of Its Results

Feedforward multilayer neural network topology was selected, because it is frequently used in the secondary structure predictions and our previous results were also obtained by using this topology. We found out that the network needs more than four hidden nodes for the real value coding [1] to handle nonlinearity in the mapping. If a shorter input vector is used, more connections are needed in the network.

We were interested in the prediction and recognition accuracies of neural networks. Prediction accuracy is $100\% \cdot TP/(TP+FP)$ and the recognition accuracy is $100\% \cdot TP/(TP+FN)$, where TP is the number of true positive cases, FN is the number of false negative cases and FP is the number of false positive cases.

Averages of results from five test sets for the real value coding are given in Table 3. Earlier [1] also binary value results were shown for comparison. As we can see, the results were almost independent of the dimension of the amino acid presentations. The results may depend more on network initializing tasks. In every test set the real value coding technique gave lower results than the binary value coding technique.

Table 3. Prediction (P) and recognition (R) accuracies for 3- and 5-dimensional real value coding and binary value coding

coding method	P (%)	R (%)
real value vector 3D	71.54	67.48
real value vector 5D	71.9	69.29
binary value vector	74.26	72.28

5   Conclusion

It is clear that the binary value coding technique gave better results in PPII secondary structure prediction. One reason for lower accuracies might be the increased nonlinearity that is well known inconvenience in structure prediction literature. When using the real value coding technique, a neural network needs more hidden nodes than with binary value coding - that was probably also effect of increased nonlinearity. Still, the number of connections in the optimal neural network structure was the same for both techniques.

Despite lower accuracies, we still believe that the direction of our research is right: In prediction work, we must take into account properties of amino acids. Already now, the method has many good properties (space saving, understandable form for humans, general nature for other secondary structure prediction and sequence alignment). We believe that there is a great amount of information in the world of molecules that can be exploited and then, our system to coding sequences can be a framework toward better sequence representation.

References

1. Siermala M., Juhola M., Vihinen M.: Neural Network Prediction of Polyproline Type II Secondary Structure. In: Hasman et al. (eds): Medical Infobahn for Europe, Proceedings of MIE2000 and GMDS2000, Vol. 77. IOS Press, Amsterdam (2000) 475-947
2. Hanke J., Raich J.: Kohonen map as a visualization tool for the analysis of protein sequences: multiple alignments, domains and segments of secondary structures. CABIOS 12 (1996) 447 – 454
3. Agresti A.: An Introduction to Categorial Data Analysis. John Wiley & Sons, New York (1996)
4. Dayhoff M., Schwartz R., Orcutt B.: A model of evolutionary change in proteins, matrices for detecting distant relationships. In: Dayhoff M. O. (ed.): Atlas of protein sequence and structure Vol. 5. National biomedical research foundation, Washington DC (1978) 345-358
5. Goldberg D.: Genetic Algorithms in Search, Optimization, and Machine Learning. Addison-Wesley, Reading (1989)
6. Berman H., Westbrook J., Feng Z., Gilliland G., Bhat T., Weissig H., Shindyalov I., Bourne P.: The Protein Data Bank. Nucleic Acids Research 28 (2000) 235-242
7. Needelman S., Wunsch C.: A general method applicable to search for similarities in amino-acid sequence of two proteins. J. Mol. Biol. 48 (1970) 443-453

Notes on Medical Decision Model Creation

Matej Šprogar[1], Peter Kokol[1], Milan Zorman[1], Vili Podgorelec[1],
Lenka Lhotska[2], and Jiří Klema[2]

[1] Laboratory for System Design, Faculty of Electrical Engineering and Computer
Science, Smetanova ulica 17, 2000 Maribor, Slovenia
{matej.sprogar,kokol}@uni-mb.si
[2] Gerstner Lab, Czech Technical University in Prague, Faculty of Electrical
Engineering, Technická 2, CZ-166 27 Prague 6, Czech Republic
lhotska@feld.cvut.cz,klema@labe.felk.cvut.cz

Abstract. To evaluate some intelligent method for decision-making we
need to compare the method against the competing methods to get some
idea of its performance and capabilities. In everyday practice this is
enough and the method, if proven good, can be used for different
problems. In medicine however we have a demand for the best solution
in all circumstances. It is therefore impossible to declare one method as
acceptable for every type or even every single problem. In this article
we would like to stress some important aspects of machine learning in
medicine, especially the creation of specific decision models. We
believe the evolutionary concept is a good approach to this as it creates
many diverse solutions.

1   Introduction

The doctor is many times not aware of the new medical procedure or medication for
some illness. It's simply because he or she can't be expected to keep up with all of the
medical advances as they come out. A similar dilemma is in the world of computer
generated intelligent models for medical decision-making. A perfect intelligent model
would know how to deal with any data yet there is only a small subset of that data
actually available for the learning process and the learning process itself has flaws.
Therefore we can only hope that the final model will behave as desired in most of the
cases.

It is impossible to draw direct connections between the medical and the computer
world. While in the real life each mistake can be lethal in the virtual world the same
mistake only affects some statistics. If the patient and doctor look for second opinion
they look for new knowledge, new experience; in AI we try to decide for the best
decision model, for example a decision tree (DT), and then use alternate ways to
construct this specific model and evaluate its quality. Because the direct qualitative
comparison of the decision-model producing methods is impossible we must compare
the produced decision models. And for that we need a dataset. Medical databases are
usually far from perfect (from the learning perspective) and this introduces new
problems in the decision making process.

J. Crespo, V. Maojo, and F. Martin (Eds.): ISMDA 2001, LNCS 2199, pp. 270-275, 2001.

2   Medical Approach to Decision Model Evaluation

Differential diagnosis is a working list of possibilities that a doctor uses in the process of diagnosing a specific disease. If in doubt the doctor/patient can ask for a second opinion. A "blind" second opinion is when medical records, test results and first physician's opinion are not made available to the second doctor; alternative is to share this information. The advantage of the "blind" approach is that it cannot be influenced by previous information. The disadvantage is that the second opinion doctor may not be able to tell you why his/her opinion is different without knowing the basis of the first doctor's opinion. A third option is to provide test results, X-rays and other information without the first doctor's written diagnosis and treatment recommendation. Most second opinion doctors prefer knowing the first opinion, but they can still provide a good second opinion if they can at least review previous medical records. This information is helpful as it often provides clues and baselines to compare to new test results [9].

2.1   Evaluating the Decision Model

The aim of using computers in medicine is to provide help for doctors to select the correct diagnosis and appropriate treatment and to discover new knowledge. Because we don't know how to code the medical knowledge of a human expert into a computer program we mostly use intelligent techniques that extract information from given data. The data describes known cases with the attributes that are found relevant by the doctors. In the whole data gathering process there are many presumptions and errors and almost every database also includes a certain amount of noise. When this data is used for the computer model new limitations arise and the result is therefore almost always only an approximation of some wishful ideal model.

The behaviour of the decision model must be inspected using different testing methods and must also be compared to other decision models. For this purpose the public access database for machine learning [7] is of great help yet the comparisons are usually inadequate – a gain of a few percent is not enough to pronounce one model superior to the other. We use an evolutionary method for decision tree construction and are aware of its advantages and deficiencies – the evolutionary process yields many different solutions, can have convergence problems, is robust on different types of databases and is theoretically capable of finding the optimal solution [5, 10]. The catch with the decision model evaluation is however in the comparison of our evolutionary trees with other trees made on public and private datasets.

The main problems with all (medical) datasets usually are (1) small size with high overfitting possibility; (2) noise; (3) missing values. The diverse public datasets include all of the above and are therefore a good testing playground to get the general feeling of our method. But we must not forget the "No free lunch [8]" theorem, where Wolpert and Macready proved that, when performance is averaged over all possible search spaces, all search algorithms perform equally well. If we regard learning methods as search methods then all the methods are equally effective. To use the decision method for medical purposes we must be sure of its strength. And because of the theorem we can't always expect to get good results on fresh datasets. In fact, we have to prove the method to be good on every new dataset, too. Now we have a problem – if we have to make a detailed evaluation of the decision model (in our case the decision tree) for a given dataset then this is a task for the experienced professional. To make an analysis of a dataset it's not enough just to use some tool and collect the results. We must compare those results with results of other methods, do a statistical analysis... This is a lot more difficult than just depend on the final accuracy score [10].

For example, the recognized and well-known C4.5 (and the successor, C5) algorithm for DT construction is a good general performer with usually high level of accuracy. But we can't expect the C5 to perform best on all datasets. The tree produced with C5 however is good reference tree that other trees can be compared with. Because of high expectations from the doctors we need the "best" results for each dataset. Therefore we have to *push* the decision model building method. This is dangerous because it's easy to cause overfitting of the model to the underlying data. We found the evolutionary computing (EC [2]) to be very effective in this respect as it easily produces a whole family of solutions (decision trees) instead of a few similar ones – this is an advantage with difficult datasets where the solutions are likely to fall into a local optimum. And because the EC can create *any* possible model it's logical to expect that the evolved model will achieve at least the same quality as the C5 produced one. With this thinking we are also close to the dilemma of evaluating the EC DT producing method itself. If EC is capable of producing *the* best DT in every case (though it will probably not) then it's possible to push it on every single dataset until it outperforms other methods... But since we are concerned with getting the best model for one particular dataset this is exactly what we want.

3   Using Intelligent Classifiers

To get the best decision tree for our dataset we decided to use something like the "second opinion" approach, which is a well-known principle in medicine. But before we give the dataset to the second professional to analyze and create a DT model, we have to decide how much information to give to this second expert. We have possibilities similar to those in the medicine and first option is to select a blind second opinion. This is because there is no biased information for that dataset, we wish for independent opinion and we certainly don't want to influence any results. The input for the second expert is therefore only the dataset accompanied with the necessary description of the data. We hope the blind second opinion will give some possibilities we wouldn't think of or some new clues that are not so obvious from our perspective. To extend the research we also asked for the second opinion from the third professional, this time he was given all details and knowledge of our work and also the results from the second expert.

The hesitation about this "second opinion" is that we can perform all the comparisons and evaluations simply by ourselves – it's faster and cheaper. The medical experience however teaches us that this is not the best way to go. The second opinion from an independent expert can tell us more about our method, our final decision model and the dataset we are using than we would discover by ourselves. The following example doesn't reveal any new knowledge; it just shows some differences we might never have seen otherwise. Presented dataset is difficult for the classification systems because a small improvement in sensitivity usually dramatically reduces the specificity score.

3.1   Mitral Valve Prolapse Dataset

This medical dataset describes the cardiac problem of mitral valve prolapse [3] in children and is a result of a major medical study. The MVP] dataset describes children and youths under age of 18. They were selected regardless of their medical records and previous examinations. A total of 631 patients are recorded in the dataset. With results from auscultation, phonocardiography, ECG and echocardiography we collected a total of 103 attributes possibly showing the presence of MVP. Three final classifications are possible: prolapse, silent prolapse and no prolapse.

3.2   Methods and Results

Predictive power is only one aspect of the decision model and therefore we prefer to use the decision tree, which is a transparent model that shows why the particular classification was made. Our tool uses genetic algorithms (GA) and can therefore produce a whole set of decision trees with different properties. We expect to find some very good trees or even optimal trees but none of this is for certain [4,5]. We used the 10-fold technique to split the dataset into training and testing subsets and then ran our tool several times on each of the learning sets until we got some converging results for that fold. Statistical scores of decision trees were quite interesting – we could observe tree's overall accuracy, sensitivity and specificity, size and average depth... Table 1 displays the best statistics encountered.

Table 1. The best results for the GA produced decision trees

	Best	Average
Overall accuracy	96.2	88.0
Sensitivity	90.1	80.7
Specificity	96.7	90.1

If the MVP would be a public database we would check our testing statistics against other published results. But this is not the case and because of the nature of GA trees, which have a wide range of scores, it's difficult to say how good this score really is. Is it possible to build an even better tree? We were able to construct more different trees all with similar scores. Because of this we concluded that we could determine MVP in several ways - the medical doctors also confirmed that later on. But we still have no clue how well the GA method performed on the MVP dataset.

To compare our results with that from the second opinion we had to create one testing set. We randomly selected 501 cases out of 631 for learning and the remaining 130 for the testing. This learning/testing pair was then given to the second/third expert. The results for this data arrangement are presented in Table 2.

3.3   Other Approaches

When we received the blind second opinion for the MVP dataset we could see that the basic idea behind the second analysis was close to ours. Instead of the GA based tool the analyst used the recognized C5 [6]. First advantage was visible when we read the remarks about the dataset – the *prolapse* diagnosis was problematic and it constantly had lower sensitivity scores. Because the scores for the *silent prolapse* were significantly better (and it's more difficult to diagnose) the other expert even suspected that the notations had been mixed in the dataset! The resulting model from the informed expert, who also used a GA-based tool, was the best of all. While the isolated GA and C5 methods had no clue of the quality of the results the informed expert could twist and push his method to achieve better results than the EC and the C5 method alone.

It is difficult to compare different tree topologies because it's the combination of the shape and attributes that makes the classification. Smaller trees tend to have better generalization capabilities while there is no perfect rule to select the order of tests in tree nodes. We are still waiting for medical explanation for all trees. We should note here that GA sometimes produced trees with layers very similar to that of C5.

Table 2. Comparison of best testing results (EC tool and 2 second opinions)

	Our results	Blind second opinion	Informed second op.
Sensitivity	63.6 (7/11)	63.6 (7/11)	72.7 (8/11)
Specificity	95.0 (113/119)	93.3 (111/119)	95.0 (113/119)
Accuracy	92.3 (120/130)	90.8 (118/130)	93.1 (121/130)

4   Discussion and Conclusions

The presented dataset, especially the chosen learning and testing set pair, is difficult for any classification method because of sensitivity and generalization problems. The informed second opinion (with the results of C5 and our EC method) could use this information to adapt the fitness function and focus more on the attributes found relevant by both methods. At the same time the minimal scores were known and the method itself could be adapted to suit the MVP problem more. This is not positive for the method itself as only a skilful professional is able to perform such modifications, but it's positive for the MVP diagnosis.

Just like the medical doctor the computer expert can't master certain specifics. The problem when evaluating certain learning methodology is that it can only be evaluated on a specific dataset. A general comparison is impossible because it consumes too much time and resources. If we dislike certain solution we have the option to build another model yet the doubt of its quality remains. The normally used comparisons of scalar measures have some disadvantages that are not so obvious. We must have the appropriate tool for a reference build in the first place. Then we need the necessary experience – an inexperienced user simply doesn't know how to set all the parameters to fully exploit such tool. Above all there is a great chance that we'll overlook a small detail that just may have a great impact on the overall score of the model.

The problem with the second opinion is that you must find a second expert to perform necessary work on a high enough level, who has the experience and knowledge to give quality feedback. In the end is the question of funding but depending on the problem it may be worth a try.

References

1. A Second Opinion Medical, An Information & Physician Verification Service: http://www.physicians-background.com (jan. 2001)
2. Banzhaf, W., Nordin, P., Keller, R. E., Francone, F. D.: Genetic Programming – An Introduction. Morgan Kaufmann Publishers Inc (1998)
3. Boudoulas, H., Kolibash, A. J., Baker, P., King, B. D., Wooley, C. F.: Mitral Valve Prolapse and the Mitral Valve Prolapse Syndrome: A Diagnostic Classification and Pathogenesis of Symptoms. American Heart Journal, 118 (1989), 796 – 818
4. Kokol, P. Et al: Decision Trees and Automatic Learning and their Use in Cardiology. Journal of Medical Systems. 19(4) (1994)
5. Podgorelec, V., Kokol, P.: Self-Adaptation of Evolutionary Constructed Decision Trees by Information Spreading. Proceedings of the International Conference on Artificial Neural Nets and Genetic Algorithms. Springer Verlag (1999) 294 – 301
6. Quinlan, J. R.: C4.5: Programs for Machine Learning. Morgan Kaufmann, San Mateo, CA (1993)
7. UCI Machine Learning: http://www.ics.uci.edu/~mlearn/Machine-Learning.html (feb. 2001)
8. Wolpert, D., Macready, W.: No Free Lunch Theorems for Optimization. IEEE Transactions on Evolutionary Computation, Vol. 1(1) (1997) 67-82
9. Yale - New Haven Hospital: Getting a Good Second Opinion. http://www.ynhh.org (2001)
10. Šprogar, M., Kokol, P., Hleb Babič, Š., Podgorelec,V., Zorman, M.: Vector Decision trees. Intelligent Data Analysis 4, IOS Press (2000) 305-321

Refining the Knowledge Base of an Otoneurological Expert System

Kati Viikki and Martti Juhola

Department of Computer and Information Sciences
P.O. Box 607, FIN-33014 University of Tampere, Finland

Abstract. This paper deals with the possibilities to refine the knowledge base of an otoneurological expert system ONE with the knowledge learned from data. The augmented knowledge base produces better results for benign positional vertigo, Menière's disease, sudden deafness, traumatic vertigo, and vestibular schwannoma. The results of this study suggest that learning from data is useful in refining the knowledge base. However, the knowledge acquired from human experts is also needed.

1   Introduction

Vertigo is a symptom that can be caused by a wide variety of diseases [5]. An otoneurological expert system ONE [2] is developed to assist the diagnostic procedure for peripheral and central diseases involving vertigo [5] and to provide a tutorial guide for medical students. Diagnostic work-up with vertiginous patients requires thorough knowledge of otoneurology [5]. An interactive expert system helps even general practitioner to request the right investigations and to submit the challenging patients to the right specialist for further evaluation [5].

The performance ability of an expert system essentially depends on its knowledge base. The knowledge representation model of ONE employs weight and fitness values. A weight value expresses the relevance of an attribute for a certain disease. A fitness value expresses how well an attribute value fits to a certain disease. The weight and fitness values stored in the knowledge base of ONE are defined on the basis of expertise of otoneurologists and information obtained from the literature [7]. According to previous studies, ONE seems to outperform another otoneurological expert system [1] and to do well also when compared to human experts [7]. However, reasoning on Menière's disease and vestibular schwannoma has been difficult for ONE [2]. Benign positional vertigo and vestibular neuritis cases with confounding values (i.e. symptoms and signs not related to the current disease) have also caused difficulties for ONE [7,14], which calls for the further refinement of its knowledge base.

The database of otoneurological cases makes ONE beneficial for medical research. It can be also utilised in the research of machine learning methods: The continued collection of patient cases has enabled the knowledge acquisition from data using decision trees [13], genetic algorithms [8], and neural networks [4]. The present study explores the effects of fitness values extracted from a data set

J. Crespo, V. Maojo, and F. Martin (Eds.): ISMDA 2001, LNCS 2199, pp. 276–281, 2001.

on reasoning results for the six largest diagnostic groups [6] in the database of ONE.

2   The Inference Mechanism of the Otoneurological Expert System ONE

The present version of ONE deals with 18 diseases and disorders involving vertigo [7]. Its inference mechanism resembles the nearest neighbour methods of pattern recognition [11] and takes into account the attributes concerning patient history, clinical tests and examinations. For each disease, a description is given in the knowledge base in the form of fitness values and weights. To each attribute, a weight value expressing the significance of the attribute for the disease is set. Fitness values set to attribute values express the correspondence between the attribute values and the disease.

The inference mechanism transforms attribute values to scores based on the fitness values and weights. Let d be a disease and $n(d)$ be the number of attributes associated with the disease d in the knowledge base. The score $S(d)$ for the disease d is calculated as

$$S(d) = \frac{\sum_{i=1}^{n(d)} x(i)w(d,i)f(d,i,j)}{\sum_{i=1}^{n(d)} x(i)w(d,i)}, \tag{1}$$

where

- $x(i)$ is 1, if the value of ith attribute is known for the disease d, otherwise 0;
- $w(d,i)$ is the weight value for the attribute i for the disease d; and
- $f(d,i,j)$ is the fitness value for the value j of the attribute i for the disease d; the fitness value varies from 0 to 1.

The diseases with the highest scores are the best fits and suggested by ONE. To handle uncertainty caused by missing values, ONE generates upper and lower bounds for the score. The lower bound is calculated using the lowest fitness values for the missing values and the upper bound using the highest fitness values for the missing values. In addition to the scoring scheme, ONE uses necessary attribute values attached to certain diseases. In order to be diagnosed as having a certain disease, the case, which is processed, has to fulfill the requirements concerning the necessary attribute values set for the disease.

3   Fitness Values Based on Frequency Distributions

In the present study, the fitness values were calculated from data. The data were collected in the Department of Otorhinolaryngology at Helsinki University Central Hospital. It contained 815 patient cases representing the six largest diagnostic groups in the database of ONE: Menière's disease ($n_{md} = 313$; 38.4%), benign positional vertigo ($n_{bp} = 146$; 17.9%), vestibular schwannoma ($n_{vs} =$

130; 16.0%), vestibular neuritis ($n_{vn} = $ 120; 14.7%), traumatic vertigo ($n_{tv} = $ 65; 8.0%), and sudden deafness ($n_{sd} = $ 41; 5.0%). From each diagnostic group, approximately 70% of cases were randomly selected to the training set. The rest 30% of cases formed the testing set.

The fitness values were calculated from the training data within the six diagnostic groups. For each attribute i, the frequency distribution was calculated. The fitness value $f(d, i, j)$ was calculated as the proportion of the frequency $fr(d, i, j)$ of the value j to the highest frequency $fr(d, i, h)$ of the distribution:

$$f(d, i, j) = \frac{fr(d, i, j)}{fr(d, i, h)}. \tag{2}$$

The fitness values for the attribute values not appearing in the cases of the training data were set to 0. In order to calculate the fitness values, the continuous attributes were discretized. The range of observed values was divided into k equal-width bins [3]. The number of bins depended on the attribute.

4   Experimental Results

Effects of weight and fitness values on the resulting scores were examined. The upper and lower bounds of the score and the necessary attribute values were not employed in these experiments. The test cases were diagnosed using four different weight and fitness value systems:

– Experiment 1: The weights and fitness values defined by experienced otoneurologists were used. In this system, weights typically varied from 0 to 5. The weight 0 means that the attribute does not concern the disease at all. Some notably large weights were also used: for sudden deafness the attribute concerning type of hearing loss with the weight 40, for traumatic vertigo the attribute head trauma with the weight 200, and for vestibular schwannoma the attribute concerning tumour in the acousticus nerve with the weight 200.
– Experiment 2: The weights defined by the otoneurologists and the fitness values learned from the training data were used.
– Experiment 3: For the relevant attributes defined by the otoneurologists, the weight values of 1 and the fitness values learned from the training data were used.
– Experiment 4: All the 170 attributes were associated with the weight 1, except those whose values were missing from all the training cases of the diagnostic group. These missing attributes had the weight 0. The used fitness values were learned from the training data.

In the Experiment 1, the test cases were diagnosed by ONE with the descriptions of the six largest diagnostic groups in its knowledge base. In the Experiments 2-4, a classification system simulating the inference mechanism of ONE was used. The system was implemented in the MATLAB computing environment [10].

Table 1. True positive rates (%) from four experiments (*TPR1 – TPR4*)

Diagnosis	N	TPR1	TPR2	TPR3	TPR4
Benign positional vertigo	44	59.1	61.4	61.4	65.9
Menière's disease	94	62.8	80.9	80.9	94.7
Sudden deafness	12	66.7	91.7	91.7	66.7
Traumatic vertigo	20	95.0	100.0	25.0	80.0
Vestibular neuritis	37	81.1	70.3	70.3	75.7
Vestibular schwannoma	39	30.8	30.8	33.3	66.7

The disease with the highest score was considered as the result. For each diagnostic group, the true positive rate (*TPR*) was calculated as the percentage of correctly inferred cases:

$$TPR = 100\frac{tpos}{pos}\%, \tag{3}$$

where *tpos* is the number of correctly inferred cases and *pos* is the number of all cases in the diagnostic group. The true positive rates from the four experiments are shown in Table 1.

The scoring scheme 4 with the weights of 1 and the fitness values learned from the training data produced the best true positive rate for benign positional vertigo, Menière's disease, and vestibular schwannoma (65.9%, 94.7%, and 66.7%, respectively). In the case of Menière's disease and vestibular schwannoma, the true positive rate was notable larger (over 30%) compared to the true positive rate of the scoring scheme 1, i.e., that obtained by ONE. Sudden deafness was inferred best with the scoring schemes 2 and 3 in which the attributes defined by the otoneurologists were used with the fitness values learned from the training data. The weights of the attributes did not affect the inference results.

For traumatic vertigo, the weights defined by otoneurologists and the fitness values learned from the training data produced the best results (*TPR* of 100.0%). An essential attribute in inferring traumatic vertigo is head trauma that had the weight of 200 in the scoring schemes 1 and 2. These schemes produced very good results. If the weight of head trauma was reduced to 1, the true positive rate decreased dramatically to 25.0%. However, when a larger group of variables were used in the Experiment 4, a good true positive rate (80.0%) was achieved again. For vestibular neuritis, the weights and fitness values defined by the otoneurologists yielded the best true positive rate of 81.1%.

5   Discussion

Possibilities to refine the knowledge base of the otoneurological expert system
ONE by acquiring knowledge from data were studied. The four different scoring
systems employed in the inference were formed using the knowledge acquired
from experts and the fitness values learned from the training data. The use of
the learned fitness values produced better results for benign positional vertigo,
Menière's disease, sudden deafness, traumatic vertigo, and vestibular schwannoma. Vestibular neuritis was an exception with the best results produced by
the weight and fitness values defined by the experts.

In the case of sudden deafness, the relevant attributes defined by the otoneurologists were important. This result coincides with the results of our earlier
study [13] concerning a subset of the current data set: Increasing the number
of attributes used in the decision tree construction produced lower true positive
rates for sudden deafness. The magnitude of weights was not important in the
case of sudden deafness, whereas the true positive rate for traumatic vertigo
decreased from 100.0% to 25.0% when the weights defined by the experts were
set to 1. This decrease can be explained by the attribute head trauma with the
weight of 200 in the scoring scheme 2. However, the use of the largest attribute
group with the weights of 1 in the Experiment 4 produced the good true positive rate (80.0%) for traumatic vertigo. For Menière's disease and vestibular
schwannoma, the scoring scheme 4 with the largest attribute group yielded the
best results, which agrees with the results of our earlier study with decision
trees [13].

The above phenomena relate to the problem of attribute or feature subset
selection [9]: Which attributes should be used to describe learning data or included in the learned models? Although a larger attribute set usually contains
more information, it does not necessarily produce better results. Future work
in the refinement of the knowledge base of ONE will include the use of feature
subset selection methods (e.g. [9,12]) to find good descriptions for the six otoneurological diseases. It will also examine the employment of different discretization
and interpolation methods (e.g. [3,15], respectively) for continuous attributes.
Yet another future aim is to develop a method for weight definition based on
data. A scoring scheme that combines the weights and the fitness values learned
from data to the knowledge acquired from human experts is our ultimate goal.

To conclude, the results of this study suggest that the knowledge learned from
data is useful in refining the knowledge base. The refinement of a knowledge base
is a complicated task, in which the knowledge acquired from human experts is
also needed.

Acknowledgements

The authors thank Prof. Ilmari Pyykkö, M.D., Erna Kentala, M.D., Yrjö Auramo, Ph.D., Matti J. Tapani, B.Sc., and Erkki Mäkinen, Ph.D., for their contribution to the study. The work of the first author was funded by Tampere

Graduate School in Information Science and Engineering (TISE), and by a grant from Ella and Georg Ehrnrooth Foundation.

References

1. Auramo, Y., Juhola, M.: Comparison of inference results of two otoneurological expert systems. Int. J. Bio-Med. Comput. **39** (1995) 327–335 276
2. Auramo, Y., Juhola, M., Pyykkö, I.: An expert system for the computer-aided diagnosis of dizziness and vertigo. Med. Inform. **18** (1993) 293–305 276
3. Dougherty, J., Kohavi, R., Sahami, M.: Supervised and unsupervised discretization of continuous features. In: Prieditis, A., Russell, S. (eds.): Machine Learning: Proceedings of the 12th International Conference. Morgan Kaufmann, San Francisco (1995) 194–202 278, 280
4. Juhola, M., Laurikkala, J., Viikki, K., Auramo, Y., Kentala, E., Pyykkö, I.: Neural network recognition of otoneurological vertigo diseases with comparison of some other classification methods. In: Horn, W., Shahar, Y., Lindberg, G., Andreassen, S., Wyatt, J. (eds.): Artificial Intelligence in Medicine. Lectures Notes in Artificial Intelligence, Vol. 1620. Springer, Berlin (1999) 217–226 276
5. Kentala, E.: A neurotologic expert system for vertigo and characteristics of six otologic diseases involving vertigo. Academic Dissertation, Department of Otorhinolaryngology, University of Helsinki, Finland (1996) 276
6. Kentala, E.: Characteristics of six otologic diseases involving vertigo. Am. J. Otol. **17** (1996) 883–892 277
7. Kentala, E., Auramo, Y., Juhola, M., Pyykkö, I.: Comparison between diagnoses of human experts and a neurotologic expert system. Ann. Otol. Rhinol. Laryngol. **107** (1998) 135–140 276, 277
8. Kentala, E., Laurikkala, J., Pyykkö, I., Juhola, M.: Discovering diagnostic rules from a neurotologic database with genetic algorithms. Ann. Otol. Rhinol. Laryngol. **108** (1999) 948–954 276
9. Kohavi, R., John, G. H.: Wrappers for feature subset selection. Artificial Intelligence **97** (1997) 273–324 280
10. MATLAB 5.3 (2000) http://www.mathworks.com/ 278
11. Mitchell, T. M.: Machine Learning. McGraw-Hill, New York (1997) 277
12. Viikki, K.: A variable grouping method based on graph theoretic techniques. Report A-2001-1, Department of Computer and Information Sciences, University of Tampere, Finland (2001) 280
13. Viikki, K., Kentala, E., Juhola, M., Pyykkö, I.: Decision tree induction in the diagnosis of otoneurological diseases. Med. Inform. **24** (1999) 277–289 276, 280
14. Viikki, K., Kentala, E., Juhola, M., Pyykkö, I.: Confounding values in decision trees constructed for six otoneurological diseases. In: Lavrač, N., Miksch, S., Kavšek, B. (eds.): Proceedings of the 5th International Workshop on Intelligent Data Analysis in Medicine and Pharmacology (IDAMAP-2000), Berlin (2000) 58–60 276
15. Wilson, D. R., Martinez, T. R.: Improved heterogeneous distance functions. Journal of Artificial Intelligence Research **6** (1997) 1–34 280

Segmentation of Color Fundus Images of the Human Retina: Detection of the Optic Disc and the Vascular Tree Using Morphological Techniques

Thomas Walter and Jean-Claude Klein

Centre de Morphologie Mathématique, Ecole nationale supérieure des Mines de Paris
35 rue St.Honoré, 77305 Fontainebleau CEDEX, France
{walter,klein}@cmm.ensmp.fr
http://cmm.ensmp.fr/~walter/

Abstract. This paper presents new algorithms based on mathematical morphology for the detection of the optic disc and the vascular tree in noisy low contrast color fundus photographs. Both features – vessels and optic disc – deliver landmarks for image registration and are indispensable to the understanding of retinal fundus images. For the detection of the optic disc, we first find the position approximately. Then we find the exact contours by means of the watershed transformation. The algorithm for vessel detection consists in contrast enhancement, application of the morphological top-hat-transform and a post-filtering step in order to distinguish the vessels from other blood containing features.

1 Introduction

1.1 Outlines

In ophthalmology, the automatic detection of blood vessels as well as the detection of the optic disc may be of considerable interest for computer assisted diagnosis. Detecting and counting lesions in the human retina like microaneurysms and exudates is a time consuming task for ophthalmologists and open to human error. That is why much effort has been done to detect lesions in the human retina automatically. Finding the main components in the fundus images helps in characterizing detected lesions and in identifying false positives. Furthermore, vessel detection is interesting for the computation of parameters related to blood flow. The detection of the optic disc may be a first step in the early detection of the glaucoma. Over and above that, the optic disc and the vessels can be considered as landmarks of the fundus images, that may be used afterwards for image registration of images taken at different times or using different methods (as shown in [1]). To perform a robust feature based image registration, it is indispensable to rely on a robust and fast algorithm for vessel detection.

J. Crespo, V. Maojo, and F. Martin (Eds.): ISMDA 2001, LNCS 2199, pp. 282–287, 2001.
© Springer-Verlag Berlin Heidelberg 2001

1.2   Some Morphological Operators

In this section we briefly define the basic morphological operators used in this paper (see [2], [3]).

Let $\mathcal{D}_f$ be a subset of $\mathbb{Z}^2$ and $T = \{t_{min}, ..., t_{max}\}$ be an ordered set of grey-levels. A grey-level image f can then be defined as a function $f : \mathcal{D}_f \subset \mathbb{Z}^2 \rightarrow T = \{t_{min}, ..., t_{max}\}$. Furthermore, let B be a subset of $\mathbb{Z}^2$ and $s \in \mathbb{N}$ a scaling factor, we can write the basic morphological operations as:

- Erosion: $\left[\varepsilon^{(sB)}(f)\right](x) = \min_{b \in sB} f(x + b)$
- Dilation: $\left[\delta^{(sB)}(f)\right](x) = \max_{b \in sB} f(x + b)$
- Opening: $\gamma^{(sB)}(f) = \delta^{(sB)} \left[\varepsilon^{(sB)}(f)\right]$
- Closing: $\phi^{(sB)}(f) = \varepsilon^{(sB)} \left[\delta^{(sB)}(f)\right]$

We call sB structuring element B of size s. Furthermore we may define the geodesic transformations of an image f (marker) and a second image g (mask):

- Geodesic erosion: $\varepsilon_g^{(n)}(f) = \varepsilon_g^{(1)} \varepsilon_g^{(n-1)}(f)$ with $\varepsilon_g^{(1)}(f) = \varepsilon^{(B)}(f) \vee g$
- Geodesic dilation: $\delta_g^{(n)}(f) = \delta_g^{(1)} \delta_g^{(n-1)}(f)$ with $\delta_g^{(1)}(f) = \delta^{(B)}(f) \wedge g$
- Opening by reconstruction: $\gamma_g^{rec}(f) = \delta_g^{(i)}(f)$ with $\delta_g^{(i)}(f) = \delta_g^{(i+1)}(f)$
- Closing by reconstruction: $\phi_g^{rec}(f) = \varepsilon_g^{(i)}(f)$ with $\varepsilon_g^{(i)}(f) = \varepsilon_g^{(i+1)}(f)$

2   Detection of the Optic Disc

2.1   Properties of the Optic Disc

The optic disc is the entrance of the vessels and the optic nerve into the retina. It appears in color fundus images as a bright yellowish or white region. Its shape is more or less circular, interrupted by the outgoing vessels. Sometimes it has the form of an ellipse because of a non-negligible angle between image plane and object plane. The size varies from patient to patient; its diameter lies between 40 and 60 pixels in 640×480 color photographs.

2.2   State of the Art

In [5] the optic disc is localized exploiting its high grey level variation. This approach has shown to work well, if there are no or only few pathologies like exudates, that also appear very bright and are also well contrasted. In [6] an area threshold is used to localize the optic disc. The contours are detected by means of the Hough transform. This approach is quite time consuming and it relies on conditions about the shape of the optic disc, that are not always met.

2.3   Algorithm Based on Morphological Operators

The Color Space Having compared several color spaces, we found the contours of the optic disc to appear most continuous and less disturbed by the outgoing vessels in the red channel f_r of the RGB color space. As this channel has a very small dynamic range and as we know that the optic disc belongs to the brightest parts of the color image, it is more reliable to work on the luminance channel f_l of the HLS color space to localize the optic disc and on f_r to find its contours.

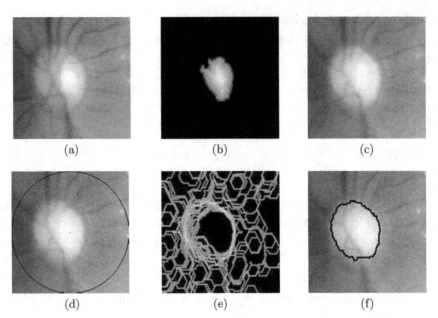

Fig. 1. The detection of the optic disc: (a) Luminance channel (b) Distance image of the biggest particle (c) red channel (d) red channel with imposed marker (e) morphological gradient (f) result of segmentation

Localizing the Optic Disc As we know approximately the size of the optic disc and as we can assume that parts of it belong to the brightest parts of the image f_l, we apply a simple area threshold to obtain a binary image b, that contains some parts of the optic disc as well as bright appearing pathologies like exudates. Exudates are not very big, and they are far from reaching the size of the optic disc. Hence, the biggest particle of the image b coincides with one part of the optic disc. Its centroid c , that can be calculated as the maximum of the discrete distance function of the biggest particle of b (shown in figure 1b) can be considered as an approximation for the locus of the optic disc.

In a first step we filter the image f_r in order to eliminate large gray level variations within the papillary region. First we "fill" the vessels, applying a simple closing $p_1 = \phi^{(s_1 B)}(f_r)$ with a hexagonal structuring element $s_1 B$ bigger than the maximal width of vessels. In order to remove large picks, we open the resulting image: $p_2 = \gamma^{(s_2 B)}(p_1)$. As this filter alters the shape of the papillary region considerably, we reconstruct it: $p_3 = \gamma^{rec}_{p_1}(p_2)$.

In order to detect the contours of the optic disc, we apply the classical watershed transformation [2] to the gradient $\Delta p_3 = \delta^{(B)} p_3 - \varepsilon^{(B)} p_3$ of the filtered image (shown in figure 1e) with c as internal marker and a circle among c with radius bigger than the diameter of the papilla as external marker (see figure 1d).

2.4   Results

We tested the algorithm on 30 color images of size 640×480 containing various pathologies. In all images, we could localize the optic disc with the proposed technique. In 27 images, we also found the exact contours. However, in some of the images, there were small parts missing or small false positives due to their low contrast. In 3 images the contrast was too low or the red channel too saturated, the algorithm failed and the result was not acceptable.

3   Detection of the Vascular Tree

3.1   Properties of the Vessels

Vessels appear darker than the background, their width is always smaller than a certain value λ, they are piecewise linear and they are connected in a tree like way. However these properties hold only approximately: Due to the presence of noise, the vessels are often disconnected, and not each pixel on a vessel appears darker than the background. The vessel borders appear often unsharp.

3.2   State of the Art

Much has been written about the detection of vessels in medical images; particularly for retinal images, matched filters [7], neuronal networks [5], a grouping algorithm of edgels [8] and a combination of linear and morphological methods [9] have been proposed. Our main objective is to conceive a fast and robust algorithm, the sensitivity being less important.

3.3   Vessel Detection Algorithm

In the following, we work on the green channel f_g of the RGB color space, because blood containing features appear most contrasted in this channel. In order to eliminate the noise and small "walls", that may disconnect the vascular tree, we apply a simple Gaussian filter, followed by an opening of size 2.

Now we apply $\vartheta g = TH\left[TM(g)\right]$ to the prefiltered image g, with the toggle-mapping $TM(g)$ (see [4])

$$h(x) = \left[TM(g)\right](x) = \begin{cases} \phi^{(s_1 B)}g(x) & \text{,if } \left[\phi^{(s_1 B)}g - g\right](x) \leq \left[g - \gamma^{(s_2 B)}g\right](x) \\ \gamma^{(s_2 B)}g(x) & \text{,if } \left[\phi^{(s_1 B)}g - g\right](x) > \left[g - \gamma^{(s_2 B)}g\right](x) \end{cases}$$

and the top-hat by closing $TH(h) = \phi^{(s_1 B)}h - h$ with s_1 equal for both operators. We choose s_1 in a way, that by applying $\phi^{(s_1 B)}$ the vessels are completely "filled". Therefore, the gray-level value $g(x)$ of a vessel pixel x is closer to the opening than to the closing, and so it will be darkened, whereas the border pixels will take the value of the closing (see figure 2). As $\phi^{(s_1 B)}h = \phi^{(s_1 B)}g$ (see [4]), all pixels that take the value of the closing in $TM(g)$, take a 0 in the top-hat-image, i.e. all holes extracted by the top-hat transform are disconnected.

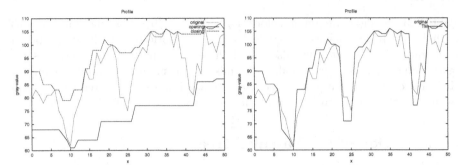

Fig. 2. The effect of the toggle-mappings: (a) shows a profile of an image with three vessels and the corresponding opening and closing (b) shows the resulting toggle-mapping

The rest is straightforward: Knowing that the vessels are piecewise linear we can calculate the supremum of openings with big linear structuring elements B_i (about 40 pixels) in different directions (we use the efficient recursive algorithms proposed in [2]). In that way we remove all features, into which the linear structuring element does not fit in any direction. As a result we obtain a set of unconnected lines. We can recover the vascular tree by an opening by reconstruction (for reconstruction operator see [2]):

$$\gamma^{sup}(\vartheta g) = \bigcup_{i=1}^{12} \gamma^{(sB_i)}(\vartheta g) \qquad\qquad R = \gamma^{rec}_{\vartheta g}\left[\gamma^{sup}(\vartheta g)\right]$$

3.4   Results

We tested the algorithm also on the 30 color images. The results are fully satisfactory in well contrasted images and still acceptable in low contrast images. Smaller vessels, if not connected to the rest of the vascular tree are often missed, which is not a drawback if vessel detection is used for image registration. There are very few false positives. However, if there are a lot of hemorrhages and microaneurysms, particularly if they are close to the vascular tree, another prefiltering step must be performed (an infimum of closings with linear structuring elements of different directions, followed by a closing by reconstruction, see [9]).

4   Conclusion

Two new algorithms for automatic segmentation of fundus images of the human retina have been presented in this paper. The optic disc and the vessels belong to the main features in the human eye, their detection is indispensable to understanding ocular fundus images. The proposed algorithms shall be used as a first step in image registration, for the identification of false positives in pathology detection and for classification of the detected pathologies.

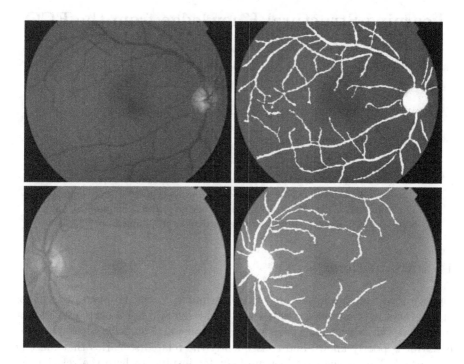

Fig. 3. The results of the segmentation algorithms

References

1. F. Zana and J.-C. Klein, A multi-modal segmentation algorithm of eye fundus images using vessel detection and hough transform, *IEEE Trans On Medical Imaging*, vol.18,no.5,1999. 282
2. P. Soille, *Morphological Image Analysis: Principles And Applications*, vol. 1, Springer-Verlag Berlin, Heidelberg, New York, 1999. 283, 284, 286
3. J. Serra, *Image analysis and mathematical morphology*, vol. 2, Academic Press, New York, 1988. 283
4. F. Meyer and J. Serra, Contrast and activity lattice, *Signal Processing*, vol. 16, no. 4, (303–317), 1989. 285
5. C. Sinthanayothin et al, Automated localisation of the optic disc, fovea and retinal blood vessels from digital colour fundus images, *British Journal of Ophtalmology*, vol. 83, no. 8, (231–238), 1999. 283, 285
6. S. Tamura et al, Zero-crossing interval correction in tracing eye-fundus blood vessels, *Pattern Recognition*, vol. 21, no. 3, (227–233), 1988. 283
7. S. Chaudhuri et al, Detection of blood vessels in retinal images using two-dimensional matched filters, *IEEE Trans On Medical Imaging*, vol. 8, no. 3, (263–269), 1989. 285
8. A. Pinz et al, Mapping the human retina, *IEEE Trans On Medical Imaging*, vol.1, no.1,(210–215),1998. 285
9. F. Zana and J.-C. Klein, Segmentation of vessel like patterns using mathematical morphology and curvature evaluation, *IEEE Trans On Medical Imaging*,2001, (to be published). 285, 286

Learning Structural Knowledge from the ECG

F. Wang[1], R. Quiniou[2], G. Carrault[1], and M.-O. Cordier[2]

[1] LTSI, Campus de Beaulieu, 35042 Rennes Cedex, France
[2] IRISA, Campus de Beaulieu, 35042 Rennes Cedex, France

Abstract. We tackle the problem of discovering, without the "manual" aid of an expert, implicit relations and temporal constraints from a collection of dated events detected on temporally structured signals. The approach associates tightly signal processing and symbolic learning methods. It is illustrated on learning cardiac arrhythmias from ECGs.

1 Introduction

Signal processing specialists are often confronted to the problem of recognizing a sequence of events corresponding to the signature of a particular process state. This difficulty may be even greater in biomedical domains where processes behavior is poorly known and consequently the related scenarios that must be recognized. This is the case in neurology, for instance, where the relation between electroencephalogram peaks (transient paroxistic events associated to the pathology) and epilepsy crises is not well explained. This is also the case in cardiology, where precursor signs of arrhythmias in sinusal beats are poorly known. Then the question is: "if a relation exists between signals and process states, how can it be automatically qualified?".

At an abstract level, the problem is to discover from a collection of events $E = \{E_1, ..., E_n\}$ occurring respectively at time $\{t_1, ..., t_n\}$ the implicit relations $\Re(E_j, E_k)$ and the temporal constraints $TC(t_j, t_k)$ between the events E_j et E_k. To illustrate the idea, look at the process trace in figure 1. The problem is to

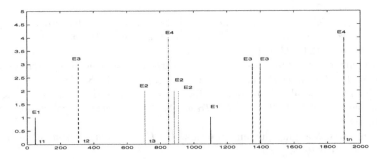

Fig. 1. Temporally structured events

J. Crespo, V. Maojo, and F. Martin (Eds.): ISMDA 2001, LNCS 2199, pp. 288–294, 2001.

discover that events of type E_1 always precede events of type E_4 with a temporal delay 700 ms $< \Delta_t < 900$ ms, independently of events of type E_2 and E_3.

We propose to associate signal processing and machine learning to discover such relations. The signal processing module abstracts the signal data into series of symbolic time-stamped events that an inductive logic programming (ILP) learner processes in order to discover relevant and discriminant high-level temporal signatures called chronicles. The resulting descriptions are used as reference patterns in an intelligent monitoring system which associates the signal processing module mentioned before and a specialized matcher [3].

We illustrate our approach on the discovery of expert rules for recognizing cardiac arrhythmias from electrocardiograms (ECG) [2]. Several attempts to learn knowledge for monitoring cardiac patients have already been performed. They use formalisms such as expert rules [1], neural networks [12], attributed grammars [11,6] or fuzzy rules [7]. The originality of our approach lies in the fact that we use symbolic events and explicit temporal constraints that makes the knowledge more readable and understandable by the clinical staff.

In the next section we develop the proposed approach and give some details about the signal processing and the machine learning techniques that are used. Then we present some results obtained in the field of cardiology.

2   Associating Signal Processing with Machine Learning

An important constraint in biomedical domain is to express knowledge at an abstraction level that is close to experts' own knowledge in order to let them assess the data. Very early, (expert) rules were recognized several advantages such as simplicity, uniformity, transparency, readability, etc. These properties make them desirable for applications such as on-line monitoring where signal processing techniques are involved but also where information presentation is an important aspect since they motivate the decisions. Rules are difficult to acquire from experts and machine learning techniques have been proposed to achieve this task. As first-order rules containing temporal constraints are the target, inductive logic programming (ILP) appears the most adequate [9].

2.1   The Signal Processing Module

The signal processing module aims at transforming the numerical input sequence into series of labeled symbolic events. More precisely, it aims $i)$ at detecting and at identifying the markers of the cardiac activity (P waves, QRS complexes), and $ii)$ at classifying waves in normal or abnormal classes. This information (occurrence time, wave duration, morphology, ...) is used to generate the symbolic event sequence that will be used by the chronicle recognition module.

The QRS detection is achieved by Gritzali's algorithm [4] which can be seen as a generalization of several detectors combining different channels. Several versions of the algorithm were tried, varying the number of ECG channels and the combination method (distributed or centralized combination).

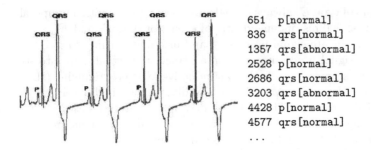

Fig. 2. Events extracted from the bigeminy ECG on the left

The P wave detection is far more complex. The new approach that is used here relies upon observing that the P, QRS and T waves in the ECG signal have different morphologies that enables a reliable classification by a neural network. After QRS complexes, high frequency noise and baseline wandering have been adaptively eliminated [5], peaks above a certain threshold that may correspond to candidate P waves are looked for. Then, a multi-layered neural network classifies the candidate waves as being a real P wave or noise.

Wave qualification into normal or abnormal is achieved by wavelet decomposition, the results of which are fed into a probabilistic neural network. After this final step, interesting waves are translated into symbolic events (see figure 2): a label, p or qrs, an occurrence time and a qualification are assigned to events.

2.2   Learning Cardiac Arrhythmias from Symbolic Events

Machine learning covers inductive techniques that aims at discovering definitions of a target concept from positive and negative examples of this concept. Inductive logic programming (ILP) is such a technique that induces concepts as first-order logical formulas. ILP has been successful at knowledge discovery in domains such as molecular biology or engineering [9]. It can be viewed as searching a clause space for hypotheses that respect a particular syntax specified by a learning bias. The selected theories, i.e. sets of clauses, must be complete (they must cover all the positive examples) and correct (they can't cover any negative example).

ICL [10] proposes a high-level concept specification language called DLAB in which the hypothesis language syntax can be defined. DLAB grammars are preprocessed in order to generate candidate hypotheses from the most general to the specific ones. We have used several DLAB specifications in order to induce set of rules enjoying such properties as readability, efficiency or robustness. A DLAB grammar consists in rule templates that fix the syntactic form of clauses defining the target concept. It makes use of operators 1-h: meaning that from 1 to h elements must be taken from the list following the operator. The special bound len, which represents the total length of the list, can also be used.

The notion of cardiac cycle is commonly used to define rhythm disorders. We used this notion for bias specifications too. A rule expressing an arrhythmia is

```
1    1-1:[
2      len-len:[p_wave(P1, 1-1:[normal, abnormal], R0),
3          qrs(R1, 1-1:[normal, abnormal], P1),
4          0-len:[rr1(R0, R1, 1-1:[short, normal, long]),
5            pr1(P1, R1, 1-1:[short, normal, long])]],
6      len-len:[p_wave(P1, 1-1:[normal, abnormal], R0),
7          pp1(P0, P1, 1-1:[short, normal, long])],
8      len-len:[qrs(R1, 1-1:[normal, abnormal], R0),
9          0-1:[rr1(R0, R1, 1-1:[short, normal, long])]]]]
```

Fig. 3. Syntactic specification of a cardiac cycle in DLAB

composed of several successive cardiac cycles. As specified in figure 3, each cycle is described as either a P wave followed by a QRS (lines 2-3), or an isolated P wave (line 6), or an isolated QRS (line 8). Additional constraints on inter-wave temporal intervals (PP, PR, RR) can be also added (lines 4-5, 7, 9).

3 Results

The goal of the experiments was to demonstrate that understandable and useful arrhythmia specifications could be learnt from ECG temporal data. A second objective was to assess the flexibility of using a declarative bias for imposing desirable properties such as readability or robustness on induced concepts.

3.1 Data

Real ECGs were taken from the *MIT-BIH* database [8]. Three classes of examples related to well-known arrhythmias were selected (left bundle branch block - lbbb, Mobitz type II - mobitz2, bigeminy) plus a normal sinus rhythm. 20 ECG lasting 10s each were extracted for each class and translated into a symbolic form by the signal processing module described above. A symbolic ECG example is a set of events wave(Evt, Type, Time, Qual, P_evt) stating that Evt is related to a wave of type Type (p or qrs), which occurred at time Time, the shape of which is Qual (normal or abnormal). P_evt designates the event that precedes Event on the ECG. It provides a temporal structure to the set of events.

3.2 Experiments

Learning Shortest Rules The first experiment was performed with a learning bias imposing only one mandatory cycle. The induced rules are supposed to be the most efficient ones for recognition as they involve the minimal number of events. The results obtained after a 10-fold cross validation (10 learning rounds on 90% of the examples and test on the remaining 10%) are shown in figure 4. The resulting accuracy (the ratio number of correctly recognized/total number of examples) was 100% for training as well as for test.

```
class(bigeminy) :-    %[17, 0, 0, 0], [0, 18, 18, 19]
   qrs(R0, abnormal, _),
   p_wave(P1, normal, R0), qrs(R1, normal, P1), rr1(R0, R1, long).
class(lbbb) :-        %[0, 18, 0, 0], [17, 0, 18, 19]
   p_wave(P0, normal, _), qrs(R0, abnormal, P0),
   p_wave(P1, normal, R0), qrs(R1, abnormal, P1), rr1(R0, R1, normal).
class(mobitz2) :-     %[0, 0, 16, 0], [17, 18, 2, 19]
   p_wave(P0, normal, _), equal(P0, R0),
   p_wave(P1, normal, R0), qrs(R1, normal, P1), pr1(P1, R1, normal).
class(mobitz2) :-     %[0, 0, 2, 0], [17, 18, 16, 19]
   p_wave(P0, normal, _), equal(P0, R0),
   p_wave(P1, normal, R0), qrs(R1, abnormal, P1), pr1(P1, R1, normal).
class(normal) :-      %[0, 0, 0, 19], [17, 18, 18, 0]
   p_wave(P0, normal, _), qrs(R0, normal, P0),
   p_wave(P1, normal, R0), qrs(R1, normal, P1), rr1(R0, R1, normal).
```

Fig. 4. Rules induced with a bias imposing 1 mandatory cycle, 2 optional cycles

The rules are expressed as Prolog clauses. For instance, the first rule says that a bigeminy can be characterized by an abnormal QRS followed by a normal P wave followed by a normal QRS and the temporal interval between the two QRSs is long. Note, that this rule characterizes also trigeminy. As no examples were given for trigeminy there is no reason that the induced rule discriminates between bigeminy and trigeminy. This illustrates the fact that most general rules are induced. The lists following the rule heads give respectively the number of examples covered by the rule and the number of examples not covered by the rule in each class (in the order bigeminy, lbbb, mobitz2 and normal).

Learning More Readable Rules As they represent recurrent phenomena, some arrhythmias are often described by experts on several cycles, e.g. 3 or 4. In this second experiment the number of mandatory cycles was set to 3. This bias causes the rules to be more specific and eventually they cover less examples. Sometimes, several rules are necessary to define a class, as for bigeminy:

```
class(bigeminy) :- % [13, 0, 0, 0], [5, 19, 17, 18]
   p_wave(P0, normal, _), qrs(R0, normal, P0),
   qrs(R1, abnormal, R0), rr1(R0, R1, short),
   p_wave(P2, normal, R1), qrs(R2, normal, P2).
class(bigeminy) :- % [5, 0, 0, 0], [13, 19, 17, 18]
   p_wave(P0, normal, _), qrs(R0, normal, P0),
   p_wave(P1, normal, R0), qrs(R1, abnormal, P1),
   p_wave(P2, normal, R1), qrs(R2, normal, P2).
```

The first rule corresponds to the usual bigeminy. The second rule illustrates an interesting phenomenon. The examples covered by this rule refers to ECGs where the ectopic beats occur between a P wave and the expected following QRS. This explains the presence of a large QRS which reflects an abnormal ventricle activation. This illustrates the power ILP that is able to discover such subtleties and use them for discrimination. Accuracy of 10-fold cross validation was still 100% for training and test in this experiment. Such good results can be explained by the fact that MIT-BIH records arenot noisy.

4   Conclusion

We have described how to associate signal processing and inductive logic programming to learn structural patterns from real signals and illustrated the approach on learning cardiac arrhythmias. Since the domain of cardiology is well known, specialists could assessed the relevance or readability of learnt results. The learnt definitions discriminate between those classes for which examples are given and only those. This explains why they are sometimes a bit strange to clinicians used to definitions that discriminates between all known arrhythmias. However, all learnt definitions were rated good and relevant.

The flexibility of the ICL bias language was demonstrated. This makes it possible to tailor the learnt definitions to the particular context, explicative or efficient monitoring, for instance. The rules could be adapted to an individual patient by learning from his own ECGs or from arrhythmias he may suffer from.

A first extension of this work concerns taking into account multiple sources of information, i.e. multichannel ECGs as well as ECGs associated with hemodynamic signals. A second extension aims at applying the same approach to less known domains such as EEG analysis or processing signals during anesthesia.

References

1. I. Bratko, I. Mozetic, and N. Lavrăc. *Kardio: A Study in Deep and Qualitative Knowledge for Expert Systems.* MIT Press, 1989. 289
2. G. Carrault, M.-O. Cordier, R. Quiniou, M. Garreau, J.-J. Bellanger, and A. Bardou. A model-based approach for learning to identify cardiac arrhythmias. In *Proc. of AIMDM'99*, LNAI, vol. 1620. Springer Verlag, 1999. 289
3. C. Dousson. Alarm driven supervision for telecommunication networks. ii- on-line chronicle recognition. *Annales des Télécommunications*, 51(9-10):501–508, 1996. 289
4. F. Gritzali. Towards a generalized scheme for QRS detection in ECG waveforms. *Signal Processing*, 15:183–192, 1988. 289
5. A. I. Hernández and G. Carrault. Annulation adaptative du QRS. In *colloque GRETSI*, pages 591–594, 1999. 290
6. G. Kókai, Z. Alexin, and T. Gyimóthy. Application of inductive logic programming for learning ECG waveforms. In *Proceedings of AIME97*, volume 1211, pages 126–129. Springer-Verlag, 1997. 289
7. M. Kundu, M. Nasipuri, and D. K. Basu. A knowledge based approach to ECG interpretation using fuzzy logic. *IEEE Trans. Sytems Man and Cybernetics*, 28(2):237–243, 1998. 289
8. G. B. Moody and R. G. Mark. The MIT-BIH arrhythmia database on cd-rom and software for use with it. In *Computers in Cardiology 1990*, pages 185–188. IEEE Computer Society Press, 1990. 291

9. S. Muggleton. Inductive logic programming: issues, results and the challenge of learning language in logic. *Artificial Intelligence*, 114(1-2):283–296, 1999. 289, 290

10. L. De Raedt and W. Van Laer. Inductive constraint logic. In *Proceedings of the 5th Workshop on Algorithmic Learning Theory*, LNAI, 1995. 290

11. E. Skordalakis. ECG analysis. In H. Bunke and A. Sanfeliu, editors, *Syntactic and Structural Pattern Recognition Theory and Applications*, pages 499–533. World Scientific, 1990. 289

12. R. L. Watrous. A patient-adaptive neural network ECG patient monitoring algorithm. *Computers in Cardiology*, pages 229–232, 1995. 289

Recurrence Quantification Analysis to Characterise the Heart Rate Variability Before the Onset of Ventricular Tachycardia

Niels Wessel[1], Norbert Marwan[1], Udo Meyerfeldt[2], Alexander Schirdewan[2],
Jürgen Kurths[1]

[1] University of Potsdam, Am Neuen Palais 10, PF 601553,
D-14415 Potsdam, Germany
{niels, marwan, jkurths}@agnld.uni-potsdam.de
[2] Franz-Volhard-Hospital, Humboldt-University, Berlin,
Wiltbergstr. 50, D-13125 Berlin, Germany
{meyerfeldt, schirdewan}@fvk-berlin.de

Abstract. Ventricular tachycardia or fibrillation (VT) as fatal cardiac arrhythmias are the main factors triggering sudden cardiac death. The objective of this recurrence quantification analysis approach is to find early signs of sustained VT in patients with an implanted cardioverter-defibrillator (ICD). These devices are able to safeguard patients by returning their hearts to a normal rhythm via strong defibrillatory shocks; additionally, they are able to store at least 1000 beat-to-beat intervals immediately before the onset of a life-threatening arrhythmia. We study these 1000 beat-to-beat intervals of 63 chronic heart failure ICD patients before the onset of a life-threatening arrhythmia and at a control time, i.e. without VT event. We find that no linear parameter shows significant differences in heart rate variability between the VT and the control time series. However, the results of the recurrence quantification analysis are promising for this classification task.

1 Introduction

Implantable cardioverter defibrillators (ICD) are a safe and effective treatment for ventricular tachycardia or fibrillation (VT) [1-3]. These fatal cardiac arrhythmias are the main factors triggering sudden cardiac death. Therefore, an accurate identification of patients who are at high risk of sudden cardiac death is an important and challenging problem. Nowadays, third generation ICD offer not only important advances in arrhythmia treatment, but also permit the correct characterisation of the rhythm leading to intervention [4,5]. Additionally, they are able to store at least 1000 beat-to-beat intervals immediately before the onset of a life-threatening arrhythmia.

In this contribution we study the heart rate variability (HRV) of chronic heart failure ICD patients before the onset of a life-threatening arrhythmia and at a control time, i.e. without VT event. HRV parameters have been used to predict the mortality risk in patients with structural heart diseases [6,7]. Linear parameters only provide

J. Crespo, V. Maojo, and F. Martin (Eds.): ISMDA 2001, LNCS 2199, pp. 295-301, 2001.

limited information about the underlying complex system, whereas nonlinear descriptions often suffer from the curse of dimensionality. This means that there are not enough points in the time series to reliably estimate these nonlinear measures. Therefore, we favour measures of complexity which are able to characterise quantitatively the dynamics even in rather short time series [8-10]. For ICD stored HRV data sets we found some evidence for predictability of VT in patients with a low number of ectopic beats [10]. In this investigation, we apply the concept of recurrence quantification analysis to find some precursors independently from the ectopy.

2   Methods

2.1   Patients

We studied the ICD stored 1000 beat-to-beat intervals before the onset of 131 VT episodes and at 74 control intervals without VT in 63 ICD patients of the Franz-Volhard-Hospital with severe congestive heart failure. No patient had received a class I or class III antiarrhythmic drug for 18±9 months prior to the study. Time series including more than one episode nonsustained VT, episode of induced VT, or ventricular pacing are excluded from the analysis. To estimate the amount of ventricular premature beats we use an adaptive filtering algorithm for preprocessing, which tends to be superior to standard algorithms [11]. The beat-to-beat intervals of the VT at the end of the time series were removed from the tachograms so that we analysed only the dynamics occurring immediately prior to VT.

2.2   Standard heart rate variability analysis

To detect early signs of life-threatening VT, we applied a multiparametric analysis. Before starting the analysis, ventricular premature beats and artifacts usually should be removed from the time series to construct the so-called "normal-to-normal" beat time series (NN). We used the adaptive filtering algorithm [11] for preprocessing of the data. As a basically analysis a certain number of standard HRV parameters from time and frequency domain were calculated (e.g. *sdNN, pNN50, LF/HF*) [12]. These standard parameters of HRV analysis are based on linear techniques. To classify dynamic changes in the time series, we present the following nonlinear concepts of recurrence quantification analysis outlined below.

2.3   Recurrence quantification analysis

Recurrence plots (RP) were firstly introduced to visualise time dependent behaviour of orbits in the phase space [13]. They represent the recurrence of the phase space trajectory to a state. The recurrence of states is a fundamental property of deterministic dynamical systems [14,15] - to quantify this effects Zbilut and Webber have introduced the *recurrence quantification analysis* (RQA) [16]. They define measures using recurrence point density, diagonal segments and paling in the recurrence plot, *recurrence rate, determinism, averaged length of diagonal structures, entropy* and *trend*. Two of these parameters turned out to be of interest in this paper: the *determinism* and *entropy*. *Determinism* is defined as the ratio of recurrence points forming diagonal structures to all recurrence points. The *entropy* denotes the Shannon entropy of the histogram of diagonal line segment lengths and reflects the complexity of the deterministic structure in the system. First promising applications of the RQA method to heart rate variability data are described in [17-19].

2.4 The intermittency approach

The described measures are using only diagonal structures in the RP. However, a RP contains more geometrical structures which may contain important information. Therefore, we introduce measures quantifying also horizontal and vertical structures, which give qualitative information about laminar behaviour and intermittency.

Analogous to the definition of averaged length of diagonal structures, we define the averaged length of vertical structures

$$TT := \sum_{v=v_{min}}^{N} v \cdot P(v) \bigg/ \sum_{v=v_{min}}^{N} P(v) \tag{1}$$

what we call *trapping time TT*. $P(v)$ is the probability distribution of vertical line of length v; the computation of TT is realised for values of v which exceed a minimal length v_{min}. This was done to avoid the major influence of sojourn points, as described in [20]. TT emphasises parts of the RP with vertical lines represent laminar states in the system: A system consisting mainly of laminar (or trapped) states has a high TT, a system without laminar states has a very low TT.

Similar the definition of the *determinism* [16], we can compute the ratio of the recurrence points forming the vertical structures, the so called *laminarity L*:

$$L := \sum_{v=v_{min}}^{N} v \cdot P(v) \bigg/ \sum_{v=1}^{N} v \cdot P(v) \tag{2}$$

The *laminarity* decreases if the RP consists of more single recurrence points than vertical structures. Finally, the Shannon-entropy of the distribution of the vertical line lengths $P(v)$ is calculated which is a measure for the variability of the vertical structures. If there are vertical structures with varying lengths, the entropy will be high; a lot of vertical structures with the same (or similar) lengths will cause a small entropy.

3 Results

3.1 Standard heart rate variability

We observed 131 VT episodes in 63 patients. Sixty-four episodes were not included because of atrial fibrillation, permanent pacing, incessant VT, incomplete storage of episodes, or storage artifacts. The remaining 67 VT episodes and 47 control series from 46 patients comprise the report. The mean VT cycle length was 310±53 ms. Comparing the HRV parameters of all 67 VT and 47 control time series, only the mean sinus rhythm cycle length showed differences, the time series leading to VT had a significantly shorter cycle length (meanNN 694.4±138.1 ms), than the control time series (meanNN 760.8±140.2 ms). The ectopy time, calculated as the sum of the coupling interval and the following pause of all premature beats, did not differ between the VT and control time series. The ectopy time of the VT group was 96.0±129.9 sec according to 14% of all 1024 beat-to-beat intervals and 68.2±98.1 sec, according to 9% of the control time series ($p > 0.05$).

3.2 Recurrence quantification analysis

All parameters described in section 2.3. were calculated for the heart rate data before VT and at a control time. Embedding dimensions were chosen from 3 to 15, the delay equal to 1, radii from 5 to 50 % for a relative scaling approach and radii ranging from 10 to 100 ms for absolute scaling. This investigation was a totally exploratory data analysis, we had to be aware of multiple testing problems in the statistical analysis. Nevertheless, we found some significant differences between both groups of time series (see table 1).

Table 1. Significant parameters in the RQA approach. The statistical analysis was based on the two-sided t-test as well the non-parametric Mann-Whitney-U-test.

Parameter	Embedding dimension	Radius	P
Absolute scaling			
Entropy	4	10	<0.05
Determinism	12	20	<0.01
Determinism	13	30	<0.05
Entropy	14	40	<0.05
Determinism	15	70	<0.05
Relative scaling			
Determinism	15	5	<0.01
Determinism	15	10	<0.01
Determinism	5;6	15	<0.05
Entropy	10	20	<0.05

As one can see, significant results were obtained only for small radii and for high embedding dimensions. Figure 1 shows a typical example for the distribution of the

RQA parameter. Significant differences were found because of zero recurrences in the control group 0. These results are in agreement with our findings in [10], intermittently decreased epochs of short HRV before VT lead to higher number of recurrences.

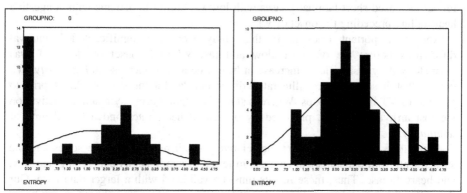

Fig. 1. The distributions of the *entropy* parameter for control group 0 as well as for VT group 1 calculated with an embedding dimension of 4 and a radius of 10 (absolute scaling).

Using the intermittency approach we could detect 8 VT time series out of all series which show extremely laminar behaviour. Non of the remaining data sets, neither control nor VT series, showed such short epochs with intermittently decreased HRV.

In a next step we tested the hypothesis if there is a correlation between the VT cycle length and some recurrence parameters before the onset of this VT. For small embedding dimensions and a fixed radius we found a increasing *laminarity* with increasing VT cycle length (see fig. 2). This means that serious VT with slow cycle length are characterised by a lower *laminarity*.

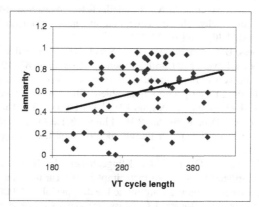

Fig. 2. The relation between the *laminarity* and the VT cycle length for an embedding dimension of 1 and a radius of 10 (absolute scaling).

4 Discussion

We identified significant differences in the dynamic behaviour of beat-to-beat intervals between the VT and control time series by means of RQA parameters. They reflect increased short laminar phases with low variability in patients with congestive heart failure preceding the onset of VT.

Another important findings in this study were the significant RR interval differences before the onset of slow and fast VT. The onset of slow VT was characterised by a significant increase in heart rate and an increase in *laminarity*. We assume that these differences illustrate a different role of autonomic regulation prior to the start of VT in both groups. Whereas slow VT began during sympathetic activation the fast arrhythmias were preceded by decreased heart rates and a low degree of *laminarity*.

Limitations of our study were the relatively small number of time series and the subsequently limited statistical analysis in terms of subdivisions concerning age, sex, and heart disease. Thus, these results must be validated with a larger data base. Our data offer the possibility of developing automatic ICD algorithms based on nonlinear dynamic HRV parameters.

Acknowledgements

We want to thank Alessandro Giuliani and Joseph Zbilut for helpful discussions.

References

1. Mirowski, M., Reid, P.R., Mower, M.M., Watkins, L., Gott, V.L., Schauble, J.F., Langer, A., Heilman, M.S., Kolenik, S.A., Fischell, R.E., Weisfeldt, M.L.: Termination of malignant ventricular tachyarrhythmias with an implanted automatic defibrillator in human beings. N Engl J Med 303 (1980) 322-324
2. Grimm, W., Flores, B.T., Marchlinski, F.E.: Shock occurence and survival in 241 patients with implantable cardioverter-defibrillator therapy. Circulation 87 (1993) 18880-18888
3. The antiarrhythmic versus implantable defibrillators (AVID) investigators: A comparison of antiarrhythmic drug therapy with implantable defibrillators in patients resuscitated from near fatal ventricular arrhythmias. N Engl J Med 337 (1997) 1576-1583
4. Hook, B.G., Callans, D.J., Kleiman, R.B., Flores, B.T., Marchlinski, F.E.: Implantable cardioverter-defibrillator therapy in the absence of significant symptoms. Circulation 87 (1993) 1897-1906
5. Gronefeld, G.C., Mauss, O., Li, Y.G., Klingenheben, T., Hohnloser, S.H.: Association between atrial fibrillation and appropriate implantable cardioverter defibrillator therapy: results from a prospective study. J Cardiovasc Electrophysiol 11 (2000) 1208-1214
6. Kleiger, R.E., Miller, J.P., Bigger, J.T., Moss, A.: Decreased heart rate variability and its association with increased mortality after acute myocardial infarction. Am J Cardiol 59 (1987) 256-262

7. Tsuji, H., Larson, M.G., Venditti, F.J. Jr, Manders, E.S., Evans, J.C., Feldman, C.L., Levy, D.: Impact of reduced heart rate variability on risk for cardiac events. The Framingham Heart Study. Circulation 94 (1996) 2850-2855

8. Kurths, J., Voss, A., Witt, A., Saparin, P., Kleiner, H.J., Wessel, N.: Quantitative analysis of heart rate variability. Chaos 5 (1995) 88-94

9. Voss, A., Kurths, J., Kleiner, H.J., Witt, A., Wessel, N., Saparin, P., Osterziel, K.J., Schurath, R., Dietz, R.: The application of methods of non-linear dynamics for the improved and predictive recognition of patients threatened by sudden cardiac death. Cardiovasc Res 31 (1996) 419-433

10. Wessel, N., Ziehmann, Ch., Kurths, J., Meyerfeldt, U., Schirdewan, A., Voss, A.: Short-term Forecasting of Life-threatening Cardiac Arrhythmias based on Symbolic Dynamics and Finite-Time Growth Rates. Phys Rev E 61 (2000) 733-739

11. Wessel, N., Voss, A., Malberg, H., Ziehmann, Ch., Voss, H.U., Schirdewan, A., Meyerfeldt, U., Kurths, J.: Nonlinear analysis of complex phenomena in cardiological data. Herzschr Elektrophys 11 (2000) 159-173

12. Heart rate variability: standards of measurement, physiological interpretation and clinical use. Task Force of the European Society of Cardiology and the North American Society of Pacing and Electrophysiology. Circulation 93 (1996) 1043-1065

13. Eckmann, J.-P., Kamphorst, S.O., Ruelle, D.: Recurrence plots of dynamical systems. Europhys Lett 4 (1987) 973-977

14. Argyris, J.H., Faust, G., Haase, M.: An exploration of Chaos. North Holland, Amsterdam, 1994

15. Ott, E.: Chaos in dynamical systems. University Press, Cambridge, 1993

16. Zbilut, J.P., Webber Jr., C.L.: Embeddings and delays as derived from quantification of recurrence plots. Phys. Lett. A 171 (1992) 199-203

17. Giuliani, A., Piccirillo, G., Marigliano, V., Colosimo, A.: A nonlinear explanation of aging-induced changes in heartbeat dynamics. Am J Physiol 275 (1998) H1455-H1461

18. Gonzalez, J. J., Cordero, J. J., Fe ria, M., Pereda, E.: Detection and sources of nonlinearity in the variability of cardiac R-R intervals and blood pressure in rats. Am J Physiol Heart Circ Physiol 279 (2000) H3040-H3046

19. Censi, F., Barbaro, V., Bartolini, P., Calcagnini, G., Michelucci, G. F., Cerutti, S.: Recurrent patterns of atrial depolarization during atrial fibrillation assessed by recurrence plot quantification. in: Annals of Biomedical Engineering 28 (2000), 61-70

20. Gao, J., Cai, H.: On the structures and quantification of recurrence plots. Physics Letters A 270 (2000), 75-87

Learning Bayesian-Network Topologies in Realistic Medical Domains

Xiaofeng Wu[1], Peter Lucas[1], Susan Kerr[2], and Roelf Dijkhuizen[2]

[1] Dept. of Computing Science, University of Aberdeen
Aberdeen, AB24 3UE, UK
{xwu,plucas}@csd.abdn.ac.uk
[2] Stroke Unit, Aberdeen Royal Infirmary
Aberdeen, AB25 2ZD, UK
Roelf.Dijkhuizen@arh.grampian.scot.nhs.uk

Abstract. In recent years, a number of algorithms have been developed for learning the structure of Bayesian networks from data. In this paper we apply some of these algorithms to a realistic medical domain—stroke. Basically, the domain of stroke is taken as a typical example of a medical domain where much data are available concerning a few hundred patients. Learning the structure of a Bayesian network is known to be hard under these conditions. In this paper, two different structure learning algorithms are compared to each other. A causal model which was constructed with the help of an expert clinician is adopted as the gold standard. The advantages and limitations of various structure-learning algorithms are discussed in the context of the experimental results obtained.

Keywords: Bayesian networks, machine learning, knowledge discovery, medical decision support systems.

1 Introduction

Predicting the outcome of patients with serious stroke is a challenging problem for clinicians as stroke is a life-threatening condition. Even though predicting both short and long-term outcome in patients with stroke is clinically very relevant, in particular for selecting optimal treatment of a patient, it is currently not supported by statistical models. There is substantial scientific evidence that both short and long-term outcome are determined by a bewildering number of different factors, such as medical history, family circumstances, and facilities for rehabilitation. The purpose of our project is to get more insight into which factors are important, and in what way these factors interact to give rise to a particular outcome.

Graphical probabilistic models, such as Bayesian networks, have become popular modelling tools for supporting decision making under uncertainty in recent years. On the one hand, they have the virtue of being sufficiently intuitive to render it possible to construct Bayesian networks with the help of domain experts.

J. Crespo, V. Maojo, and F. Martin (Eds.): ISMDA 2001, LNCS 2199, pp. 302–307, 2001.

Both their structure, or *topology*, and an associated joint probability distribution can be elicited from experts [6]. On the other hand, both topology and joint probability distribution can be learnt from data [2]. Experience with structure-learning methods so far indicates that learning is feasible for large datasets with few missing data. In medicine, however, datasets usually only include a few hundred cases, and they normally also contain at least some missing data. This is considered characteristic for a *realistic medical domain*. The question therefore arises how far one gets with learning Bayesian network topologies from data in the context of realistic medical domains. In this paper, we attempt to answer this question by adopting stroke as an example domain, taking a Bayesian network, which was developed on the basis of a causal model designed with the help of a medical specialist, as a point of reference.

The remainder of the paper is organised as follows. Section 2 introduces previous research in learning Bayesian networks from data. In Section 3, we describe the subject of stroke, and present the methods used in our study. Section 4 presents the results obtained by using different structural learning methods. In Section 5, we will discuss what has been achieved, and relate these results to the problem of learning Bayesian-network structure in the medical domain.

2 Previous Research

A frequently used procedure for Bayesian network structure construction from data is the K2 algorithm [2]. Given a database D, this algorithm searches for the Bayesian network structure G^* with maximal $\Pr(G, D)$, which is determined as described below [2]. Let $\mathcal{V}$ be a set of n discrete variables, where a variable $V_i \in \mathcal{V}$ has r_i possible value assignments: $v_1^i, \ldots, v_{r_i}^i$. Let D contain m cases, where each case contains a value assignment for each variable in $\mathcal{V}$. Let G contain just the variables in $\mathcal{V}$, and $\mathcal{B}_{\Pr}$ the associated set of conditional probability distributions. Each node $V_i \in V(G)$ has a set of parents $\pi(V_i)$. Let w_{ij} denote the jth unique instantiation of $\pi(V_i)$ relative to D. Suppose there are q_i such unique instantiations of $\pi(V_i)$. Define N_{ijk} to be the number of cases in D in which variable V_i has the value v_k^i and $\pi(V_i)$ is instantiated as w_{ij}. Let $N_{ij} = \sum_{k=1}^{r_i} N_{ijk}$. If given a Bayesian network model, assuming that the cases occur independently and the density function $f(\Pr | G)$ is uniform, then it follows that

$$\Pr(G, D) = \Pr(G) \prod_{i=1}^{n} \prod_{j=1}^{q_i} \frac{(r_i - 1)!}{(N_{ij} + r_i - 1)!} \prod_{k=1}^{r_i} N_{ijk}!$$

The K2 algorithm assumes that an ordering on the variables is available and that all structures are equally likely. For every node V_i it searches for the set of parent nodes that maximises the following function:

$$g(i, \pi(V_i)) = \prod_{j=1}^{q_i} \frac{(r_i - 1)!}{(N_{ij} + r_i - 1)!} \prod_{k=1}^{r_i} N_{ijk}!$$

K2 starts by assuming that a node lacks parents, after which in every step it adds incrementally that parent whose addition most increases the probability of the resulting structure. K2 stops adding parents to the nodes when the addition of a single parent cannot increase the probability. It is a typical *search & scoring method*. Other algorithms include the one implemented in the Bayesian Knowledge Discoverer (BKD) system [7] and the MDL algorithm [4].

A learning method which takes an entirely different approach is *dependency analysis*. In this method, we can get a collection of conditional independence statements from a Bayesian network by using the Markov condition. These conditional independence statements also imply other conditional independence statements using the independence axioms [6]. By using a concept called direction dependent separation, or *d*-separation, all the valid conditional independence relations can also be directly derived from the topology of a Bayesian network. The so-called information-theoretical algorithm implements dependency analysis [1].

In this paper, we study the practical usefulness of the above two methods for constructing topologies in the stroke domain.

3   Patients and Methods

A dataset with data of 327 patients with stroke was collected by the clinicians. Originally, the dataset contained 140 attributes, among others admission information and personal detail. Of these attributes, 29 variables were selected based on a study of the literature on stroke, indicating which of the factors might be relevant in assessing the outcome of stroke.

We have constructed a causal model with the help of a clinical expert in the subject of stroke, and used this causal model to guide the development by hand of an associated Bayesian network. The resulting Bayesian network is shown in Fig. 1. As the search algorithms described above are not perfect, and most medical datasets are not large, the relations among variables can hardly be expected to be discovered completely and correctly. It is even harder for our stroke dataset, because there were much missing data in the dataset. This explains why we studied the extent to which the developed causal model was able to guide the process of learning the topology of Bayesian networks.

A simple similarity measure, which is the *structure similarity measure*, was defined to assess the quality of a once learnt structure in comparison to a reference topology. Let C be the $n \times n$ adjacency matrix representation of a directed graph G (i.e. $c_{ij} = 1$ if $V_i \longrightarrow V_j$; otherwise $c_{ij} = 0$), with $|V(G)| = n$. Let $s(C) = \sum_{i,j} c_{ij}$ be the sum of all components of matrix C. Furthermore, we define the conjunction $\bigwedge$ of two adjacency matrices C and C' as: $D = C \bigwedge C'$, with $d_{ij} = c_{ij} \wedge c'_{ij}$. Then, the *structure similarity measure* for two graphs G and G' is defined as $\delta(G, G') = \frac{s(C \bigwedge C')}{s(C)}$, where C is the adjacency matrix associated with G and C' is the adjacency matrix associated with G'. For example, consider the two Bayesian network structures with three nodes V_i, $i = 1, 2, 3$, and associated adjacency matrices shown in Fig. 2. It is easily seen that in this case $\delta(G, G') = 0.5$.

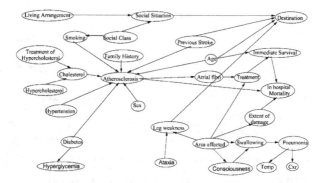

Fig. 1. Bayesian network built with the help of an expert clinician

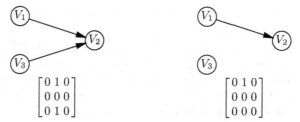

Fig. 2. Two Bayesian network structures with associated adjacency matrices

In many situations, the direction of an arc between two nodes is not important, as essentially the same d-separation information is expressed. However, the similarity measure $\delta(G, G')$ does not reflect this, and may therefore result in a measure which is lower than it actually should be. For example, the structures $V_1 \longrightarrow V_2 \longrightarrow V_3$ and $V_1 \longleftarrow V_2 \longrightarrow V_3$ are equivalent, yet $\delta(G, G') = 0.5$. To take this into account, we define another similarity measure. In this measure, we make use of the operator $\bigotimes$; we have that $D = C \bigotimes C'$ with d_{ij} defined as follows: $d_{ij} = \begin{cases} 0.5 & \text{if } c_{ij} \wedge c'_{ji} = 1 \\ c_{ij} \wedge c'_{ij} & \text{otherwise} \end{cases}$. The resulting measure, called the *undirected structure similarity measure* is defined as $\epsilon(G, G') = \frac{s(C \bigotimes C')}{s(C)}$. Of course, not in all situations are the directions of the arcs unimportant, so the ϵ measure yields an upper-bound to an accurate similarity measure.

So far, we have considered measures which focus on the structure of a Bayesian network. However, one could argue that it is the probability distribution which will matter most in the end. In order to measure the discrepancy between an independency statement as encoded in the probability distribution of a reference topology, say $P(\mathcal{V})$, and the learnt structure from a dataset, say $P'(\mathcal{V})$, one can use the Kullback-Leibler divergence measure [3]. In essence, this discrepancy is measured for the entire joint probability distribution of two Bayesian networks, where one of the probability distributions is taken as the true distribution. Here we take the expert-based network topology with probabilities learnt from data

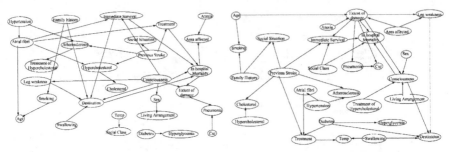

(a) Bayesian Network learnt without domain knowledge   (b) Bayesian Network learnt with domain knowledge

Fig. 3. Two learnt Bayesian Network structures

as the true one. The *Kullback-Leibler divergence measure* $I(P, P')$ is defined as $I(P, P') = \sum_{\mathcal{V}} P(\mathcal{V}) \log \frac{P(\mathcal{V})}{P'(\mathcal{V})}$.

Two different Bayesian network structures were generated from the stroke dataset. The first one, shown in Fig. 3(a), was constructed using BKD, without using any domain knowledge to guide the learning process. The other structure was learnt by BNPowersoft [1], taking a total order among the variables as a starting point, which was derived from the causal model. The resulting graph structure is shown in Fig. 3(b).

4   Results

The Bayesian-network topologies learnt using BKD and BNPowersoft are compared to each other in this section, taking the causal model designed with the help of the expert as a point of reference. BKD yielded a structure, essentially discovering 37 arcs, of which 30 additional and 27 missing in comparison to the expert's causal model. BNPowersoft was able discover 39 arcs, of which 23 additional and 25 missing.

Next, we applied the above methods to measure the similarities between the reference topology and the learnt structures. The results are shown in Table 1.

As is shown in the table, all of the three measures are better for the structure learnt by BNPowersoft. The main reason for this is that we utilised expert knowledge before the structure was learnt using BNPowersoft. So, it appears

Table 1. Comparison between structure learning results

Method	Structure learnt with BKD	Structure learnt with BNPowersoft	Ratio
δ	0.20	0.486	2.43
ϵ	0.45	0.729	1.62
I	0.66	0.320	2.06

that the quality of the learnt network improves significantly when guided by expert knowledge. We have tried to use objective methods to verify that statement. Interestingly, the ratio for the Kullback-Leibler divergence measures lies in between the ratios obtained for the two structural methods, which simply compared the structures of the graphs. Computing the Kullback-Leibler divergence is quite expensive, as one needs to go through all probability tables. Computing the structure similarity measures is cheap and straightforward, and seems to convey sufficient information.

5 Discussion

In this paper, we have investigated the relative merits of machine-learning approaches versus knowledge acquisition and modelling in the clinical context of realistic medical domains. The advantages of machine-learning approaches are obvious in that they save time compared to explicit modelling. But it is also obvious that precision cannot be guaranteed, as is demonstrated by our results. This situation is typical when using a small dataset in constructing Bayesian networks. Because there were also a lot of missing data in the stroke dataset, the results became unavoidably worse.

Despite the fact that the learning algorithms are of limited value for a dataset such as our stroke dataset, they did discover some important causal relationships between variables. It may be expected that better results are obtained when the dataset grows larger, whereas improving the learning algorithms by making them somewhat less approximate may also help. Furthermore, the quality of a learnt Bayesian network is greatly improved when utilizing expert knowledge in the context of learning. Certainly for a realistic medical domain it will be essential to exploit expert knowledge as much as possible when learning Bayesian networks from data.

References

1. J. Cheng, D. Bell. Learning Bayesian networks from data: an efficient approach based on information theory. *Proceeding of the sixth ACM International Conference on Information and Knowledge Management*, 1997. 304, 306
2. G. F. Cooper, E. Herskovitz. A Bayesian method for the induction of probabilistic networks from data. *Machine Learning* 1992; 9: 309–347. 303
3. S. Kullback, R. Leibler. On information and sufficiency. *Annals of Mathematical Statistics* 1951; 22: 79–86. 305
4. W. Lam, F. Bacchus. Learning Bayesian belief networks: an approach based on the MDL principle. *Computational Intelligence* 1994; 10: 269–293. 304
5. S. L. Lauritzen, D. J. Spiegelhalter. Local computations with probabilities on graphical structures and their application to expert systems. *Journal of the Royal Statistical Society (Series B)* 1987; 50: 157–224.
6. J. Pearl. *Probabilistic Reasoning in Intelligent Systems: Networks of Plausible Inference.* San Francisco: Morgan Kaufmann, 1998. 303, 304
7. M. Ramoni, P. Sebastiani. *Discovering Bayesian Networks in Incomplete Databases.* Report KMI-TR-46, KMI, Open University, 1997. 304

Author Index

Lecture Notes in Computer Science

For information about Vols. 1–2126
please contact your bookseller or Springer-Verlag